The Essential Herbert M. Shelton

Herbert M. Shelton

ISBN 1425454216

*H*EALTH

FOR

*A*LL

Contents: Orthopathy—Physiological Lawfulness; Disease—A Vital Process; Organic Unity—Its Relation to Cure; Toxemia; Health First; Bronchitis; Hay fever; Ductless Glands; Goiter; Colitis; Ulcers; Arthritis, Rheumatism, and Gout; High Blood Pressure; Neuralgia; Neuritis; Gluttony a Neurosis; Exercise and the Heart; Index, plus much more!

Herbert M. Shelton

ISBN 1-56459-978-7

Warning—Disclaimer

"We smile at primitive ignorance while we submit anxiously to the expensive therapeutics of our own day." — Will Durant in *History of Civilization*.

Torturing Them
to
Cure Them

"There is nothing men will not do, the
nothing they have not done, to recover
health and save their lives. They have subm
to be half-drowned and half-choked with g
to be buried up to their chins in earth, t
seared with hot irons like galley slaves, t
crimped with knives like codfish, to have ne
thrust into their flesh and bonfires kindle
their skins, to swallow all sorts of abominat
and to pay for all this as if to be singed
scalded were a costly privilege, as if bl
were a blessing and leeches a luxury."—Dr. O
Wendell Holmes.

Introduction

The chapters in this little book were published originally in the form of articles in *Dr. Shelton's Hygienic Review*. This accounts for the unusual amount of repetition contained herein. However, many years in teaching people right living have shown us the great need for reiteration so that it has not seemed wise to attempt to eliminate any of the repetition.

Psychologists say that a thing must be repeated at least three times before the average person grasps it. Our experience has convinced us that when new, radical and revolutionary truths are presented they must be repeated many times and in many ways before the average person grasps them. Understanding comes slowly and not at once.

We have reached a time when about all one requires to practice medicine is a white coat and a supply of sulfanilamide; but we have not reached a time (and never will) when the causes of illness can be ignored. This little book is unique in that it dwells particularly upon causes. We have laid great stress upon the causes of suffering, for only when these are known and removed can health be restored and future suffering avoided.

Dr. Shelton's Health School was founded in 1928. During the succeeding years of its existence people have come here from Ireland, Scotland, Australia, New Zealand, Hawaii, Canada, Mexico, Costa Rica, Nicaragua, Venezuela, Brazil, Cuba and all parts of the United States. Babies, children, old men and women and all ages between these extremes have come to the *Health School* for care and education.

For the most part we have received only the scraps and derelicts. Few have come to us who could find "relief" elsewhere. Most of our clients have been sick for years, some of them for thirty and forty years, and have tried all the "regular" and "irregular" cures they could hear of before coming to the *Health School*.

They have been poisoned, blistered, carved, electrocuted, vaccinated, inoculated and irradiated by medical men; had their legs pulled by osteopaths, their backs punched by chiropractors; have been frozen, baked, pounded and mauled by physio-therapists; have had their colons laundered times without number by the colonic irrigators; have been dieted and treated by psychologists and spiritual healers; they have tried patent medicines, herbs, "drugless" laxatives, and visited the hot springs, mineral springs, etc. Many of them have come to the *Health School* as a last resort and with little hope that we could help them.

A great variety of so-called diseases have come to the *Health School*. Many of the sufferers had been declared to be *incurable*.

The plan of care described in the pages of this book is the plan of care we have used with such gratifying success, in the types of cases described above. The thousands of former sufferers scattered over the earth who are now enjoying good health amply testify to the efficacy of *Hygienic* methods.

Not every one who has come to the *Health School* has recovered health. Those who have failed to regain health may be grouped in three categories, as follows:

(1) A few have come to the *Health School* who were already dying. They were too badly damaged in some of their more vital organs to live.

(2) Some have come early enough to have recovered full health, but for one reason or another, they have not remained long enough to accomplish their aim. They have not had enough time; or they have lacked money; or they have been unwilling to carry out the program long enough to cure themselves.

(3) Not a few more have been foolish enough to spend their time and money for care and instruction and have not carried out instructions. They have violated their instructions in many ways. These have wanted to buy health, they have been unwilling to deserve it. They would not or could not understand that they could not "eat their cake and keep it."

It is the hope of the author that this little book will fall into the hands of those who are sufficiently intelligent to use it wisely and well. To such, the information it contains will prove of inestimable value. To others it may be only a curiosity. "The wise will understand."

Orthopathy —
Physiological Lawfulness

Every part of man's body is *designed* for a particular function, and is controlled by laws that are as immutable as the law of gravitation. These laws are *designed* to govern the body's actions and preserve its integrity.

Every involuntary power exhibited in man's body constantly and ceaselessly obeys these laws. In the very nature of things it could not be otherwise. The organs must perform the functions for which they are *designed*. They must obey the laws of their constitution. They can no more do otherwise than the earth can reverse its motion, or stones cast themselves upward. When cohesive attraction splits rocks and magnetism arranges needles parallel to the equator, then may we expect to see organs of man's body disobey the laws of their constitution and perform functions for which they are not *designed*.

So long as our organs act, they must act lawfully. The action must be *upward* and *right*. Their action can never be *downward* and *wrong*. In disease as in health, all the actions of the body are according to immutable law. Every organ and function performs the work for which it is *designed*. Every action is correct, *upward*, and designed to save, improve and perpetuate life.

There are no amendments to the constitution of Nature. None of her laws have been repealed. They cannot be broken, but men may break themselves in the attempt to break them. The damage is to the man, and not to the law. And it is only in our voluntary actions that we are capable of setting ourselves in opposition to the laws of our being. Every time that we do this, the laws inflict a certain penalty. There is no escape from the penalty.

This is a Universe of law and order. Every law is the expression of a force behind it. Every force must act lawfully, being unable to act in any other way. The laws and forces controlling the body are the same in disease as in health, and their action is always for the same purpose — harmony, betterment, improvement.

Disease action, no less than health action, is *right action;* yet it occasions suffering because of adverse conditions that have been imposed upon the body. So, by the term *Orthopathy* we mean *right suffering*. The individual suffers, not because the action of the body is wrong, but because the body, under control of law, is struggling in the only way it can struggle, to free itself from impending dangers resulting from bad habits — misuse and abuse.

Let no man deceive you; let no man lead you astray. The actions of the body are always right, and in disease are as true to the pole-star of health as the needle is to the pole-star of direction. The so-called symptoms of disease which puzzle eminent physicians, are not destructive processes; they are not evils to be resisted, combatted, suppressed, subdued, or subverted. They are merely external evidences of a body's striving under control of law to preserve its integrity and existence; and the physician who regards them as anything else, reveals his abject ignorance of the most fundamental facts of life. Shun him as you would a poison.

Disease — a Vital Process

Vital actions may be grouped under two heads as follows:

1. *Normal*— the regular ordinary actions of life in the conduct of its ordinary functions, commonly called physiological; and

2. *Abnormal*—such modifications of the regular or ordinary actions of life as are essential to meet, overcome, destroy or adjust the body to abnormal, unusual, or harmful conditions and agents; and usually called pathological.

The first we call *health;* the second we call *disease.* It is necessary, however, if we are to clearly understand what disease is and, as a consequence of this understanding, properly care for the sick, that we recognize the essential unity of the actions of the body in *health* and its actions in *disease;* that back of both groups of actions are the same powers of life and the same effort to preserve and enhance life.

Physical, chemical, thermal, electrical, and vital agents are capable of damaging the body. Their effects may be grouped as chemical and mechanical. Doctors and laymen alike commonly confuse the effects of injurious agents with the efforts of the living organism to meet and overcome or destroy them and to repair damages. If we briefly glance at a few of these agents and their effects it may help us to separate the one from the other.

Cut the body of a living man and there is pain, bleeding, fibrin-formation, blood-clot, redness, swelling, healing, and sloughing of the scab. Cut the body of a dead man and none of these things follow. Strike your finger with a hammer and there is pain, hemorrhage into the tissues, blood-clot, inflammation, healing, and removal of debris. Strike the fingers of a dead man and none of these things follow. The cut is the only effect of the knife. The bruise is the only effect of the hammer. All of the above enumerated ensuing phenomena are examples of the reaction of the living body to physical or mechanical injury.

Put muriatic acid on a dead body and it destroys the flesh it comes in contact with. Put it on a live body and it does the same thing. Put quick-lime on a dead body and it destroys the flesh. Put it on a live body and it does the same. These are examples of the action (chemical) of harmful chemical substances upon the body. These destroy. But whereas, their action is followed by nothing but further decay in the dead body; in the living organism their action is followed by pain, inflammation, and healing. Put a mustard plaster on the body of a dead man and nothing happens. Put it on a live body and redness, smarting and blistering follow. Apply such a plaster to a feeble, pale, anemic, or dropsical person and it blisters with difficulty or not at all. Give a dose of salts to a dead man and nothing happens; give it to a vigorous man and violent diarrhea occurs; give it to a feeble man and a feeble diarrhea results.

Blistering and diarrhea are defensive reactions tending to protect the body from the damaging effects of the drugs. These are examples of the response or reaction of the living organism to drug substances.

From these last two examples we deduce the following law, which may be exemplified by numerous instances from the sick room: *The actions of the living organism in the presence of a drug are the responses of its own powers to the drug and are proportioned to the degree of its vital vigor.*

Flesh may be burned with fire or destroyed with electricity or consumed by parasites (vital agents). In these as in all other cases the body reacts to defend and repair itself. Its reactions are mere modifications of the ordinary or normal processes of life and no new or extra-vital super-additions to these powers and processes. Disease, like health, is a manifestation of life.

These modifications of functions are looked upon by the various conventional, orthodox "schools of healing" as foes of life. The efforts of the body to defend and repair itself are looked upon by them as the very things that endanger life. They have confounded vital action with the actions of pathogenic agents and influences. Their practice, based upon this false premise, is largely one of suppressing symptoms.

A physician, head of a sanitarium with which I was once connected, said to me in speaking of a vaginal discharge in a case of uterine cancer: "I'll stop that discharge yet." A few mornings later, it was Sunday, while walking over the sanitarium grounds with my wife, I met him. He said as he came up: "I finally got that discharge stopped; I did it with an ice-bag." He passed on and I remarked to my wife: "That is compounded murder." One hour later the patient was in a septic coma and in another half hour she was dead.

The value of drainage in wounds and abscesses is recognized, but its value in uterine cancer is not. When he suppressed the drainage in this case he sealed his patient's death warrant. The pent-up "secretion" killed the patient. In the same manner the discharge in a cold, which is also drainage, is suppressed and the suppression is called cure, even where this results in chronic disease.

Only a true understanding of the nature of disease will enable doctors to cease fighting with the body in the mad delusion that they are fighting a monster called disease; only this will stop doctors from killing their patients in their vain efforts to cure them. When once the curative nature of so-called disease is recognized it will then be understood that the only valuable thing the doctor can do is to assure his patient the best possible hygienic conditions under which to carry on these curative processes and to remove the causes that have made the curative actions necessary.

Disease only exists where it is necessary and it lasts as long as there's need for it. If it is suppressed in one place it arises in another. If its acute phases are suppressed it becomes chronic. It never ends (except where the sufferer is killed) until its need ends.

Organic Unity —
Its Relation to Cure

The only correct way of viewing the body is to view it as a whole. The organs of the body are co-equal factors in a vital reciprocity. Division of labor, as seen in the complex organism, is an internal adaptation. In an evolving organism the differentiating process is accompanied by integration of the parts (organs and tissues), the whole remaining a unit.

Borrowing a phrase from biology, the separate organs of the body collectively constitute a "web of life," in which all must do their work and labor together; all, alike, being made of one "stuff," though "modified" and "specialized" to form a hierarchy of organs—an organism. The greater organic complexity of the higher animals means increased symbiotic support for the higher functions performed by these animals.

The specialization of organs in the body is for mutual service and general welfare and involves industry, frugality and regularity on the part of each and every organ. The co-operate efforts of the totality of organs making up the body tend to produce a resultant equal to their combined value and greatly enrich each organ thereby. An organ is richer the more it contributes to the sum of organic (body) well-being.

In order to a wide physiological usefulness there must be a rhythmic performance of well regulated functions and a permanent and complex system of division of labor with systematic co-operation between the organs of the body resulting in such mutual "stimulation" and mutual enhancement as to produce and maintain a stable relation and, in general, such fortification of the body as to lead to considerable permanence and to a high degree of efficiency and integrity of the compound organism.

Physiological wealth is due to the co-operative efforts of all of the organs of the body. The better each organ does the work for which it is specialized, the better can every other organ perform the work for which it is constituted and the better will be the valuable substances that are stored up in the organism for domestic and reproductive uses.

The first requisite of organic solidarity is loyalty to the principle of co-operation. The concord existing between the various organs and systems of the body must be adequately maintained. In a broad, general sense, every part of the body acts for the good of the whole, rather than for its own selfish advantage. Good functional behavior and loyality to the organism on the part of each organ of the body are fundamental and constitutional virtues.

The blood, glands and nervous system have the chief responsibility of directing and co-ordinating the functions of the organism. There is here a deputing of inter-dependent functions, involving the necessity for a loyal discharge of duties, to special organs and systems. Such a case of division of labor, plus the loyal disposition for mutual accommodation and mutual support, is a splendid example of what H. Reinheimer has called *"internal symbiosis."*

Every gland depends upon the co-operation of the others, while the whole organism is dependent, for its well-being, upon the subtle and co-ordinated inter-organic "stimulation," requiring a high degree of subordination of the parts to the common good. For, an organism is a complex of differentiated, co-ordinated, unified, integrated and semi-independent entities (organs), which reciprocate with and compensate each other in the performance of duties. The organic units of such an organism have been specialized in order that they may better perform the particular specialized duties imposed upon them. As specialists, they are forced to rely upon the integrity and industry of the other organs of the body. Without co-operation nothing can be achieved.

Specialization in medicine, which looks upon each organ of the body as an independent isonomy and treats individual organs or parts without the least regard for this inter-organic dependence and co-operation, is a false principle. Surgical interference with the integrity of the organism upsets the nicety of physiological balance upon which the highest physiological efficiency depends.

The organic community goes forward as a whole. Nothing short of a general integrity, based on the evolved harmony between physiological partners, will avail. We must rely upon the laws and conditions governing the interdependent operations of the organs of the body and not upon interferences with the functions of one organ.

Instead of trying to compel Nature to conform to our petty ends, we should adapt ourselves to her larger purposes and greater ends. We must put our physiological house in order; not by myriads of local treatments, as physicians with a financial interest in our suffering are bent upon doing, but by duly adjusting ourselves to the ordered harmony of Nature upon which every organ and function in the body depends for its very existence.

We cannot expect Nature to alter herself and accommodate herself to our morbid appetencies and selfish ends. We must conform to her. Law and order cannot be set aside for your special benefit, or for mine.

Whatever occurs presupposes the existence of preceding forces and conditions which determine the course of subsequent events. Degenerative elements within the organism exist only because they have been produced by antecedent causes. The elements introduced by degenerative tendencies become variously blended with and superimposed upon the elements of health. Our preference for water-tight compartments causes us to look for breaks in the degenerative process and prevents us from recognizing the unity of disease.

Not only have we created many diseases, but we also have failed to differentiate between the degeneration on the one hand and the vital struggle against the degeneration and its causes on the other. Thus defensive and reparative physiological action is classed with degeneration as disease. We have failed to distinguish between physiology and pathology; between life and death. As a direct consequence we direct our supposed remedial measures, not at the causes of degeneration, but at the vital efforts to restore health. This is true not only of the older schools of medicine, but of the newer or drugless schools as well.

In every essential particular, except in their respective modalities, the newer schools of so-called healing are Allopathic from the ground up. Their whole conception of life, health, disease, causation, cure and treatment is allopathic: which means that their conceptions are essentially those of the savage medicine man. Cures, miracles, magical potencies, thaumaturgic incantations, "drugs, fake anodynes and consolatory buncombe," metaphysical nonsense, spiritual rubbish and psychological tom-foolery take the place of rational care.

To hammer, maul, twist, pull, electrocute, freeze, roast, stew and blister the body and ignore causes; to resort to mental, physical, mechanical, electrical, thermal and chemical means of stimulating and inhibiting the functions of the body and neglect to conform to the ordered harmony of Nature — such treatment cannot always be palmed off on the public as Nature Cure. Great numbers of people are outgrowing spurious "natural methods" and the doctor who does not keep ahead of these people will ultimately be left behind.

The so-called science of medicine is composed of a super-abundance of unsolved muddles. Only by years of sad failure do doctors learn to free themselves from the blind, unreasoning confidence instilled into them during their college training. Many of them, unfortunately, due to commercialism, brain laziness or credulity, never free themselves from their blind faith in the power of "remedies" to cure.

Those of us who profess a belief in the principle that only Nature cures are going to have to accord to Nature the opportunity as well as the power of cure. When we do so, our success will be much greater. We have too many "cures" to substitute for Nature Cure.

The intelligent portions of our population are growing tired of being fooled by pseudo-discoveries and pseudo-remedies constantly dangled before the eyes of a gullible public by the professionals. There are still plenty of men and women who "would rather die than think" and who will continue to pursue the fool's policy of buying for a few dollars, a "patch-up-cure" to relieve them of the penalties attached to their continued indulgencies. This group is daily growing fewer in number as knowledge of correct principles spreads.

Toxemia

Toxemia is the presence in the blood, lymph, secretions and cells of any substance, from any source, which, in sufficient quantity, will impair organic functions. Toxemia means the presence of too great a percentage of toxins in the tissues and fluids of the body. There is a normal amount of toxins in the body at all times. These become foes of life only when they are permitted to accumulate beyond the normal limit.

Toxins result from the normal breaking down of tissues in the body in the ordinary activities of life. The normal processes of elimination expel these toxins as rapidly as they form. This keeps the blood and lymph pure and sweet and good health is the result.

If elimination is impaired or checked, so that the toxins are not thrown out of the body as rapidly as they arise, they are retained in the body and accumulate there, producing toxemia. Toxemia in this form is the poisoning of the body by its own retained excretions.

Efficient elimination is maintained by an abundant supply of nerve energy (vitality). Nerve energy is lowered by any act of life that uses up nerve energy in excess of the body's power to recuperate or regenerate its forces. Any mode of living that brings on this state of lowered nerve force—enervation—necessarily checks elimination and this permits the body to poison itself by the retention of its own waste.

By enervation is meant a state of functional weakness and lowered nerve force. The functions of the various organs of man's body are all under control of the nervous system and are strong or weak, as the case may be, depending on whether the amount of nervous energy on hand is abundant or low. Our supply of nerve force fluctuates, varying in amount from day to day, from hour to hour, depending on the quality and quantity of our activities — mental, emotional, physical and physiological — and the nature of our surroundings.

Nerve energy is expended by all forms of activity and recuperated and conserved by rest and sleep. Under normal conditions nature compels sufficient rest and sleep to thoroughly recuperate from the daily expenditures. Under modern conditions, with everyone striving for wealth, social position, power and prominence, men and women disregard nature's signal for rest — fatigue — and force themselves on with stimulants. Gradually, a little each day, they expend their energy reserves, and then their standard of physiological efficiency is lowered.

Impaired function always follows enervation. Function deteriorates and, as a result, serious deficiencies arise. With nerve energy lowered, there is more or less of impairment of all of the functions of the body, but the weaker organs suffer most. Checked elimination, faulty digestion, impaired secretion and excretion, inhibition of glandular activity, etc., result from lack of nervous energy.

Drainage is the term applied to the physiological processes by which all waste and toxic matter are carried away from the cells and eliminated from the body. It is the means by which internal cleanliness is maintained.

The tremendous importance of such cleanliness may be realized when it is known that if the urine is suppressed for fifty-two hours death results; the carbon dioxide exhaled in one day would kill many times over, if retained; if a wound is pent up, so that drainage is stopped, septicemia and probably death soon result.

The normal functions of life give rise to toxic residues which poison the body if not rapidly eliminated. Ailments are due to the crowding of toxic waste into the tissues.

If the bowels, kidneys, liver, or lungs fail in their functions, the accumulation of autogenic poisons takes place. These organs are under nervous control and their efficiency is determined by the integrity of the nervous system.

Elimination, is a fundamental function of the living body and, if not prevented by faulty habits, will keep pace with the normal daily intake of the body. It is only when elimination has been impaired that the body begins to suffer from a toxic-overload.

Enervation also lowers the ability of the body to digest food. The food undergoes decomposition in the digestive tract and gives rise to whole series of virulent poisons, more or less of which are absorbed into the blood stream, there to poison the cells and tissues of the body. Defective functioning of the gastro-intestinal tract and the consequent fouling of the food supply, and the poisoning of the tissues by sepsis absorbed from the intestine, plays a big part in the production of disease. This is one of the most common forms of poisoning with which the body has to deal. Recurring intermittent poisoning is far oftener due to over-ingestion of food, not necessarily bad food, than to other causes.

The digestive juices of the healthy person are capable of destroying the toxins which may occasionally form in the digestive tract, but due to the common habits of over eating, eating wrong combinations of food, eating hurriedly and without properly masticating the food, eating when there is fever, or discomfort, the digestive organs become weakened and their secretions are so impaired that they are no longer able to protect. They lose their immunizing power and permit poisoning to occur. Finally there comes a time when the systemic intoxication over-flows and resistance is crushed, natural immunities are wiped out and acute disease results.

Carbohydrate decomposition (fermentation) and protein decomposition (putrefaction) give rise to different kinds of toxins and produce different types of. *disease*. Proteins give rise to the most virulent toxins. Protein poisoning, if tolerated, makes for degenerative rather than progressive adaptation in life, since the poisoning will cut off the organism from constructive physiological advance.

Toxemia tends to produce more enervation and to increase the toxin absorption and retention, but is not self-creating or self-evolving. A "vicious circle" is formed from which the body seeks to escape from time to time by means of an acute *disease* or crisis. Intoxication holds sway everywhere; even where no acute *disease* exists; constant chronic poisoning of the organism takes place under the influence of enervating habits.

The chief source of toxemia is the retention and accumulation within the body, due to faulty elimination, of the end-products of metabolism — cell waste. The next source, in order of importance, is absorption of decomposition products from the intestinal tract, the result of impaired digestion, secretion and excretion.

Toxemia is the product of fermentation and decomposition and of the retained end products of metabolism, of worry, spite, hate, fear, jealousy, fault finding, promiscuous love, sexual excesses, overwork, overstimulation, overeating, dissipations and excesses and too much haste for the almighty dollar. The deficiencies and excesses of which the whole human race is unconsciously guilty may be properly regarded as the basic cause of *disease*. These are the things that enervate and enervation lowers functional ability. Toxemia clogs the organism, every cell, tissue, organ, nerve fibre, the blood and lymph stream, until one after another of the organs of the body break down.

The toxic state of the body produced by checked elimination and faulty digestion forms the bed rock upon which all *disease* is founded. The toxins act as irritants in the body. The irritation is followed by congestion, inflammation, and suppuration (tissue decomposition and pus formation), while the resulting so-called *disease* is named according to its location in the body.

Nausea, vomiting, anorexia (loss of appetite), pain, fever, chills, inflammation, diarrhea, constipation, headache, and other acute febrile symptoms of *disease*, are effects largely of the poisoning resulting from the decomposition of food in the intestine. Such a crisis represents an effort of the body to eliminate the poisons and dispose of the decomposing food.

If the wrong eating and living habits are continued after the crisis is passed, there begins the development of a chronic condition. The crises become progressively less shocking (less severe), as the body builds a toleration for the poisons slowly absorbed from the intestine. As this poisoning continues, a process of degeneration begins in the body, which will be more marked in the weaker organs than in the others. As one organ or tissue after another breaks down before this chronic poisoning, Greek labels are attached to the resulting conditions, and the patient has new *diseases*. If the kidneys break down, the *disease* will be named Bright's *disease*; if it is the pancreas that breaks down, the *disease* will be named diabetes; if it is the lungs that succumb to the poisons the trouble will be labeled tuberculosis; etc., etc.

Poisoning and overstimulation result in organic change and, what was at first a mere functional disorder, becomes a structural derangement. — an organic *disease*. The resulting so-called *disease*, as previously pointed out, is named according to the organ that is crippled; but no organ suffers alone. The whole body is more or less affected.

In diabetes, the pancreas is not the only organ involved. It is preceded by and accompanied with impairment and destruction in other and often more important organs. The causes which produce diabetes do not concentrate their "attack" and spend their full force upon the pancreas alone. In other words, diabetes is only one of "several *diseases*" with which the patient suffers. In Bright's *disease*, the kidneys are not the only organs involved. In. tuberculosis, the lung *disease* is only part of the *disease* of the body. All so-called chronic and organic *diseases* are merely local developments out of a general systemic derangement.

When the organs of the body begin to break down and falter in their functions, it is easy and natural for the wreck of one organ to be followed by the wreck of another. All of the organs have been crippled more or less by the common causes of organic impairment and many of them are already on the verge of a breakdown. The *disease* is named according to to the organ that breaks down first and when other organs break down, the resulting so-called *diseases* are called complications. Complications have three sets of causes — *The Primary Causes* are those impairing and crippling influences (enervation, toxemia, and food deficiencies) which have been in operation throughout the system for years and, through their persistence, accumulation and extension, are responsible for the general impairment of the system: *Secondary Causes* are those which are the results of the organic impairment (for instance, the chief secondary cause in a simple or "uncomplicated" diabetes, is the nutritional perversion — crippled carbohydrate metabolism — resulting from the *disease* of the pancreas): *Tertiary Causes* are therapeutic procedures — this is to say, the evils wrought in the body by the agents and methods employed to "combat the *disease*" help to further weaken and destroy the body.

In a general way, this gives you an idea of the unity and continuity of *disease*. *Disease* does not exist without cause. It begins where cause begins and persists where cause persists. The initial beginnings of the so-called "degenerative *diseases* of later life" are laid in infancy, sometimes before birth, the degeneration continuing as an unbroken process throughout the life of the individual. Only the end points of the degeneration, and not its early stages, are commonly recognized.

The suffix "itis" means inflammation. Tonsilitis is inflammation of the tonsils; metritis is inflammation of the womb, gastritis is inflammation of the stomach, appendicitis is inflammation of the appendix, etc. The names merely denote the locations of the inflammation — they do not reveal the cause of the trouble, nor do they indicate the means of recovery. Only a true knowledge of cause enables one to institute proper remedial measures.

To treat the lungs for a *disease* called pneumonia, the kidneys for a *disease* called Bright's *disease*, the bronchial tubes for a *disease* called asthma, the intestine for a *disease* called enteritis, the colon for a *disease* called colitis, etc., and all the while ignore the underlying *Toxemia* and *Enervation* and the habits of living and eating that have produced them, is not only useless treatment, it is actually damaging to the patient.

The body is broken down by bad habits. If you work too hard or too much, or eat too much, or eat inadequate foods, or bathe too long or too often, or drink too much, or enjoy too much; if you dissipate and indulge in harmful practices; if you are over-stimulated in any manner, by any means, you build weakness and *disease*.

Anger, fear, grief, sorrow, jealousy, envy, spite, hatred, prejudice, lust, lying, stealing, deceit, dishonesty and all forms of dishonor and disloyalty to truth, break down the body and impair health.

These and similar bad habits can and do result in *disease* — all forms — and recovery from *disease* necessitates the correction of all of these destructive habits. You must be educated out of your bad habits and educated into new ones. The formation and fixation of new and wholesome habits is essential.

Doctors of all schools are attempting to *cure disease* without correcting enervating habits. Volume after volume is published upon the subject of *disease* and *cure*, in which the authors discuss specific *cures*, while ignoring a manner of living that makes recovery impossible.

Prevailing methods of treating these conditions are all based on a study of the changes that occur in the various organs and not upon the causes of the changes. *Toxemia* and the checked elimination that gives rise to it are ignored. The *Enervation* that produced the checked elimination is unrecognized. The *Faulty Mode of Living* that produced the enervation is not corrected. The treatment is directed at the effects, at the symptoms. Symptoms are such only and not causes. If we choke a hungry dog we stop his whining, but he is still hungry. If we "kill" pain by drugs or other methods we silence the out-cries of nature, but the causes of the pain are not touched. This is the reason that so many patients are regarded as incurable.

There is no cure short of correction of cause. The toxemia must be eliminated, nervous energies must be restored to normal; the enervating mode of living must be corrected. The methods of treating *disease* that are in vogue are not calculated to produce a single one of these necessary changes. On the contrary, almost without exception, they further enervate and add to the toxemia. Many of them encourage the wrong course of living.

Foci of Infection

What is called the *Modern Science of Medicine* is given to fads and faddishness. It changes fads with great rapidity, although seldom entirely abandoning an old one when taking up a new one. When it was agreed to accept microbes as the cause of disease they spent years in trying to find a germ for each so-called disease, old and new, in the nosologies. This led to the immunization fad and the attempt to find a serum or a vaccine to prevent every so-called disease and to an effort to cure every so-called disease with serums and vaccines.

Later the discovery of the importance of the ductless (endocrine) glands, previously declared to be useless survivals (vestiges) of man's hypothetical anthropoid stage, led to a frenzied effort to prove all so-called diseases to be the results of endocrine embalance and to the fad of treating all diseases with gland extracts, powdered glands, operations on the glands, etc.

Then came the discovery of vitamins and of deficiency diseases and the effort to prove all diseases to be due to vitamin deficiencies and the fad of giving vitamins for what have you. Even the harmful effects of chronic alcoholism were declared to be due to vitamin deficiency and not to alcohol.

These three fads now vie with each other for first place in the medical show window. They are forced to compete for honors with surgery and the new drugs that are frequently announced.

A few years ago some medical nit wit hit upon the idea of using snake venom to *cure* some so-called disease. "Success" crowned his efforts and soon snake venom was reported to be *successful* in the treatment of a wide variety of "diseases." For a time it seemed that the snake venom was destined to become the long sought panacea.

Perhaps snake venom would have achieved the enviable distinction of being a cure-all had not artificial fever come into the lime light with remarkable *cures* for a wide variety of "diseases." Another cure-all seemed to be in the making.

But, alas! and alack! Every time "medical science" thinks it has a cure-all in its hands, another contender for the place bobs up to distract attention. Artificial fever had to yield the front page to sulfanilamide. Just now this new poison bids fair to reach the pinacle that snake venom just missed.

"Frozen sleep" came in a couple of years ago and made a good start for stardom but fell by the wayside. Its promotors must have picked a poor press agent.

None of these modern cure-alls have ever succeeded to such wide-spread use or *cured* as high a percentage of cases as the old fad of blood-letting that persisted for two thousand years. Hippocrates, the *Father of Medicine*, seems to have started this fad and it persisted to the days of our fathers.

Some years ago a medical fad was started and its heyday of popularity lasted longer than that of many of the modern fads, while it is still in great favor with the sons of Hippocrates. I refer to the fad of tracing all so-called diseases to some focus (plural, *foci*) of infection and *curing* the *disease* by removing the "focus of infection." They sought to explain most diseases on a basis of focal infections and sought to *cure* them by removing organs.

What is a focus of infection? It is a center from which infection is spread. What is infection? It is defined as the invasion of the body by pathogenic microbes; although, the "focal infection" faddists often made it mean either "germ infection" or "pus infection," by which they meant pus absorption from an abscess.

Heart disease, insanity, indigestion, kidney disease, anemia, rheumatism or arthritis, neuritis, epilepsy, and many other conditions were traced to "foci of infection."

Teeth were pulled, tonsils were extracted, sinuses were drained, gall bladders were cut out, appendices were excised, ovaries and tubes were extirpated, prostate glands and seminal vesicles were removed to *cure* "disease" elsewhere in the body. The fad for removing "foci of infection" became a national menace. The frenzy became so great that whatever "disease" a man or woman had, called for an operation.

An organ did not have to be abscessed to be removed as a focus of infection. Tons of sound teeth were sacrificed in the search for pus foci. Dr. Walter C. Alvarez, of the Mayo Clinic, writing in the *Journal of the American Medical Association*, in 1920, says that, "In practice they pull the teeth first, and if the patient returns unbenefitted they can then look to see what is the matter with him."

Many epileptics gave up a mouth full of teeth without benefit. Thousands of sufferers from rheumatic arthritis suffered the loss of all their teeth without help. The tragedy of the procedure lay not so much in the fact that badly ulcerated teeth were removed but that perfectly good teeth were sacrificed indiscriminately.

Tonsils were slaughtered as freely as the teeth. In the army hospitals during the "war to end war," tonsils were carried out each day by the buckets full. Adenoids, which are also tonsils, came out as freely.

All of the other organs mentioned above were freely sacrificed on the altar of the focal infection fad, and the end is not yet. The practice is still profitable and the public is still gullible.

It is everywhere admitted that "radical treatment of foci of infection (extraction of teeth, removal of tonsils, gall bladder, appendix, ovaries, etc.,) is frequently of little or no benefit, and, besides this, many cases are seen in which no focus can be found." Dr. Alvarez says in the article previously quoted from, "In view of the fact that the most thorough removal of focal infection often fails to cure arthritis and other diseases, let us be more honest and conservative with our patients."

It is not only true that the removal of one or several "foci of infection" fails to *cure*, but it is equally true that many apparently healthy people possess "foci of infection" that appear to cause no harm. Dr. Alvarez says: "certainly the thousands of people who for the last thirty or forty years have been chewing contentedly on dead teeth (without signs of root infection) should be grateful that these radical ideas did not prevail when they were young."

T. Swann Harding said in an article a few years ago: "But several things must be remembered. Time and again powerful and healthy looking men appear with large alveolar abscesses they have carried for years. They maintain that they have never had a headache, a twinge of rheumatism, nor needed a physician."

Doctors lack a knowledge of the true cause of disease and this, plus their snapshot and indiscriminate diagnoses, caused them to send their patients to the dentist for teeth extraction or to the surgeon for removal of other organs. Classical medical "knowledge" required searching for and removing "focal infections."

Often a patient had several "foci of infection" removed in the course of a *disease*, all to no avail. Here are the highlights of a case of polyarthritis in a woman that came under our observation in 1929. Almost every movable joint in her body was affected. She had been in this condition for six long and weary years, growing progressively worse during the time. During this period she had been under the care of several physicians and in three or four hospitals.

The trouble started in one ankle. The physicians began by removing one ovary and the appendix. Later, she having grown worse, they removed her tonsils. She grew still worse and other joints became affected. They now removed sixteen teeth. She grew still worse. They removed her gall bladder. This was followed by increased disease. As a final effort at saving her they performed a pan-hysterectomy, which means they removed her womb, both tubes and the remaining ovary. After this last operation she grew still worse. Her physicians then told her that they had removed every cause of her trouble and that they could not understand why she did not get well. They could do nothing else for her.

What can an inflamed or enlarged tonsil have to do with the causation of pathology elsewhere in the body? Primarily nothing. To have tonsillar trouble we must have something else first and removing the tonsils does not remove this something else. Can you believe that enlarged tonsils and adenoids are their own cause? If they are not their own cause, then removing them does not remove their cause.

If abscessed teeth cause rheumatism, what causes abscessed teeth? If the teeth are not the cause of their own abscesses, then removing the teeth does not remove cause.

If there is pus in the gums, are the gums, themselves, the cause of it? If the gums are not cause how can "checking" the "disease" in the gum-tissue cause "disease" elsewhere to disappear?

We do not deny that abscesses do form, nor that pus is sometimes absorbed, nor that its absorption is fraught with harm. Have we not seen the harm produced by cowpox pus?

So-called immunization by vaccination and serumization is a form of infection. Infection from vaccination is no more to be desired than auto-infection from "foci." No mode of infection is better than another.

– 31

All infections are a form of septic poisoning. They are products of protein putrefaction. Call it vaccine (pus), intestinal infection, pus pockets, gonorrhea, "syphilis," etc., it all results from protein putrefaction.

Pus formation in the body may contribute to "disease" elsewhere in the body, if resistance is so low as to invite general disintegration. But its removal does not remove cause nor is it necessary to remove the organ in order to clear up the abscess. Removing the "focus of infection" only puts a temporary check upon the overwhelming absorption, it never removes the real cause, which cause is responsible for the abscess in the first place.

Suppose the germ theory is correct. Suppose germs have infected the tonsils. Suppose from this "focus" they have entered the circulation and reached the knee, ankle, and shoulder. Suppose arthritis exists in each of these joints. Each infected joint is now a secondary "focus of infection." From each of these joints germs may sally forth to infect other joints or other organs. This being true, can the arthritis be *cured* by removing the tonsils? Will it not be necessary to remove each infected joint also? If·it is the heart that is infected will the disease be *cured* without removing the heart? Is it not necessary to remove all "foci of infection?"

Tilden very correctly says: "To treat foci of infection as the sole originating cause of these diseases (heart disease, arthritis, etc.); and to ignore the big things in the life-habits of the patient that break down resistance and debase nutrition, is to strain at a gnat and swallow a camel. If the ardor displayed in ferreting out minute collections of pus in the body were exercised upon locating and correcting definitely harmful habits, the advantage to the patient and to the community would be immeasurable."

HEALTH FIRST

So-called research has supplied the world of men with unnecessary occasions for fear and has done this deliberately in order to cause them to abandon self-help and self-reliance and place their trust in a half-baked mere hope of a science.

The researchers have wickedly and falsely heralded the fear-engendering story that the world is teeming with a host of vicious microscopical and ultra-microscopical beings against which no amount of integrity is a shield, and the ravages of which we can escape only by placing ourselves in bondage — a servitude born of fear — to the man with the squirt-gun and the hollow needle.

Serologists say to us: "Live as you please, eat any offal or putrid carcass to which your carnivorous taste may incline you, practice any vicious habits to which your cultivated cravings may lead you, violate any and all of the laws of your being, dissipate and go to excess as you will; we will wring from the bodies of our animal victims in the laboratory, serums to immunize you against the necessary consequences of your misconduct."

They ask us to abnegate genuine hopes of achieving wholeness for fortuitious promises of "magic," of vicarious salvation. They omit to mention that serums, the production of which is a lucrative business, are most likely to result in a whole long train of evils of their own, which are often more lasting than their promised benefits are supposed to be.

Dependence upon artificial means of preservation has caused too much neglect of natural preservation which, alone, can insure strength of the individual and health of the race. Every so-called disease is preceded by a more or less lengthy period of preparation, during which hygienic errors are repeated and though counterbalanced by natural resistance, there finally comes a time when the resulting systemic intoxication overflows and resistance is crushed, natural immunities are wiped out, and it is only then, if ever, that microbes can do any damage.

Microbes are spread throughout Nature. Human groups swarm with tubercle bacilli. They are found in many kinds of food. In spite of this not everyone develops tuberculosis. The robust and vigorous laugh at these little fellows. Only those who are weakened by unwholesome living, poor nutrition and faulty emotional conduct can become a prey of "bad germs."

Infection, whether parasitical or bacterial, is not a matter of accident, but of "soil," Bad "soil" conditions are due to bad behaviour — all bad actions producing bad reactions upon the body. Microbial pullulations are possible only where there is a failure of organic resistance. Failure of organic resistance is the immediate cause of infection, otherwise the least contact with microbes would suffice to produce infection.

The soil is more important than the "germ." Infection and degeneration can set in only when the soil is badly fertilized by inappropriate nutrition. An organism that has degenerated into a mere bouillon culture has brought itself to this state by its own transgressions. Liability to infection is in keeping with degeneration. To be pronouncedly liable to infection is to be always perilously near infection and the incidence of infection is only too likely to follow in the wake of liability.

What tells most in parasitic as in bacterial infections is the loss of resisting power due to behavior that weakens the power of the body. The parasite is a notorious weakling. For a higher organism to evidence a pronounced liability to parasitic imposition, proves that it has indulged in weakening habits.

We assume that the body alters its general means of defense according to different requirements and as demanded by the character of every new relation. With an occurrence of an infection, the body is forced to reorganize its means of defense. Whether we have a "make-shift" immunity or a normal immunity must depend upon how we order our life thereafter. "Make-shift" immunity is one that is unattended by a concomitant reduction of liability. Serologists experiment with "make-shift" immunities and tamper with old established bonds sacred to integrity and norm-immunity.

Mere destruction of alleged pathogenic organisms is no safeguard of health and unless the intrinsic morbidity is removed by radical remedial measures, other organisms and other symptoms will soon supplant those artificially suppressed. A few minutes reflection will reveal the physical impossibility of reaching all the parasites, actual and prospective, with poisons, or of "curing" and preventing "disease" by the injection of all manner of serums for alleged "immunization" against the legions of "infective diseases" that our general morbidity engenders.

The inherent integrity of the organism is our own best safeguard. The respective potencies of the physiological means of defense are derived from the enviroment — from food, air, water and sunshine. The defensive power of the epithelial tissues is dependent upon proper nutrition.

Nutrition also determines whether the bacteria shall be parasitical or symbiotic in their relations to us. Bacterial toxins are metabolic products of bacterial activity, their character being determined by the habits of feeding of the patient.

Resistance, being a matter of integrity, depends upon behavior. It is impossible to destroy all germ life and it would be fatal to all other forms of life if it were done. It is impossible for us to avoid all contact with bacterial organisms. It therefore behooves us to build and maintain our defenses against any possible damage which they may be responsible for. This is best done, not by artificial means, which leave an aftermath of troubles of their own, but by natural means, which restore and maintain integrity, which prevent and remedy our general morbidity. Wholeness, health, is our best safeguard and this depends upon a few simple natural conditions.

Half-Way Houses of Science

Dr. Manson, hero of *The Citadel*, had adopted as his principle of practice; *take nothing for granted*. He insisted on going to the "bottom" of everything — thorough examination and all that sort of stuff. On one occasion, in the early part of his career, he was called in by an older physician to assist in certifying a man for the asylum. Manson refused to sign the certificate without first (true to his principle) examining the patient, despite the assurances of the older physician that the evidence was clear that the patient was suffering with acute homocidal mania.

Examining the man he found physical changes such as "coarsened features," swollen face, thickened nostrils, waxy skin, etc., and mental symptoms that indicated insanity. But Dr. Manson was not satisfied. "Why, why, he kept asking himself, *why* should Hughes talk like this? Supposing the man had gone out of his mind, what was the cause of it all? He had always been a happy, contented man — no worries, easy going, amicable. Why, without apparent reason had he changed to this?

"There must be a reason, Manson thought doggedly; symptoms don't just happen of themselves. Staring at the swollen beauties before him, puzzling, puzzling for some solution of the conundrum, he instinctively reached out and touched the swollen face, noting subconsciously as he did so, that the pressure of his finger left no dent in the oedematous cheek.

"All at once, electrically, a terminal vibrated in his brain. Why didn't the swelling pit on pressure? Because — now it was his heart which jumped — because it was not true oedema, but myxoedema. He had it, by God, he had it. No no, he must not rush. Firmly he caught hold of himself. He must not be a plunger, wildly leaping to conclusions. He must go cautiously, slowly, be sure!

"Curbing himself, he lifted Emry's hands, yes the skin was dry and rough, the fingers slightly thickened at the ends. Temperature — it was subnormal. Methodically he finished the examination, fighting back each successive wave of elation. Every sign and every symptom — they fitted as superbly as a complex jigsaw puzzle. The clumsy, slow mentation, the attacks of irritability culminating in an outburst of homocidal violence. Oh! the triumph of the complete picture was sublime."

The triumph! What triumph? "He had diagnosed the case." The patient is "sick in mind because he's sick in body. He's suffering from thyroid deficiency — an absolutely straight case of myxoedema."

What did it all amount to? Just this — the young doctor sought out all the signs and symptoms of pathology he could find, grouped them together, and to the ensemble attached a name. That is diagnosis. To diagnose is to find and name the symptom-complex present. It is not to find cause. Diagnosis ignores cause. It seeks only for pathology.

Will it be answered that thyroid deficiency was the cause? Not so. It was but a link in a chain. What caused the thyroid deficiency? It never entered the head of Dr. Manson, nor of his creator, Dr. Cronin, that thyroid deficiency has a cause. Medical men are so accustomed to starting with an established pathology as cause that this case did not go beyond the thyroid pathology.

The treatment was, accordingly, directed, not at the true cause, but at the thyroid deficiency. The patient was given thyroid extract. "There was a period of quavering anxiety, several days of agonized suspense, before Hughes began to respond to the treatment. But once it had started, that response was magical. Emry was out of bed in a fortnight, and back at his work at the end of two months."

A beautiful story but —! Every doctor of experience knows that these cases don't end in this manner. Even if temporary apparent benefit does follow the administration of the thyroid extract, it can last only so long as the thyroid extract is given; given perhaps, in increasing doses. Giving the glandular product does not remove the cause of glandular impairment. At best, it is only a doubtful palliative.

As soon as the glandular product is stopped, and sometimes while it is still being used, the patient begins to slip back into his prior condition. For the thyroid is still impaired. The impairing causes are still at work. The crutch gone, the cripple can only hobble along again.

Dr. Cronin has his patient treated *scientifically*. Dr. Manson is nothing if not *scientific*. He was *thorough* in his examination and up to date in his treatment. Also he followed the *scientific* pattern in stopping at a half-way point in his search for cause. He did not go back of the thyroid deficiency to find its cause. And only by finding and removing primary causes can he prevent the recurrence of his patient's troubles.

Thyroid deficiency does not cause itself. It does not just happen without cause. The lack of thyroid function is not the cause of the lack of thyroid function. The deficiency of thyroid secretion is not the cause of the deficiency of thyroid secretion. To give thyroid extract from sheep or hog will not start up thyroid function. Indeed it tends to lessen thyroid function. However scientific the procedure may be, it is wholly inadequate to the removal of the real cause or causes of trouble in this case.

Allergy

The press of the country has recently been full of items and articles about what is called *allergy*, which is defined as an abnormal sensitivity to substances which are harmless to most people. Hay fever, asthma and hives are among the most common forms of suffering that are said to be due to allergy. Migraine headache is also classed as an allergic phenomenon.

The *American Weekly*, which is the Sunday magazine supplement of the Hearst papers, for Sunday, Sept. 20, carries a lengthy article on allergy under the title: "Maybe Its Your Wife Who Makes You Sick."

We learn from the article that most microscopic fragments of a woman's hair, specks of skin, or powder, and dandruff scales may cause cold symptoms, sneezing and other discomforts, and that cold water (as in cold bathing) can bring on allergic reactions.

The author of the article informs us that between 10,000,000 and 13,000,000 people in the United States (about one in ten of our population) have hay fever or other allergic symptoms. Many of these "have been suffering since early Spring from the pollen of successive plants which have come into bloom such as the grasses, trees and weeds, the peak of misery has come to them since the middle of August." In August, ragweed and cedar trees begin to shed their pollens.

The writer tells us that while the rich can get away to less-pollen infested regions, or install air-conditioning plants with pollen filters, in their homes and go "into virtual retirement during the annual hay fever season," most of the victims of hay fever have been tied to their jobs and to their everyday way of life and have sneezed and suffered and cursed their fate." Others, he reminds us "have tried the nose filters which cut down the amount of offending pollen inhaled at each living breath."

The article contains a brief outline of a fantastic and chimerical theory of the cause of allergy, which seems to be taken from a recent book, *Your Allergy and What To Do About It*, by Dr. Milton B. Cohen and his daughter, June Cohen.

Briefly stated, this theory is, that the body manufactures antibodies (bacteriolysins) to destroy germs and the toxins these produce. Once the body has discovered the ability to produce antibodies it will react to any foreign substance — whether "dangerous living disease germs," or "substances that are inanimate and of themselves harmless" — by the production of antibodies, and thus make us sick. Let me quote the following from the article:

Whatever the reason it is unfortunate that in certain people some non-living harmless things cause the cells of the body to release a substance which is poisonous. This kind of poisoning, resulting from the action of antibodies on harmless non-living things, is called an allergic reaction.

In hay fever the harmless thing attacked with ferocity by the body is the pollen of various plants, particularly ragweed.

"What has been said about the development of immunity from a disease like typhoid fever, applies in the development of an allergy except that it is the second — rather than the first — exposure to the allergic material which creates the symptoms.

Let us go back to Mr. Smith again — or to you — and see what happens if it develops that you are allergic to eggs. You eat some eggs and absorb some of the protein called albumen into your blood stream. This is a foreign protein. Ordinarily it would do nothing, for it is non-living and will not grow and propagate itself.

However, the antibodies of the body against this foreign protein begin to be created. But by the time they have been created the albumen has disappeared and they have nothing to con-

- 41 -

tend with. They are ready to fight but have no opponent.

When a dose of egg albumen is absorbed a second time, however, your cells are ready to act for they have attached to them the antibodies that attack egg albumen. Pouncing on their harmless foes, they produce poisons which cause the well known allergic shock. This type of reaction can occur in anyone, says Dr. Cohen.

In one of his syndicated articles Dr. Irving S. Cutter, says: "almost any plant along the roadside or in the woods may affect you or me." Seems man does not belong on the earth. His whole environment seems to be opposed to him.

Now, "for the first time," says the article in the *American Weekly*, "Science really knows what happens when you have 'allergies'." We are to understand that the above absurdities constitute this knowledge possessed by "science." There is no science about it — it is a mass of baseless speculation. No doubt the new theory will stimulate the production of cures that do not cure, but the so-called victims of allergy will not be helped.

No plan of care based on the theory that hay fever, asthma, hives, migraine, eczema, etc., are allergic manifestations has ever provided more than a temporary and questionable palliation. Dr. Cohen is "barking up the wrong tree," if he imagines he has tracked down the cause of allergy (sensitivity). His speculations follow the well-known medical pattern and this pattern has always been barren of worthy results.

Sensitivity is not cause. It is but a link in a chain. Even assuming that his fanciful theory is correct, it must be recognized that the production of antibodies to fight harmless things is abnormal, and this abnormality is not causeless.

Let us quote again from the article in the American Weekly:

There is a famous case reported to the American Medical Association in which a husband went into a severe, and real, fit of coughing from asthma whenever his wife came near him. His physician reported:

"His attacks are of the severe asthmatic type, which require epinephrine for relief, and this he must take nightly if his wife is at home. For a few years it has been impossible for them to sleep in the same bed at night. It has been suggested that the wife's hair might be the offending cause. Is this likely?"

The A. M. A. suggested a continuation of skin tests for allergic and offending materials and said that several hundred materials ought to be studied as the possible cause. That was over a year ago. No report on the case has been brought to public attention since that time.

How futile this study of "several hundred materials" to find what the "offending materials" are! It has been repeated in thousands of cases and nothing more than evanescent and, more often than otherwise, harmful palliation has come from it.

It is more important to know what makes one sensitive than to know what he is sensitive to. Let us dismiss the nonsense with which Dr. and June Cohen have filled a book and look for a minute at a case of hay fever. Examining the case we discover that the lining membrane of the nose is inflamed, hence very sensitive to irritation. It is inflammation that renders the membrane abnormally sensitive — that is, sensitive to the normal elements of man's environment.

Continuing with our investigation we learn that the sufferer has chronic catarrh, had it, in fact, for several years before hay fever symptoms developed. We find that when the hay fever season is over and the symptoms characteristic of this trouble are no longer present, the sufferer still has catarrh. Frequent colds are suffered through the winter.

Carrying our investigation still deeper we find indigestion (gastritis) with constant fermentation and putrefaction in the digestive tract. The first development of acute gastritis came in infancy following a period of over-eating, or following upon the heels of too much excitement or other enervating influences. Due to wrong care and imprudent feeding, gastritis became chronic, frequent nose colds were followed by chronic nasal catarrh and, finally, hay fever.

The sufferer from asthma has followed practically the same line of pathological evolution, except that frequent chest colds, bronchitis, have finally developed into chronic bronchitis with the same inflammatory sensitization of the bronchial membranes that is' seen in the nasal membrane in hay fever.

To get rid of asthma and hay fever, get rid of the chronic catarrh that forms their foundation. To get rid of the catarrh, remove its cause. Toxemia is its cause and toxemia has many causes.

Six years ago a resident of Brooklyn, New York, who had spent five years in Arizona in a vain effort to cure asthma with the magic of climate, came to the *Health School*. After he had been here less than three weeks the editor's boy entered the solarium, where the man was having a sunbath. The boy was carrying a cat. The man took the cat in his hands and stroked it a few times then handed it back to the boy. He took a deep breath and then, with a sigh of relief said, "Before I came here, if that cat had merely entered the room where I was, I would have had an attack of asthma."

How much better to get rid of the cause of sensitivity than to spend your whole life running from cats, dogs, horses, flowers and trees! Even if you can afford to air condition your home and put in special pollen filters, do you want to spend all the rest of your life in the house? Or, do you want to wear a filter on your nose for the next ten to sixty years? Can you afford to leave your work or your business each "hay fever season" and go away to the mountains or to the sea?

Only the idle rich can afford most of these programs, and these, by palliating their symptoms and ignoring their causes, allow their whole bodies to give down before these causes. While the writer in the *American Weekly* assures us that "it is sheer luck which makes them (hay fever sufferers) suffer their tortures where normal people are completely well and untouched," we assert that abnormality has definite and ascertainable causes.

In 1918 the editor cared for his first patient with hay fever. It was summer in San Antonio and she was suffering with a severe form of hay fever. She had so suffered for several years prior thereto.

She made a speedy recovery right in her own home, with no attention given to pollens, cats, dogs, feather pillows, face powders, or her husband's dandruff. She has remained free of hay fever to this day and has spent the whole of the intervening twenty-two years in San Antonio. All cases of bronchial asthma and of hay asthma may recover in the same permanent manner by overcoming their chronic toxemia. How do we know this? We know because we have seen it done in hundreds of cases, even in cases of asthma that had persisted for twenty years.

What about "egg allergy?" It is due to impaired digestion, or to eating beyond digestive capacity. The normal digestive tract, if not over-loaded, will not permit any undigested egg protein to enter the blood stream.

All proteins must be digested before they can be used by the body. After they are digested they are transformed, during their passage through the intestinal wall, into human (therefore no longer foreign) proteins. All proteins are foreign proteins and are poisonous if they get into the body without undergoing these digestive and transforming processes.

All serums are foreign proteins and all of them produce anaphylatic shock, which is just another name for serum poisoning, or protein poisoning. The "allergic" symptoms produced by serums are worse than any ever produced by eggs that are eaten.

We do not consider eggs good human food and do not advocate their use, but we know that when toxemia is eliminated and nerve energy restored. so that digestion and metabolism are normal. the former sensitivity to eggs ceases to annoy. To restore good health ends all the annoying symptoms and reactions that are based on impaired health.

The normal man is adjusted to his natural environment. The normal elements in man's natural environment become sources of discomfort only after resistance has been broken down. When resistance is restored to normal the former discomforts come to an immediate end.

The Fallacy of Diagnosis

"Correct prescription, according to allopathic standards, can be based only on correct diagnosis. The old school of medicine recognizes hundreds of different diseases, each one an entity by itself, arising from specific causes — mostly disease germs. From this it follows that each specific disease must be treated by specific drugs, vaccines, serums and antitoxins, or by specially devised operations. It is evident that the wrong remedy applied in a given case will not only prove useless, but may cause serious injury; yet if fifty per cent of all the diagnoses rendered in our best equipped hospitals are erroneous, how can the doctor apply the right remedy? Will somebody please explain?" — H. Lindlahr, M. D.

In his book, *"Fads, Frauds and Physicians,"* T. Swann Harding, says:

"But the physician declared that no layman can diagnose his own condition correctly. As a matter of fact Dr. Charles Mayo made the proud boast before a surgical congress in Washton, D. C., in 1927, that the Mayo Clinic had attained the phenomenal record of fifty per cent correct diagnoses. This included of course necropsies who died but about whose ailment the Clinic was diagnostically correct. Certainly few would contend that the snap diagnoses of average general practitioners working alone are right in more than one case out of five. The error on cancer diagnosis with the best facilities at hand is 30 to 40 per cent."

Of laboratory diagnosis, Mr. Harding has the following to say:

"The point is that there has long been and still is a great deal of bunk in clinical laboratory work and the reports thereof. Inexperienced technicians are used too extensively as time savers; 'routine' or 'complete' tests are required by doctors who do not know what the words signify; expensive special blood counts, blood chemistry examinations, and other tests are requested by physicians over and over again on the theory that a correct diagnosis will somehow happen, like Topsy, and very frequently all this costly (to the patient) clinical examination is gone through with before the patient is examined physically by the physician."

Mr. Harding is not telling us anything new about the medical profession, yet he would be one of the first to decry the other "healing" professions because they "cannot diagnose disease."

To the layman the physician is a trained specialist who can tell "one" disease from "another" with a commendable degree of accuracy. The layman has been taught that so-called diseases are specific entities with symptoms and pathology that are so clean cut and individualistic that he who runs may read. He does not realize how much alike these "diseases" are and how arbitrary is the differential diagnosis of so-called diseases. Therefore, the first thing he asks of the physician is: "Doctor, what have I?"

Group medicine is the present vogue. Clinical groups are formed composed of specialists for every system of the body. The sick man or woman goes to one of these clinics and is run through the hands of fifteen to twenty specialists each one of which examines and analyzes his department of the human body.

Each specialist determines the condition of those organs and parts of the body that have been made the object of his specialty and names the deviations from normal which he finds. That is the disease. After the patient has been through the hands of twenty of these specialists, he emerges from the clinic with from twenty to thirty diseases.

What have the specialists really discovered? They have found symptoms. The nose and throat man finds rhinitis, sinusitis and tonsilitis;

the gastro-enterologist finds chronic gastritis, enteritis, colitis, proctitis and cholangitis; the genito-urinary man finds cystitis and metritis; etc, etc. Everyone of these local so-called diseases are but local manifestations of a general catarrhal condition. They are mere symptoms, effects — successive and concomitant developments out of common antecedents. Instead of recognizing the unity of these many so-called diseases, "*scientific medicine*" singles out individual organs or parts for special treatment or for surgical removal.

The group now get their heads together and decide what the outcome of your many diseases will be (a prognosis). Their opinions are based on the usual results of their own methods of treating and abusing the local states. Once the patient deserts them and their methods and turns to other methods, their prognosis ceases to have any value. Outside of their own drugged sphere, doctors have no right to opinions.

Ours is a world of amazing multiplicity. It is a world of endless changes, increasing divergencies and ever widening differentiations. So broad and boundless is the multiplicity around us that it has been aptly described as a "perpetually multiplying multiplicity."

Back of all this boundless multiplicity is an ultimate *unity*. The sciences approach perfection as they approach the unity of first principles. The *unity* and *continuity* of phenomena have become the corner stones of science. No system of thought or practice which fails to recognize these principles can ever become a science. The order and continuity exhibited throughout nature's processes demonstrate her underlying unity and lawfulness.

Health (physiology) and disease (pathology) do not fall outside the principle of the unity of phenomena. However diversified "diseases" may appear, there are many diseases in appearance only. As an explanation of variations in living phenomena, health and disease are convenient terms, but they are not ultimate realities.

The "modern science of medicine" knows nothing of these principles, but still believes in multitudes of unitary causes, multiple un-unified phenomena, myriads of specific diseases, and in the need for multiple remedies for "diseases." Hence, its confusion, its uncertainty, its gropings, and its failures. It is not science. It is not modern. In its many departments it is a storehouse of facts, but its facts are not correlated and unified. These facts are like beads without a string — scattered all over the floor. Medicine today is where chemistry was before the discovery of the laws of chemistry; it is comparable to astronomy before Newton and Kepler. It is on a par with astrology and alchemy. Indeed medicine men are still searching for an elixir vitae, a panacea, a philosopher's stone.

Law and order are lacking in all of the various schools of so-called healing. They one and all believe in cures, miracles, magical potencies, thaumaturgic incantations, unitary causes and specific cures. In all save their modalities, the drugless schools are allopathic from the ground up. Their whole conception of life, health, disease, cure, treatment, etc., is allopathic; and this means in turn, that their conceptions are essentially the same as those of the troglodyte medicine man.

Diseases are regarded as active entities, inherent, definite, causitive entities, producing, by themselves, observed effects. Treatment is ostensibly a warfare upon disease. Actually it is a war upon the body and the forces of life.

There are two general processes in so-called disease — namely (1) a process of degeneration brought about by the concerted action of all the impairing influences which come in contact with the body, and (2) the vital self-defensive struggles to throw off these impairing influences and to repair the damages they have produced in the body. The degeneration represents a retrograde metamorphosis or downward evolution, and tends towards dissolution. The defensive reactions or processes are one with the reactions and processes of health — they are vital or physiological processes, intensified or modified to meet the emergency, and tend to save life.

"All acute diseases are crises of toxemic saturation," to use Dr. Tilden's words, and should all be 'treated' without reference to names. Back of the symptoms, the symptom-complex, the 'specific disease,' the endless transition, flux, diversity, complication, differentiation and multiplicity of manifestation, lies the eternal and universal principle of unity.

The human body is a complex organic unity, is a "unitary community," as Virchow said, in which all parts cooperate towards the accomplishment of an inner and immanent purpose, — namely, the unfolding and maintenance of a perfect physiological standard. Its movements in "disease," as in "health," are the outworking of inward powers of adaptation which seek always to adapt the living organism to its environment. For the energy of the body, always and everywhere very unlike in its modes, is ever the same in principle and purpose.

While any whole is evolving there is always going on subsidiary evolution of the parts into which it divides itself. This is true of the totality of things made up of parts within parts, from the greatest down to the smallest. We see this plainly in any physically cohering aggregate, such as the animal body. While it is growing larger and assuming its general form, each of its organs is doing the same. We recognize these organs as necessary groupings and differentiations to facilitate the adjustments of the organism, and we recognize, also, that these organs are not different existences, but are component parts of one unified, correlated and interdependent organism. We know that the evolution of the organism and the evolution of its various parts do not represent several kinds of evolutions, but one evolution going on everywhere after the same manner.

Properly applied, analogical reasoning is capable of helping us to understand many things and may be of service to us in arriving at the truth. However, no analogy can go on all-fours and it is necessary, in considering any analogy between the development of the body and the development of disease, to keep in mind that disease, is not an organism, not an entity, but merely a widening and increasing condition.

Evolution, like many other terms loosely employed by science, has no definite meaning. Pathological evolution, as I have defined it, is the mode of educing the extension and completion of the process of degeneration and may fairly be applied to the aggregate of so-called diseases, always presupposing that the reverse metamorphosis cannot take place without the continual activity of causation.

The more I study the manner of the evolution of disease, the more I am impressed with its unity, even in full view of its multiplicity of forms and manifoldness of stages. All the diseases of the nosology are but an aggregate of evolutional results, which, while they appear to the superficial observer as specific and independent entities are parts of one unified whole. Disease in many parts of the body does not represent many different kinds of evolutions, nor yet, many diversified causes, but one evolution going on everywhere after the same manner. "Diseases" do not exist *sui generis*.

In each type of disease, as in the aggregate of types, the multiplication of effects has continually aided the transition from a more homogeneous to a more heterogeneous state. In a succession of "diseases" from a "lower" (simple) to a "higher" (complex) type, and a consentaneous greater degree of complication, many factors cooperate in effecting the pathological evolution. There are varieties but not species in disease.

Dr. Rabagliati thinks that there are "two great lines of the development or evolution of diseases." Tracing these he says:

"In one the sequence of events is indigestion, heartburn, acidity, the occurrence of watery blebs or blisters on the lips or tongue, sore throat (tonsilitis) acne of the skin, rheumatism (initis, I have ventured to call it — congestion of connective tissue generally, lymph-congestion rather than blood-congestion), constipation, bronchitis and broncho-pneumonia, pneumonia itself, scanty high-colored urination often accompanied by a heavy deposit on standing, insomnia, eczema, and apoplexy or cancer. In the other we have indigestion, fullness and weight after eating, faintness, relieved immediately by frequent eating, and remotely aggravated by the same, enlargement of glands in the neck, the watery blebs on the neck mentioned above, free urination without deposit of precipitate, tendency to free perspiration or sweating, the occurrence of diseases in a joint such as the knee, hip, elbow or ankle, anemia (thripthemia, or catatribemia rather it should be called), pallour and attenuation, feeling of general or frequent fatigue, *pelosis*, or proneness to become black and blue on receipt of very slight or unremembered injuries, flushing followed by coldness, lameness of hands, rheumatism, diarrhea, pleurisy and tuberculosis."

In view of the unity and continuity of pathology, we say that diagnosis is not only faulty in application, but it is fundamentally wrong in principle. It consists in finding the non-existent and in differentiating the undifferentiated.

Rational Care of the Sick

It should be the business of everyone of us to understand the natural resources of a healthy life and an abundant vitality, and to make use of the most appropriate and most powerful natural agencies as the simplest and most effective means of restoring and renewing health, strength and youth.

He who wants to rebuild and renew his body, when the old frame has, for years past, been accumulating toxins, rather than attempt to patch up the body, will prefer the natural to the artificial remedies.

At this point I am reminded of the thousands who yearly journey long distances to the renowned mineral springs and mineral wells to imbibe their mineral-laden waters in the hope of renewing their health and strengthening their bodies — only to be disappointed.

There are more minerals in fruits and vegetables than in most mineral waters and these have the advantage of being usable by the body. The crude minerals in the water represent only so much irritating dirt; the minerals in the fruits and vegetables are necessary food elements. The minerals in the water always and necessarily injure the body; the minerals in the fruits and vegetables always and necessarily contribute to the renewal of the body.

The common use of charcoal by those who suffer with gas and indigestion supplies us with another striking example of our vicious habit of puttering with palliatives instead of making radical corrections of the causes of our troubles.

Charcoal attracts to itself and condenses many gases and vapors, for which reason it is employed to relieve flatulence and the discomforts of indigestion and constipation. It should be very obvious to the reader, however, that such treatment permits the causative factors to remain untouched. The charcoal does not remedy the indigestion and constipation; but by affording some transitory relief from the discomforts of these, it encourages the neglect of the causes of these troubles and thus becomes a positive evil rather than a benefit.

In like manner, bicarbonate of soda is commonly employed where there is a sour stomach due to fermentation. Many thousands of sufferers from indigestion employ soda several times a day for the short respite from discomfort which it brings to them. They do nothing to remedy the causes of their chronic indigestion.

Besides affording temporary relief from discomfort and thus encouraging neglect of the causes of their troubles, soda has other and positively evil effects, such as neutralizing the hydrochloric acid of the stomach, destroying the pepsin of the gastric juice and destroying the vitamins in the food. Its use, even as a temporary expediency, is never advisable.

These conditions have no natural tendency to disappear, but, on the contrary, become worse and worse, as time passes unless their causes are corrected or removed. If we wish to prevent an incurable organic condition from developing, these functional disturbances must be prevented or remedied and not suffered to continue while we content ourselves with enervating palliatives.

Barrelsful of pepsin and pancreatin have been given to dyspeptics — they are still suffering. Oceans of "bitters" are swallowed yearly to improve digestion. These not only do not increase gastric secretion, but they actually lessen the secretion of gastric juice. Alcohol is used by many as a stimulant to digestion. It precipitates the pepsin and thus destroys the activity of the gastric juice.

It is said that "seventy tons of aperient pills are used in England annually without curing the English constipation." We not infrequently meet with those who have been taking laxatives and cathartics regularly for from ten to fifty years and are still constipated. But they continue to use their "cures," and when one cure ceases to cure they resort to another.

Constipation is treated with methods that invariably make the condition worse. Laxatives, cathartics, enemas, irrigations, rectal dilators, wheat bran, agar agar, psyllium seed, herb compounds and other agents and methods which have no influence at all upon the causes of impaired bowel function, but which do weaken the colon, are employed by almost everybody in America. The users of these methods do not overcome their constipation. Instead, the constipation becomes increasingly obstinate and the colon becomes weaker and weaker until it sags or "falls" and ultimately lacks power to function at all.

Tonsils are removed, teeth extracted. the appendix excised, ovaries cut out, the gall bladder extirpated — in short, organs are wantonly and needlessly sacrificed — while the causes of the troubles in these and other organs of the body are left to continue their impairing work. Thyroid enlargement is cut away and, if the patient does not die from the operation, due to the persistence of the original causes of the goitre, the remaining portion of the thyroid enlarges.

Tumors are removed and their causes left untouched. Other tumors develop subsequently at the same or another site. Essentially benign tumors become malignant as a result of the operation. We are told that the causes of tumors and cancers are unknown and this enables us constantly to overlook the fact that anything which acts prejudicially to the general health is a factor in the production of these things.

Glandular extracts are administered, or the glands are irradiated or electrocuted or drugged, while the causes of glandular impairment are ignored. If the glands are working over time, they are inhibited; if they are not working enough, they are stimulated. But the factors that are responsible for their excessive or deficient function are permitted to continue to impair the glands and other organs of the body.

Thus I might go on and on with this recital of the tinkering and patch-work methods in vogue — methods of stimulating or depressing the organs of the body and poisoning its cells and tissues, in a foolish effort to compel it to behave in a healthy manner in spite of impairing causes that are either ignored or unrecognized. But no useful purpose would be served by such a recital.

The whole plan of modern treatment of disease is irrational and injurious. To relieve pain, for instance, certainly no agent or practice should be employed that tends to deprive the nerves of the power to produce it — to feel. Not the pain, but its causes or occasions should be removed. It is equally as rational to administer opium to relieve the pain in a corn and leave the ill-fitting shoe on the foot, as it is to give it to relieve pain elsewhere in the body and not remove the exciting cause.

The history of those who come to us shows that their weak spot is nervous depletion with functional weakness of both the digestive organs and the emunctories. Prior treatment received by these people has all been of a character to extend and perpetuate the abnormalities.

Physicians have made great advances in the determination of pathology and of differential disease states, but this has caused them to attach too much importance to special points of pathology, which, therefore, receive exclusive therapeutic attention. Pathology, in general and in particular is progressive in character, both in degree and in form. It not only passes through various stages of development, but tends to develop in different directions from the same beginnings.

Beginning with nervous depletion, digestive derangement and impaired elimination, the pathology develops, step by step as one organ and function after another or one tissue after another is strongly affected by the general weakening, poisoning and starving of the body. But the different forms thus assumed — the "different diseases" thus developed — do not necessarily call for a corresponding difference in remedial care. They certainly do not call for the enervating palliation and symptomatic suppression everywhere in vogue.

By the continuity of disease I mean that related sequence of progressive effects which binds all so-called disease units together so that the innumerable "diseases" are not single independent "diseases," but integral parts of the whole process. We must forever discard the superstition that each so-called disease is an isolated entity risen into existence out of nothing, either to continue until it destroys its victim, upon which it feeds parasitically, or else be driven back into nothingness by the conjurations and potencies of the doctor.

Only the processes of nature (working with natural agents and forces) can resupply lost or diminished nervous energy and rebuild damaged nervous structure. This can be done only by agents and substances, the innate qualities of which supply the current demands of the vital powers.

True remedies are those only the constant tendency of which is to restore the healthy state. Agents that excite or depress nervous activity; narcotics that deprive the nerves of the power to tell us, by aching, of trouble; cathartics that lash tired, overworked bowels into vigorous and exhausting action — these are not remedies. The true anodyne is not the drug that all but stops the nervous activity, but the process that removes the cause of the pain. So-called drug anodynes are, in reality, odynes.

The hygienist, is, therefore, bound to preserve, with the utmost care, the vital powers of his patient; to provide every condition favorable to recovery; and to avoid every measure in practice which has proven to be deleterious or dangerous to the organism. For, under no circumstances and at no stage of any so-called disease, is there need to make any use of means which tend to injure either immediately or remotely, the permanent health of the sick person. The future integrity of the organism must not be sacrificed upon the altar of the therapeutic god — *Immediate Transient Respite from Discomfort.*

Natural methods are those agents and influences that bear some vital or nutritive relation to the living body. Artificial methods are those agents and influences that bear an anti-vital and poisonous relation to the living organism. The first either supplies nutriment or promotes nutrition; the second excites and destroys. *Natural methods rebuild and renew; artificial methods exhaust and tear down. We should not find it difficult to make our choice between these two groups of methods.*

REFORM VS. CURE

We live in an age when the sensational and the sensual are much stronger than the spiritual and the ideal. Men's higher natures are in more or less complete subjection to their appetites and desires. The animal is in the ascendency and is thoroughly perverted. People are bent on the gratifications of today and give no thought to the *judgment* that is coming.

With occasional exceptions, those around us are governed by low and groveling appetites, and swelling, surging desires and passions. In most men the mind is a bond-slave to a diseased body; the higher faculties of the mind are subordinated to the propensities, and convictions are allowed to yield to desires. The will and the higher powers of the mind are not in control. Aims are low, gratifications lower, excesses and dissipations subjects of boasting and swaggering; and degradation and defilement are the common lot of all. All classes of men are to a greater or lesser degree slaves to their bodily appetites and passions.

The result of all this is physical, mental and moral decay, corruption, disease and death. Poor health is the almost universal rule; good health the exception but seldom seen. To man of today, health, perfect, uninterrupted, and joyous health, is a myth and a total stranger. They have read of it, they have even talked of it, but it visits them only in their dreams and they think of it only as having existed in some long forgotten Golden Age or Edenic Paradise. To them life is an unending round of pains and sufferings. This is all true because man has not learned and will not learn the *Hygienic Way*.

When man becomes sick he seeks a *physician* — one who by the magic power of some drug or serum, vaccine or operation, or else some machine, or apparatus, or metaphysical formula, can *cure* him — to dose away and treat away the evil effects of such a mode of living and permit him, at the same time, to continue such living. He wants to be *cured* of his dyspepsia, rheumatism, catarrh, general debility, etc., and then be permitted to go on ignorant and undisciplined, unrestricted and untrained, to make himself sick all over again. Such methods only deal with *effects* and leave untouched the *causes* by which the evils they attempt to combat are produced. Patients thus *cured* return, like the sow that was cleansed, to their wallowing in the mire. For, it will be observed that, in all this treatment, there is no lesson taught, no discipline enforced, no condition instituted that is of any value in health or in a subsequent state of disease; the intellect of the patient is left a blank, his body a scene of devastation. He returns to the manner of living that produced his disease, in the first place, and in this he is encouraged by physicians and relatives, by nurses and friends, and by conventional examples, which he sees all around him every day. The result is he is again sick before long and the process of *curing* him is repeated.

The Hygienic Review has no sympathy with this old delusion of *cure* and no regard for the curing professions that foster this fallacy for their own financial gain. The mission of the *Review* is to impress upon its readers the folly, the shame, and the crime of being sick, that they shall feel as guilty when they become sick as when they have committed theft; to teach its readers, as far as it can, how to subdue appetites, change habits, confirm principles, and arouse to renewed activity those elements of goodness in man's nature which now actuate but feebly the human soul. The mission of the *Hygienic Review* is to teach its readers, if they can be taught, how they may not only overcome all their weaknesses and diseases, and thus be truly cured, but how to remain free from disease and weakness throughout life.

It seeks to guide those liable to suffer from disease to a true knowledge of themselves, and to the cause of their miseries, and finds a cure for these in the discipline and correction of faulty and perverted voluntary habits of everyday life.

The *Hygienic Review* would impart to its readers the knowledge that Nature cures disease, and that she does it by the wise application of those same means which she employs to maintain beings in a healthy state.

The *Hygienic Review* would reawaken your instinctive repugnance to poisonous medicines and fan it into an intense disgust. It would caution you against the clap-traps and catch-pennies by which the unwary and unknowing are led to their undoing. In their place it would substitute an intense enthusiasm for a simple, natural, wholesome and well-ordered life — a life so pure from stain that the blessing of uninterrupted good health shall settle down upon the brow of all.

Avoiding and Remedying Colds

Coryza or rhinitis, commonly known as a cold, costs the American people an enormous sum of money each year. The cost in loss of time from work and in doctor's bills runs into several millions of dollars. The cost in lowered efficiency and lessened productive power is also very great. If for no other reason than that of saving money the people of America should be interested in the cause and prevention of colds.

The cold is one of the simplest maladies with which man suffers. It is also one of the most common of his affections. It has been one of his most frequent difficulties throughout recorded history. Yet only within the last few years has any effort been made to determine the nature and cause of colds. During these few years many "research" workers have spent huge sums of money and expended much time and energy in their effort to discover the cause of colds.

Today they know as much, or nearly so, as when they began their work. The cause of the cold is still a deep, dark mystery. They come, they run their course, they pass and the patient and physician know neither why nor how.

Failure to find the cause of colds is due to the fact that the "research" workers are bent over their microscopes trying to find the little germ-devils that are responsible for the mischief. They assumed in advance that colds are caused by germs and a germ they must find.

Although the guilty germ-devil has not been apprehended it is assumed that he is there just the same and those who are seeking for a cure for the cold are trying to locate a serum that will exorcise the legion of germ-devils that have obsessed the bodies of those who suffer with colds. Many serums have been tried but all of them have failed.

Failure is writ large on both the efforts to find the cause and on the efforts to find the cure. This is so for the reason that cause is being sought for in realms where it does not exist and because a voodooistic method of cure can never succeed.

The causes of colds are known; have been known for a long time. Likewise the proper method of dealing with a cold is known. This knowledge has been in our possession for years. The "research" work that has been carried on and which is now being carried on is worse than wasted.

Enervation and toxemia are omnipresent where there is any departure from the normal standard of health. These are antecedent to the development of any so-called disease.

Enervation is a state of lowered nervous energy and always acts to lower physiological efficiency. Excretion or elimination is checked, digestion is impaired and resistance to any and all disease influences is lowered by enervation.

Enervation is brought on by a mode of living that uses up nervous energy in excess of the daily supply. Anything that lowers the powers of life, any excess or overstimulation, produces this state. Lack of rest and sleep are potent causes of enervation. Nervous strain, grief, anxiety, worry and other such emotions help to lower nervous energy.

Toxemia is an excess of toxins in the blood. These result primarily from the activities of life; are the normal end-products (waste) of the activities of the cells of man's body. Normally they are excreted, but when enervation has crippled the processes of elimination more or less of them are retained and accumulate in the tissues and lymph. This is to say, toxemia is due to the retention in the body of the poisons that the normal body is throwing off every minute of its life, day or night, asleep or awake, from the cradle to the grave.

Under a full tide of nervous energy, sound organs of elimination are able to keep these wastes or toxins down to a healthful minimum and thus maintain health. But when these have been weakened and their functional efficiency has been reduced by enervation, they are not successful in maintaining the normal purity of the fluids of the body.

A common source of toxins is the digestive tract. Either from over eating, or from impaired digestion, due to enervation, food decomposes in the stomach and intestine and some of the resulting toxins are absorbed into the blood.

Under ordinary circumstances, the liver destroys these toxins and the kidneys eliminate them. But when the functions of these organs have been crippled by enervation, or when the toxins are thrown into the blood in such quantities that these organs are overwhelmed, the body is forced to find some other manner of disposing of them.

When the membranes of the nose and throat are selected as the channels through which to leak out the surplus food and excess of waste and toxins, we call the process a cold. The common cold is a process of vicarious elimination — it is a safety valve, a cleansing or curative measure.

The two great causes of colds are *repletion* and *exhaustion* (enervation). Repletion, or plethora, tends to overtax the functions of life and poison the body and necessitates an unusual house cleaning process.

Excesses of sugar, starches and milk are the chief causes of catarrhal conditions, of which the cold is one. Eating when exhausted, when worried, or over excited, or under any similar circumstance, when the digestive powers are lowered and the eliminative functions are impaired, results in poisoning and necessitates recourse to an unusual means of elimination.

Colds, then, are not something that we "catch," or that catch us. Instead of catching something we are getting rid of something and that something is too hot and feverish to be called a cold. The nose running and drooling are simply nature's effort to get rid of excess.

Colds do not, as is popularly taught, lay the foundation for other more serious diseases. They are efforts to prevent development of more serious conditions. The condition of the body that makes a cold or a series of colds necessary, may, and often does, due to the persistence of its causes, demand other and more acute eliminating measures to remedy; but the cold, which is a process of compensatory elimination, did not lay the foundation for the subsequent process.

Tuberculosis no more develops out of a cold than the hair on a man's head develops out of the hair on his face. The persistence of the condition the body seeks to remedy by means of the cold, may finally result in tuberculosis, but the cold, as a process of elimination, is distinct from the toxic condition of the body which it seeks to remove.

The prevailing view is that colds are caused by germs and that the less virulent germs (of colds) first break down the body's resistance, after which, the more virulent germs (of infantile paralysis, measles, tuberculosis, etc.), are able to invade the body and play havoc therein. This view seems absurd and lacks verification.

Colds often begin early in life as mild maladies confined practically to the nose and lasting but a short time. As life continues and the impairing influences to which it is subjected weaken the body more and more, colds extend down the throat into the chest. Each cold seems to be down a little deeper, to hang on a little longer and to give more trouble. This marks the weakening and deterioration of the body. Finally, the causes against which the cold is a defense, so completely undermine the body that some serious disease develops.

Viewed superficially, the frequent colds seem to have resulted in the more serious malady;

but actually, the colds have prevented the more serious condition from developing much earlier. The colds have saved life and preserved health against great odds. Chronic disease is due to chronic provocation and not to the intermittent processes of vicarious elimination.

It is always desirable to prevent disease — to have good health. But, due to our mode of living, bodily conditions develop that make disease necessary and, under these conditions, colds and other such eliminating processes should be welcomed, not feared. They are life-savers, not destructive processes.

Many so-called diseases begin with a cold and this has helped to lead us to believe that colds prepare the way for "other diseases." Nothing could be farther from the truth. The cold, in such a case, is only one part of a general house-cleaning process in which several tissues or organs cooperate in eliminating the toxemia.

Colds have a habit of developing after feast days, such as Thanksgiving and Christmas. They may develop at any time, however, when over-eating or enervation have resulted in a need for them.

Although it is commonly thought that exposure to cold and dampness causes colds, some of the most severe colds develop in summer and in periods of drought. Colds are more common in damp, cloudy, cold weather, because we eat more, are less active and stay more indoors in poorly ventilated rooms. During the summer we eat less and are out doors and in the sun more. On the other hand, in summer, Nature tends to dispose of food excess by means of diarrhea.

No amount of exposure results in colds in those who are in good health and who take proper care of themselves. A healthy man may be so badly frozen that he is unconscious and then, if he is warmed and cared for so that he does not die, he does not develop a cold. In some parts of this country it is nothing unusual for certain religious sects to break the ice and baptize new converts, but no colds result. Men go hunting in winter, fall through the ice and get wet, and then tramp long distances to the nearest farm house and do not develop colds.

I do not mean to convey the thought that undue exposure of this kind will not be followed by a cold in those who are already enervated and toxemic. Such exposure will place a sufficient check upon elimination in these people to result in a cold or some other acute eliminating process.

Now that we understand what a cold is and what its causes are, we are prepared for a rational plan of prevention and a sane method of care. Colds are prevented, that is, made unnecessary, by living in such a way that a high standard of health is maintained. Moderate eating of wholesome foods, daily exercise, fresh air, sun baths, plenty of rest and sleep — these are the elements out of which health is compounded.

No cure for colds is needed. The cold is a curative process. It should not be suppressed, or checked, or "cut short." It should be allowed to complete the work of purification — "let it run its course" — without hindrance.

By this I do not mean that there is nothing that we can do, when we have a cold, that is helpful. There is much that can be done and that should be done. Colds last from a few hours to a few weeks. The average cold lasts three or four days. Colds are self-limited. For these reasons, almost anything seems to be a cure. If we resort to pulling the ears, or twisting the toes to cure a cold, these measures would seemingly be successful.

However, when a cold develops that persists for several weeks, all of the vaunted "cures" that people swear by fail. These are the colds that weigh the cures in the balance and find them wanting. In all cases where the cold does not last over three or four days, anything and everything appears to cure. In cases where the cold lasts several weeks, nothing appears to cure.

It is precisely in these long-drawn-out colds that the simple Natural Methods prove their true worth. Put to the acid test in such conditions, they do not suppress the symptoms, but hasten the elimination of the toxic-overload back of the cold. Let us see what these methods are.

There is no more rapid means of getting rid of excess than fasting. The individual suffering with a cold should immediately stop all food except water; or else, he should confine himself to fruit juices. Eating intensifies and prolongs a cold. All the water desired may be taken. There is no reason to force water upon the system in the absence of thirst, but one should drink all the water demanded by instinct.

Whenever it is possible, if the sufferer will go to bed and rest, the process of elimination will be speeded up through all channels and the toxins will be eliminated from the body in shorter time. Rest is especially important for those who are run down or exhausted.

Where one can not get away from his or her duties and go to bed, every effort should be made to secure as much extra rest and sleep as circumstances permit. Go to bed early, and get all the rest possible through the day. Take things easy.

Keep warm. Chilling checks elimination and prolongs the cold. Do not roast yourself. Do not stay in an ill-ventilated room. Have plenty of fresh air in the room day and night, but keep warm.

Rest, warmth, fasting — these are the natural measures which insure speedy consummation of the process of vicarious elimination that is a cold, and a return to normal health. If these measures are inaugurated at the beginning, no cold will ever persist for weeks, as many do under the prevailing plans of care.

There are many ways of suppressing a cold which are often successful or partially so, but suppression, which means thwarting Nature's efforts to eliminate an excess of toxins, is not desirable. Such measures tend to produce chronic disease. Not only do they have directly injurious consequences of their own, but they lock up, as it were, the toxins in the body and these produce more or less permanent damage to one or more of the organs of the body. The cold should be allowed to run its course, shortened only by such purely natural measures as positively promote the elimination of toxins. If this is done, the cold will always be followed by improved health.

What Caused the Quints'
Tonsillar Troubles?

The Quints were cared for "scientifically." All the wisdom of *Modern Medical Science* was expended in caring for them. Trained nurses were substituted for their mother and they were well protected from all possible *sources of infection*. The government backed the program with unlimited funds. Nothing was left undone that *science* and wealth could do. Their whole lives were ordered in conformity with the best *science* has to offer.

Yet, at an early age they all became sick. At first they had colds, which *science* could not cure. Their condition grew steadily worse until their tonsils became involved and, finally, the glands of their necks. *Medical Science* stood helplessly by and watched a simple cold grow progressively worse and, then, had nothing better to offer than the removal of the girls' tonsils.

Science has failed! Science has not succeeded in making and keeping the girls healthy. Science has proved unable to stop a simple cold or to cure a simple sore throat. Science has begun the melancholy program of cutting out the tell-tale effects of its plan of care. The first operation has been performed; will the appendix, or the gall-bladder, or the cervical glands be next; or, will science next extract a few teeth?

If the trouble is an infection, that is, if it is due to the invasion of the body by germs, including the streptococcus, and these have already spread to the glands of the neck, which glands are the same kind of structures as the tonsils and adenoids, will removing the tonsils and adenoids prevent future trouble? In order to remove the "infection" will it not be necessary to also remove the glands of the neck? If any other structures have become involved, will these not have to be removed also? Each infected gland becomes a secondary "focus of infection."

Will removal of the tonsils and the adenoids remove cause? If not, if cause is allowed to continue operations, will it not continue to produce effects? It is begging the question to say that germs are the cause. Germs are everywhere. Children live in an atmosphere of germs and should be sick all the time if these are the cause of disease. At most, germs may become an auxiliary cause, they can never be primary.

If germs are the cause of disease, and, if man did not possess resistance to them, no child could live more than a few days after birth. The mouth and throat of every infant, child and adult, harbors at all times millions of germs of many kinds — tubercle bacilli, diphtheria bacilli, hemolitic streptococci, etc. Scientific investigation discloses the fact that fifty per cent. of normal throats harbor streptococci. In ninety per cent. of normal persons they are harbored in the tonsils; in eighty per cent. of normal persons they are found in the depths of the tonsils; and in one-hundred per cent. of normal persons they are found in the crypts of the tonsils. These same germs reach the stomach through the medium of food and drink. Is it not remarkable that any of us are alive?

We must go beyond the ubiquitous germ to find the cause of the suffering of the Quints. For, unless there is a condition of the body varying from health, germs can do nothing. The healthy body is proof against germs of all kinds.

The state of the body immediately preceding the appearance of the germs — the state of the body that allows the germs to operate — is, therefore, the important one. This it is that determines the possibility of "infection," and no operation can possibly remove this body-state. Without this state of lowered resistance disease never could appear, germs or no germs. When germs invade the living organism it is a sign that the organism is weakened and in a state of lowered resistance.

Whatever lowers resistance, whatever produces the state of the body that allows the germs to operate, is the true, the basic, cause of disease.

The germs are merely adventitious — secondary. The real remedy is to remove the cause of lowered resistance and build resistance. Cutting out important defense organs — the tonsils, adenoids and other lymphoid structures in the throat, neck and elsewhere, are parts of the body's first line defenses — does not increase resistance. Indeed, the depressing effects of the anæsthetic, loss of blood, shock of the operation, post-operative anodynes (pain killers), the "nerve sedatives" (depressants) given both before and after the operation, and the fear and apprehension created by the prospect of the operation, all tend to further reduce resistance. They enervate and enervation is lowered resistance.

Even though the Quints survived their operations, they are not restored to health; for the operations will not have removed cause. Like millions of others who have had their tonsils and adenoids removed, a little later it will be found necessary to remove another "focus of infection," and still another, and another. Cutting out effects, palliating symptoms, no matter how skillfully and scientifically done, never removes cause, and until cause is removed there is no cure.

What has tonsilitis to do with other diseases? That diseased tonsils harbor septic material is not denied. But the condition, in order to persist, must be daily, yes hourly, fed on the products of decomposition. Unless the cause of the tonsillar trouble is constantly added to, it speedily spends its force and the tonsils return to normal. If cause is not removed, the removal of the tonsils will not restore health. Disease continues connected to its basal cause, irritating the doctor by causing his best prognoses to go awry.

Disease is not its own cause. Tonsilitis is an effect. Treatment directed to these effects can never be anything more than doubtful palliation. The tonsils may be successfully removed but the patient is not cured, because cause is untouched.

All of this will become more clear to the reader if we trace the development of disease and point out its real causes. The functions of the body depend on nerve energy for their performance. Every function in the body is efficient or not, depending on the amount of nerve energy reaching its organ. When nerve energy is abundant, function is efficient, and we have health; when nerve energy is low, functions lag and there begins the development of disease.

The body is not an inexhaustible store-house of energy that may be drawn upon without limit. Everything that we do uses up energy; even living uses up energy. All goes well so long as we do not use up more nerve energy during the hours of activity than we regenerate or recuperate during hours of repose. But if our mode of living is such that we daily use up energy in excess of our daily recuperation, our supply of energy is gradually lessened, producing enervation.

Enervation lowers function — it reduces secretion and excretion. Impaired excretion (elimination) permits the gradual accumulation of retained body waste — end-products of metabolism. These wastes are poisonous and act as stimulants (irritants) and thus produce more enervation. Thus, the retained toxin becomes an ally of enervating habits by over-stimulating the body. Over stimulation always produces enervation. We have a vicious circle established and the longer it runs, the farther and farther is the individual carried away from the standard of good health.

A normal person develops enough waste products in a few hours to produce death, if they are not eliminated. Full nerve energy is necessary for normal elimination, and such a state cannot be maintained while enervating habits are practiced. Impaired elimination permits the day by day accumulation of the uneliminated catabolic waste — toxin — producing toxemia.

Waste is a constant product; auto-generated at all times. Toxemia is the common state of mankind and, due to enervation, from wrong life, man oscillates, from the cradle to the grave, between a mild toxemia and a state of toxic saturation. Toxins vary from slight irritants to virulent and deadly poisons. The amount and virulence of toxins determines the danger. They may produce anything from a simple catarrh or redness of the skin, to measles and tonsilitis, or to diphtheria, small-pox, and bubonic plague.

Toxins circulating in the blood come in contact with every tissue and pervert nutrition. When the toxic saturation becomes great enough to cause reaction, vicarious or compensatory elimination takes place through some point of the mucous membrane — usually of the respiratory or digestive tracts. These crises we call disease — colds, catarrhs, etc. — and name according to the location of the eliminative fontanel.

Chronic toxemia means a state of inebriety, and, like chronic alcohol poisoning, leads to tissue and organic changes, producing old age and organic and degenerative diseases. At all times the body is in a state of toxic overstimulation, and all the time an imperceptible organic change is taking place in all the tissues throughout the body.

Enervation also checks secretion — digestive secretions and endocrine secretions are inadequate. This results, not alone in indigestion and subsequent poisoning, but in nutritional perversion from insufficient secretions of the ductless glands.

Gastro-intestinal putrefaction and fermentation, instead of digestion, take place and the poisoning, added to metabolic toxemia and retained urea, produces a pan-toxemia that may result in serious diseases. Intestinal putrescence evolves ptomaine poisoning, which puts a deadlock on elimination; then vicarious elimination through the mucous and serous membranes becomes necessary to save life. Putrefactive poisoning — poisoning from decomposing proteins, especially animal proteins — is especially virulent, and, when added to toxemia, as a complication, forms the basis of the virulent types of disease.

The simplest and commonest type of disease is a cold (catarrh) which usually disappears, with or without treatment, in a week, or less. Indeed, if the toxemia is mild and not accompanied by infection from putrescence absorbed from the bowels, the cold should be gone in two days. It is common to think that when the symptoms have disappeared the patient is restored to health. Not so. If he had not been much below the near-health standard, he would not have developed a cold. The cold (crisis) is past, but its cause is still present, and in a short time the symptoms will reappear and he will have "another" cold.

A toleration for metabolic toxins can be built, just as a toleration for morphine, nicotine, caffeine, etc., can be built. This really means that the warning voice of self-protection can gradually be put to sleep while the body is slowly, gradually, insidiously undermined. After toleration is established, crises occur only when the toxins accumulate beyond the point of toleration. Those who carry toxins to the point of toleration will develop occasional or frequent crises.

If the habits that cause the enervation are continued, the toxins will reaccumulate after each crisis — each process of vicarious elimination — or disease, and many crises will occur before organic change takes place.

Toxemia is a constant product and exerts a constant influence. It muddies all the waters of life, contaminates everything it touches, and lowers the vitality of all the tissues. When toxemia has brought about a chemical change in the tissues of the body — —when a favorable soil has been produced by enervation and toxemia — then, and not until then, germs, which are omnipresent, may become an auxiliary, but never a primary cause.

Inflammation of the tonsils is due to toxemia. Chronic inflammation is due to toxemia complicated by chronic intestinal auto-intoxication. Intestinal auto-intoxication is due to indigestion — fermentation and putrefaction of food — as a result of eating beyond digestive capacity, or eating such food mixtures as overtax the digestive enzymes.

The involvement of the cervical glands of the Quints reveals that they suffered from excessive protein intake. Chronic putrescence (sepsis) resulting from protein putrescence in the intestine, involves the lymph-adenoid tissues, producing adenitis, and ultimately, tuberculosis. The cess-pools under the diaphragms of these children are the real sources of their infections, and the removal of the lymphatic structures, while leaving the cess-pools untouched, will not restore health. Treating symptoms as cause is worse than folly.

Their pictures show the Quints to be quite plump. The plump and rotund individual may feel and look well, but he will break down in the most vulnerable part of his organism as soon as sufficient toxemia and intestinal poisoning have accumulated. Their plumpness indicates overfeeding, and overfeeding is a most potent cause of enervation. Indeed, it is one of the most common causes in children. Overfeeding is also a source of poisoning. The slow destruction of the life of the blood by toxic material resulting from an over-crowded nutrition is a common cause of trouble in both children and adults.

We have previously pointed out that when we have normal nerve energy, organic functioning is normal — we have health; and that when we are enervated — nerve energy is lowered — organic functioning is impaired and we develop disease. What are the causes of enervation? There are hundreds of these; in this article I intend to deal only with those most common in the lives of children, ignoring, for our present purposes, the many additional enervating influences affecting the lives of adults.

Parents should know the causes of enervation in children; for, otherwise, they cannot care for them properly. Children are often born weak — enervated — and any care the Quints received should have taken into consideration their relative weakness from birth. It should be known that the enervated child cannot digest food — any kind of food — as well as when not enervated. The effort to build strength in weak children by feeding "plenty of good nourishing food" defeats its own purpose. Such feeding enervates and poisons.

A bugbear of nearly all mothers and most doctors is the undernourished child. In America are many thousand of thin, undeveloped children, who, under the advice of doctors, are eating three big meals a day and guzzling milk and fruit juices or other foods between meals, because of "undernourishment." Some of these children put on weight — fat — while most of them remain "undernourished." All of them suffer frequent colds, sore throats, and other diseases; many of them have poor vision, defective hearing, enlarged glands, and other evidences of poisoning and enervation, while the death rate among them is high.

Feeding beyond digestive capacity enervates and poisons — it does not nourish. Yet, we customarily begin our overfeeding on the day of birth and continue it throughout life. Few infants pass the first month of life without a cold or other toxemic crisis.

Babies are handled too much, they are dressed too warmly, they are excited too much, they are overstimulated too much and too often in many mental and physical ways. They are fed when tired. When a child is very tired it should be put to bed without food, or, at most, given fruit juice only.

Children play too hard, and when they do this they become very nervous, cross, and, even hysterical. The parent who sees his child becoming nervous, loud and boisterous, should have him stop playing and lie down until rested. Intense play is a form of mental and emotional overstimulation that produces enervation.

A child that overplays, overeats, overenjoys, or that overdoes in any way will wear out its nerve energy. If he does anything to excess he will become enervated. His health standard will be lowered and from that time on he will be liable to be made sick by any and all unusual influences — a Thanksgiving or Christmas dinner, cold, heat, fatigue, excitement, etc. — that put an added check upon secretion and excretion.

Many children are over-sunned. We tend to go to the extremes in everything we do. We not only overeat, we overdo in every way. Sunshine is good for baby. Fine! Give him as much as possible! So baby and child are overstimulated and profroundly enervated by too much sun-bathing.

Children become enervated by insufficient rest and sleep. It is during repose that energy is recuperated, and when rest and sleep do not balance expenditures in activity, enervation results. Enervation is the sum of all our expenditures, normal and abnormal. When the total daily expenditure exceeds the daily recuperation, we become enervated. There is only a certain store of nerve energy available for all the activities of the body and if this is dissipated, functions cannot be carried on efficiently. Enervating influences beyond the compensatory capacity of the organism, produce toxemia, and toxemia produces disease.

If we do not build disease by taxing the organism to its very limit; if conservation of energy and not its dissipation, is the guiding principle of life; if moderation instead of excess is practiced: there will be no enervation and, consequently, no toxemia. Good health will stand like a Gibraltar amid all the influences that help to prostrate the enervated and toxemic. Epidemics will pass us by and there will be no apparent excuse for cutting out diseased organs (effects), while ignoring completely the causes of the disease. It should be worth something to know that your children can be made and kept healthy.

Bronchitis

Bronchitis means inflammation of the bronchial tubes. In this article we shall deal only with catarrhal bronchitis. This is inflammation of the mucous membrane lining the bronchial tube. The lung tissue itself is not involved. Bronchitis may be either *acute, sub-acute,* or *chronic*.

Acute bronchitis is often called a chest cold, and a "cold" it is. Its chief symptom is rapid breathing, a sharp, dry cough, and fever. The temperature runs about 101 to 102 degrees Fahrenheit. There is likely to be a sense of constriction about the chest, with soreness under the breast bone and pain when coughing. In infants, breathing may be so rapid and difficult that they become cyanotic (blue); in older children the rapid breathing is not likely to distress them. Considerable mucus may be coughed up and expectorated or swallowed.

Chronic bronchitis is the result of chronic provocation and the suppression of acute bronchitis. Coughing and expectoration may be the only symptom present in this condition, or there may be considerable irritation and soreness in the chest and even some difficulty in breathing.

In the majority of cases, acute bronchitis lasts but a few days to two weeks; chronic bronchitis may persist for years ultimately terminating in asthma.

When the human organism is impaired and elimination is checked, some portion of the mucous membrane of the body forms the common point of vicarious elimination. The stomach is the most abused organ of the body, hence indigestion, or catarrh of the stomach — *gastritis* — is one of the first crises in toxemia — diseases.

The abuse of the stomach begins almost immediately after birth. Fondling and overfeeding enervate the child. The meddlesome midwifery of *"Modern Medical Science"* enervates both mother and child, rendering the mother's milk, it it does not suppress it altogether, unfit as food. Indigestion appears often in babies soon after birth and then begins a program of infant feeding and care that rivals in its variety of means of torture those of the Inquisition. Here in infancy is laid the foundation for the almost universal gastro-intestinal catarrh, which, as it extends on and on, involves more or less, all of the mucous membranes of the body and gives rise to all the so-called catarrhal diseases.

Indigestion is not often repeated before the membranes of the throat and air passages become involved in the toxemic crises — colds (coryza), influenza (la grippe), tonsillitis, quinsy, pharyngitis, laryngitis, bronchitis, sinusitis, etc., develop. Although named from their locations as distinct diseases, they are merely crises in toxemia.

The mucous membranes lining the intestines and collateral organs — gall duct, gall bladder, pancreas, etc. — as well as the respiratory passages, the reproductive organs, the bladder, etc., may all be called upon to do vicarious duty. That is, they may all be forced into work as channels of compensatory elimination. The name of the toxemic crisis will be determined by the location of the compensatory process.

They are all crises of toxemia, complicated by exogenous toxins, usually intestinal infections — ranging from simple fermentation of carbohydrates to septic decomposition of animal proteins. Colds, scarlet fever, diphtheria, simple or septic measles, discreet and confluent small pox, pneumonia, typhoid and typhus fever, etc., represent a pan-infection, complicating a primary, or metabolic, toxemia.

When toxemia and intestinal intoxication are great enough to produce reaction (arouse resistance) certain organs or parts are commandeered to do vicarious elimination. When any special area of mucous membrane is forced into repeated or continual crises, chronic inflammation is established. When organs, due to repeated stressing by crises, take on organic change, we have so-called organic diseases.

When inflammation becomes chronic, coryza becomes rhinitis, with the usual organic changes in the membrane, such as adenoids, hay fever, polyps, ozena, etc.; tonsilitis and pharyngitis become enlarged tonsils, and the catarrh extends to the Eustachian tubes, inner ear, mastoid cells, etc.; laryngitis and bronchitis extend to the lymphatics and adenitis develops and, in those with a tendency to tuberculosis, enlarged cervical glands and tuberculosis of the pharnyx, larnyx. or lungs; gastritis evolves induration, ulceration, and fungation — cancer; duodenitis takes on ulceration; catarrh extends into the gall-duct, gall-bladder and liver and gall-stones or "other diseases" follow; pancreatitis develops when the catarrh extends up the pancreatic duct and, then, diabetes and "other diseases" of the pancreas; in the colon and rectum ulcerative colitis and proctitis develop; in the kidneys of gouty subjects stones form; in the vagina and womb, ulcers and cancer; in the male, prostatitis and prostatic enlargement.

Such is the unity and the evolution of disease. Diseases stem from a common cause and have a common starting point. Germs are declared to be cause. They are, at most, complicating factors. They are never true causes; are never primary.

Bronchitis is a *catarrhal disease*. Bronchorrhea — diarrhea of the bronchi — is a catarrhal condition. *Catarrhal diseases* are crises of toxemia — they are one of Nature's ways of eliminating excessive accumulations of toxins. Chronic catarrh, wherever located, is nothing more than a continuous elimination through the mucous membrane.

Behind every catarrh is a toxic state. Catarrh is impossible in the absence of toxemia. Toxemia is produced by anything and everything that enervates the body. Too much starch, sugar, cream, butter, and milk are frequent causes.

Acute bronchitis is a crisis in toxemia. It means that the mucous membrane lining the bronchial tubes has been requisitioned to do vicarious duty — that toxemia is being sent out through this membrane acting as a channel of compensatory elimination. Chronic bronchitis is the aftermath of frequent acute bronchial crises.

In describing the treatment of bronchitis, Wheeler's *Handbook of Medicine* says: "In the first stage employ the bronchitis kettle, containing a solution of eucalyptus or pinol; administer a brisk saline purge, and a diaphoretic mixture • • •. The cough may be relieved (*suppressed*) by Dover's powder, or by heroin, but opiates tend to depress the respiratory centre, and should not be used if there is much cyanosis (blueness). When expectoration has become more copious, ammonia, and iodide of potassium, with paregoric may be given. The strength must be supported (destroyed) by tonics (atonics), hypophosphites, etc. Later, the mineral acids are of use in diminishing the amount of expectoration."

This treatment is symptomatic, suppressive and injurious. Any patient who is subjected to a bombardment like that described above will inevitably be left more enervated than before. and will have a foundation laid for a more severe crisis later. Treatment of this type is employed without the slightest suspicion that bronchitis has a cause, or that the symptoms are curative processes. It is the outgrowth of voodooism. Sane men and women do not employ such devilish methods.

The *Hygienic* care of the sufferer with bronchitis is simplicity itself. It does not busy itself with treating and suppressing symptoms and trying to *support* the strength of the patient by employing substances that always weaken in the end.

Fasting, rest and warmth are all that are required until the crisis has passed. There should be no effort to check the cough and diminish the expectoration except by removing the need for these — that is, by eliminating the toxemia.

Bear in mind that the crisis — the *disease* — is a curative process. It is not something to be cured. The purpose of hygienic care is merely to supply the body with the most favorable condition under which to carry forward its curative work.

Fresh air in the sick room is highly important. This should be supplied without allowing the patient to become chilled.

In young children, rest and quiet are particularly important. Babies should not be disturbed. Looking at the child's tongue, counting its pulse, taking its temperature, and similar procedures, frequently repeated, disturb and exhaust the child. The tongue is coated, the pulse is rapid, there is fever. You know these things and do not have to be forever confirming them. It is more important that the child rest.

Stop all food at once in infant, child or adult and give nothing but water until the symptoms have subsided. Feed fruit juices and fruit at first, and only gradually add other foods to the diet.

Chronic bronchitis will often require a long fast. It should persist, whenever possible, until the bronchial catarrh has ceased. Rest in bed is essential during the fast. Daily sunbaths and a few minutes of exercise each day are also important. Proper feeding and general care after the fast will assure an evolution into good health and will preserve health thereafter.

Sinusitis

Sinusitis is inflammation of the nasal sinuses. The suffix, *itis*, means inflammation. When placed at the end of the name of any part of the body it signifies inflammation of that part. Hence, tonsilitis is inflammation of the tonsils; appendicitis is inflammation of the appendix, metritis is inflammation of the womb, cystitis is inflammation of the bladder, cholecystitis is inflammation of the gall-bladder, hepatitis is inflammation of the liver, pancreatitis is inflammation of the pancreas, gastritis is inflammation of the stomach, enteritis is inflammation of the small intestine, colitis is inflammation of the colon, phrenitis is inflammation of the brain, cerebro-spinal meningitis is inflammation of the meninges of the brain and cord, carditis is inflammation of the heart, pneumonitis (pneumonia) is inflammation of the lungs, osteitis is inflammation of the bone, etc., etc.

The sinuses, or accessory air chambers, are the hollow interiors of the bones of the face. In the lower forehead just above the roof of the nose are located the frontal sinuses, along the roof of the nostrils are the ethmoid sinuses; opening at the rear are the sphenoid sinuses; while the antrums open on the sides. All of these sinuses, together with the nose form a series of communicating air chambers and are all lined with mucous membrane.

All of the hollow organs of the body that communicate either directly or indirectly with the outside world are lined with mucous membrane. The whole digestive tract from mouth to anus, including the gall-bladder and gall ducts are so lined. The whole respiratory tract — nose, sinuses, trachea, bronchi, etc. — the auditory canals; the genito-urinary tracts; and the eyes are all lined with this type of inner skin.

At any point in the body where there is a mucous surface, catarrh is a possibility. Catarrh is inflammation of a mucous membrane with a discharge of an abnormal amount of mucus of an abnormal character. It is always the same in whatever part of the mucous lining of the body it is located. A cold is an acute catarrh of the nose and throat. The same condition in the stomach will be labeled gastritis; while the same condition in the womb is called endometritis.

Sinusitis, or so-called infection of the sinuses, is a catarrhal inflammation of one or more of the accessory air chambers mentioned above. Like any other catarrhal condition any where else in the body, it may be either acute or chronic. Acute sinusitis is often seen in colds as a part of the cold; chronic sinusitis is often associated with chronic catarrh of the nose and throat and is merely part of the same condition. It frequently accompanies hay fever and asthma, sometimes developing in advance of these troubles, sometimes developing subsequent to their appearance, but in all cases being merely part of the catarrhal condition present in the eyes, nose, throat and deeper respiratory structures.

It is nothing uncommon to find patients who suffer with sinus troubles to also have gastritis, or colitis, or metritis, or cystitis. Indeed sinusitis almost never exists alone; there is almost certain to be catarrhal conditions elsewhere. By this we do not intend to convey the impression that the sinusitis causes the colitis or the metritis, or vice versa; but, rather, that all of these local conditions are but successive and concomitant developments out of a common or systemic condition. They are all caused by the same thing — they do not cause each other.

The understanding reader who has followed us this far is now prepared to understand that irrespective of name and location, catarrh is a unit, that names and locations are unimportant. Such a reader will grasp the significance of this fact and see at once how it simplifies much that seems complicated and mysterious.

In sinusitis there is the same formation of mucus, the same thickening of the lining of the membrane, and the same formation of polyps that are seen in chronic catarrh of the nose. If the catarrh is in the frontal sinuses there will be a continuous discharge from the nose; if in the sphenoid sinus the mucus trickles down into the throat. In all cases the condition is very annoying, often painful and, as now cared for, apparently hopeless.

The sinuses do not drain as well as the nose, so that the mucus tends to remain longer in them and to decompose. Sometimes they actually become obstructed so that all drainage is stopped. Pains, headaches, and other annoying symptoms result.

Sinusitis develops only after frequent toxic crises, in the form of colds, have developed and the catarrhal condition has spread into more and more of the body's mucous surfaces. It rests on a basis of enervation and toxemia and gastro-intestinal catarrh.

The regular treatment of "sinus infection" is far from satisfactory and sufferers go on suffering year after year watching their sinus trouble grow worse all the while. This is true for the reason that these methods of treatment are directed at the symptoms while ignoring cause.

There is a story of an incident which occurred at an institution for the feeble-minded. The superintendent, noticing water in the basement one morning, told one of the inmates to go down and clean it up. Returning in the afternoon, he found the man in the basement working with a mop, with the water still running. He shouted down to the man:

"You idiot, why don't you turn off the tap"?

Looking up with a grin, the man replied: "Nobody ain't payin' me to turn 'er off; I'm gettin' two-bits an hour to mop 'er up."

Besides operations, which chisel out the sinuses, the popular plan of treating sinusitis consists of opening and draining the sinuses and washing them out with strong antiseptic douches. Such procedures have as much curative value as "blowing the nose" in a cold. It cleans the surface but does not touch the underlying causitive condition nor the remote or producing causes.

Doctors are being paid to mop up the discharge (the already excreted material) instead of being paid to turn off the source of supply. Patients pay them, not to correct causes, but to palliate symptoms. Drain the sinuses and they fill up again. Drain them again and they will refill. Keep up this process as long as you will, it will never remedy the trouble. Until the cause of catarrh is removed the sinusitis will continue to exist and will grow gradually worse. No plan of treating these cases that ignores cause can be successful.

Catarrh is an expression of "starch poisoning" caused by the consumption of an excess of carbohydrates—sugars, starches, milk—and faulty elimination. Catarrh is a drainage process, a process of vicarious or compensatory elimination, by which the toxic overload and carbohydrate excess are eliminated. The process would cease after the excess is eliminated were it not for the fact that excesses are daily consumed and faulty elimination fails to take care of them. In other words the "disease" is chronic due to chronic provocation.

Sinus troubles are better or worse as the general condition improves or retrogresses and as living habits vary, but they are never recovered from until their causes are removed or corrected.

However hopeless these cases appear under medical care, they can positively be recovered from in all cases. The natural processes of care for such cases are simple and easily fitted to the individual case by an experienced Hygienist.

They involve two general procedures: (1) Remove or correct all causes, and (2) Build positive health.

Two groups of causes are recognized: (1) The remote causes; that is, those habits and influences of life that have impaired the functions of the body and produced enervation and toxemia and introduced the carbohydrate excess into the body; and (2) The immediate causes; that is, the functional impairment, toxemia and plethora which have resulted from the operation of the remote causes.

Both the immediate and remote causes must be corrected or removed and the processes of doing these are different with the two groups of causes, and require the direction of a skilled Hygienist in their application.

Experience and skill are required to ferret out and correct or remove all of the remote causes, for these are legion. To correct a few causes and leave the others in operation will not suffice to remedy the condition. The removal of the immediate cause is accomplished by a cleansing and recuperating plan that only an experienced Hygienist can fit to the needs of each case.

Positive health is built by the proper use of the elements of Natural Hygiene—air, water, food, sunshine, rest, exercise, etc. These must be used to meet the particular needs of each case. The skilled Hygienist will have no difficulty in adapting these to individual needs. Blanket prescriptions and cover-all treatments are not wise and are doomed to failure.

To build health is easy after the causes that have impaired health and are maintaining the impairment are removed. However, in practically all cases, there exist conditions that require special modifications of the health building program in order to fit it to the needs and capacities of the individual. All care must be individualized. Skill and experience are required for this. Not a method of treatment, but a mode of living is the way to get rid of sinusitis at all stages of its development. Permanent recovery is possible in all cases.

Bronchial Asthma

Bronchial asthma is defined as "a disease marked by intermittent dyspnea (difficult breathing), cough, and a sense of constriction, due to spasmodic contraction of the bronchi (bronchial spasm) and a swelling of the bronchial mucous membrane. The paroxysms last from a few minutes to several days."

Reading medical text books dealing with asthma and going over the entire lot of causes ascribed to it, one is surprised at the paucity of ideas as to the real fundamental causes, which he meets. As a rule, the text-books describe bronchial asthma as an "expiratory dyspnea that appears paroxysmally" due to "some reflex irritation of the nasal, pharyngeal, and bronchial mucous membranes." If the reader imagines that these big words indicate that the text-book writer knows what he is writing about, let us assure him that actually all this jargon is intended to conceal ignorance and stupidity.

The medical view of asthma presents an absurd situation primarily because of its entire lack of knowledge of its etiology and pathology. If its literature on the subject is a "hopelessly chaotic jumble," as one medical author puts it, he is also correct in saying that the treatment of the disease is "still more hopeless." The profession considers the disease to be incurable, although acknowledging that some do "outgrow the condition."

Most medical writers of the present ascribe bronchial asthma to "protein hypersensitiveness." These writers do not pretend to know the cause of the hypersensitiveness, or allergy, as it is called.

Asthmatics are roughly divided into two classes:

(1) Those sensitive to ingested substances — oysters, meat, eggs, etc.

(2) Those sensitive to air-carried irritants

— pollens, emanations from horses, cats, dogs, feathers, dust, etc.

Those sensitive to air-carried allergens rarely absorb a quantity sufficient to give rise to general symptoms, whereas, in sensitization (allergy) to food, symptoms of general reaction are common. In some, the general sensitiveness to food causes a chronic irritation of all the organs of the body, but that organ or part of the body which is the weakest link in the chain will be the one to develop disease first. If the tendency is to asthma, then the chronic irritation produced by allergens will evolve asthmatic symptoms if and when the poison so produced is sufficient to cause reaction.

Protein hypersensitiveness (allergy) is merely another name for protein poisoning, or what amounts to the same thing, protein stuffing, in those of a neurotic diathesis.

The immediate cause of the bronchial spasm is an irritation of the nerve-endings of the vagus nerve which supplies the bronchi. In some cases even water taken into the stomach will so irritate the vagus nerve in the stomach that a direct reflex irritation of the vagus nerve in the lungs induces an asthmatic paroxysm. In the same way, drugs, some foods, gas and indigestion occasion reflex irritation of the nerve-endings in the bronchi and bring on a paroxysm of asthma.

Breathing cold air, dust, pollens, gases, foul odors, and other such things, produces a direct irritation of the nerve-endings in the lungs and brings on the paroxysm.

If water, irritating foods, drugs, indigestion, cold air, dust, pollens, foul odors, gases, etc., were primary and direct causes of asthma, nobody would be free of this condition. The real, the basic, cause of asthma is that which sensitizes the nerves and the bronchial membranes. It is this underlying cause, which is unknown to medical men, and their ignorance of this cause that converts their treatment of asthma into a farce and a tragedy.

Asthma rests on a basis of toxemia and gastro-intestinal catarrh. If asthmatics were not enervated and if their bodies were not filled with toxins to the saturation point, they would not be hypersensitive to proteins and other substances.

Asthma always means a catarrhal condition. But not all who have catarrh develop asthma. Only those with neurotic tendencies will have asthma. The non-neurotic may develop a very severe chronic catarrh and never have asthma.

There should be no difficulty in understanding the condition. The asthmatic is an asthmatic long before the broncho-spasm puts a label on him and if once we grasp the fact that in every case of asthma there is a preceding history of disobedience of the laws of life, we are in line for rational care and ultimate complete recovery.

. By uncontrolled impulses or emotions, business and domestic worries and other worries, lack of poise and self-control, sexual drain, overeating, improper eating, lack of sleep, sleeping without ventilation, overstimulation, etc., a state of enervation is built which checks secretions and excretions, and builds toxemia. Enervation plus wrong eating — too much food, wrong combinations of food, etc. — favor gastro-intestinal decomposition and this adds the enervating influence of auto-infection to the prior weakening habits.

Asthma is brought on in the first place from excessive table indulgence, plus many other nerve leaks. The enervating effects of overfeeding and physicking may produce asthma in children. The abominable habit of physicking children during infancy and early childhood is responsible for many other conditions besides asthma.

The asthmatic crisis is a toxic storm which occurs when the machinery of elimination is no longer equal to the load put upon it. From acute asthma the case is hurried to the chronic state. Then emphysema, bronchectasis and tuberculosis are logically expected to follow.

In consequence of the contraction of the finer bronchial tubes and the air-cells of the lungs, air cannot be got into the lungs, and the entire volume of blood cannot be sufficiently oxygenated and purified. The difficulty in breathing prevents rest and sleep, often making it impossible for the sufferer to recline. The palliative treatment commonly employed adds greatly to enervation and thus to toxemia. The original causes are not corrected. Under such conditions, how can recovery be hoped for?

Asthmatics who come to the *Health School* have tried all of the advertised cures and have frequently been operated on for "focal infections," presumably arising in the nose, sinuses, teeth, throat, gall-bladder, appendix, ovaries, and other suspected organs. Most of them are minus their tonsils, and one man had a long, ugly trench across his forehead, just above the eyes, where his frontal sinuses had been chiseled out.

Tonsil, adenoid, mastoid and sinus operations are ridiculous in asthma, yet they are frequently resorted to. Usually these operations are performed after the sufferers have been deluged with adrenalin, stramonium and morphine. When drugs and operations have failed the patient, he is sent to Texas, New Mexico, Arizona, Utah, California, Kansas, or Colorado. In these states the climate is supposed to cure him.

Asthmatics who are apparently helped by a change of climate discover that they are not cured, when, upon returning home, they find that they still have asthma. If we may judge from our experience, age, sex, occupation and climate have nothing to do with asthma, for it develops in both sexes, all ages, all occupations and in all climates. Changing climate, if one does nothing else, does not restore health.

The author of a standard medical text-book quotes two hundred and thirteen different authorities and recommends two hundred and thirteen different ways of treating asthma, and not one of these methods of treatment is valuable.

During the paroxysm any drug that is powerful enough to "act" on the nerves of the bronchi, in spite of the existing toxemia, and induce relaxation of the bronchial spasm, if injected into the body, will afford temporary relief. This relief is only palliative, as the toxemia, food poisoning and irritation are still present, and as soon as the effect of the drug wears off, the asthma recurs. Every dose of the drug, whatever its nature, leaves the patient still more sensitive to food poisoning and lowers the general resistance of the body.

Physicians who merely treat asthma symptomatically (and they all do) use certain drugs which either "act" on the nerve endings of the vagus or on the muscle fibers of the bronchi. The at present most popular drug is adrenalin, an extract made from the adrenal glands of animals. This drug will, in most cases, afford almost instant relief and almost every asthmatic who comes to the *Health School* has had adrenalin. Some of them have had it for years, while not a few take it several times daily.

Adrenalin does not cure asthma. On the contrary, its use greatly increases the liability to paroxysms of asthma and we find these cases to be the most difficult to restore to health. The continued employment of adrenalin produces a great lowering of the vitality of the general system, and in time, the whole muscular system, including the heart and arteries, suffers great loss in tone.

Stramonium, morphine and caffeine (coffee) give temporary relief for a time, but after a few repetitions they can no longer relieve, except in lethal doses, while the use of morphine in asthma has produced many morphine addicts.

The use of vaccines (allergies) to produce "immunity" is also quite popular. The so-called protein immunity thus produced (in a few cases) wears off, and it is a common occurrence for such cases to have a recurrence of asthma at a later date. A large part of the asthmatics who come to the *Health School* have been *cured* and *immunized* by this method, and every case is worse off from such treatment, as no attempt has been made to rid the body of the real cause, while the evil effects of this method of treatment have been added to it.

Asthma rests on a basis of toxemia and catarrh, and the dog, cat, horse, feather pillow, pollen, etc., have nothing to do with its causation. "Hot dogs" are the only "dogs" we know of that have anything to do with producing asthma.

When the underlying toxic condition is eliminated, all forms of sensitization disappear. When the asthmatic gets rid of toxemia he does not have to worry about sensitization. He automatically gets rids of this when he gets rid of the true cause — toxemia. It is, perhaps, true that all asthmatics will retain to some extent their sensitiveness to certain foods, chemicals, heat, cold, etc., as they originally had that tendency or diathesis when they were born, but by following the few simple rules of right living which are taught at the *Health School*, they may always avoid a recurrence of asthma.

In asthma there is an abnormally sensitive peripheral organ — the ethmoid area of the nose — and this is often operated upon or seared. This abnormal sensitivity should be regarded as an effect of the chronic overload of toxemia and not as a cause of asthma. Crippling the nose does not cure asthma.

It was pointed out above that the immediate cause of the bronchial spasm called asthma is an irritation, direct or reflex, of the nerve-endings of the vagus nerve which supplies the bronchi.

A hypertonicity or vago-tonic condition is induced by the irritating effect of the poisons of tox-emia upon the vagus nerves and in this way the bronchi are thrown into a spasm. The asthmatic sufferer is in a chronic state of delicate balance between absorption and elimination. Anything that helps to throw the balance in favor of elimination helps to relieve him; anything that throws it the other way increases his distress. This is the reason it is so necessary to avoid all those practices that enervate and intoxicate the whole organism. Allowing the feet to become cold is often enough to bring on a paroxysm of asthma, and a paroxysm is often relieved merely by warming the feet.

Few asthmatics have much idea of their limitations in eating, working, enjoying, etc., and, as a consequence of their over-indulgence, are constantly adding to their trouble. If they are to get well and remain well, they must learn self-control.

All sufferers from bronchial asthma can recover good health and be permanently free of asthma thereafter. How? Eliminate toxemia, restore nerve energy and correct the mode of living. The whole thing is so simple and so certain that only the foolish will continue to suffer.

Hay Fever

Of a similar character to bronchial asthma is hay fever. Indeed the only difference between the two affections is the location of the affected membranes.

Hay fever is a chronic catarrhal inflammation of the mucous membrane (schneiderian membrane) of the nose, often involving the lining membranes of the eyes, throat (pharynx), Eustachian tubes, larynx, and bronchial tubes. It may well be described as a severe cold running on day after day, with no let-up and often growing worse, for the longer it persists in the acute stage, the more sentive the mucous membrane becomes.

The catarrh is continuous but is peculiarly subject to pronounced increase in severity of symptoms in the months of May, June, July and August. In May the condition is called rose-cold; in July and August, hay-fever.

Hay fever, asthma and so-called sinus infection often co-exist. In one case the hay fever develops first, asthma next and sinus trouble last; in another case the asthma develops first, or the sinus trouble develops first. The order of their development makes no difference.

The medical profession fosters the view that because roses and strawberries come in May and pollens abound in July and August, they should be correlated as cause and effect. This view, like that held concerning asthma, overlooks the underlying cause of the sensitivity of the membranes.

Although it is true that dust, pollen, emanations from horses, cats, dogs, birds, etc., and even cold air, will drive hay-fever sufferers into intolerable suffering, this does not prove them to be causes of hay fever. Anything that irritates a sensitive mucous membrane occasions a rush of blood to the point of irritation and the pouring out of an exudate to flush away the irritant.

Within recent years enterprising doctors have discovered that some hay-fever subjects are allergic to their sweet-hearts and suffer an exacerbation (aggravation) of symptoms every-time they visit their lovers. In a few instances the source of irritation was found in the lip-stick, rouge, and face powder, or even in the perfume, but in other instances emanations from the lover's hair were blamed.

The mistake has been made of considering normal elements in man's environment — pollen, and emanations from animals — as causes of hay fever; whereas, the true cause, the basic cause, is the cause of the sensitization of membranes which normally are not sensitive to pollens, etc.

Hay fever is simply a peculiar type of chronic catarrh which only a small percentage of catarrhal subjects develop. Two people have catarrh to the same extent; one develops hay fever, the other does not. The sensitive individual is neurotic, the other is not. Both are highly toxic. Hay fever is chronic catarrh in a neurotic subject.

Only neurotic individuals — those subject to nervous diseases — will develop the individualizing sensitization that distinguishes hay fever from ordinary catarrh. The non-neurotic sufferer from catarrh will be influenced little or none by the inhalation of dust, pollen, smoke, pungent odors, or cold air. "Hot dogs" are the only dogs of which I know that may help to cause hay fever.

Hay fever rests on a basis of enervation and toxemia. The hay fever sufferer is made highly toxic by his enervating habits which inhibit full elimination of normal body wastes. The subject builds his disease daily by keeping his stomach deranged with his meats, potatoes, breads, pies, cakes, pastries, butter, breakfast foods, and even with his luscious fruits covered with cream and sugar. These things over stimulate him and pro-duce a toxic state of his blood which further adds to his enervation and produces nervousness and sensitiveness as well as catarrh.

By an enervating mode of living elimination is checked resulting in toxin retention, and accumulation. When the toxin accumulation reaches the saturation point, crises occur. This means that certain areas of the mucous membrane are requisitioned to do vicarious duty in excreting toxins. The crises are named rhinitis, tonsilitis, coryza, bronchitis, etc., depending on the area of mucous membrane used for compensatory activity. When catarrh becomes chronic, organic change takes place and if this is in the nose we have polyps, hay-fever, etc.

Medical treatment of hay fever is no more satisfactory than that of asthma. Osler advises "thorough local treatment of the nose, particularly the destruction of the vessels and sinuses over the sensitive areas." He says: "Owing to the peculiar nature of the disease and the constant reinfection of the mucous membranes by pollen on exposure to the outside air, it is advised to sleep with the windows closed and to apply the serate in the morning before rising both to eyes and nose, and again during the day if the slightest irritation is felt in the conjunctivæ or nasal mucous membrane."

Can anything be more absurd? Yes. Perhaps the latest practice of zinc-plating the lining of the nose is more absurd. The zinc-plating affords some protection against pollen, as does the mechanical filter now on sale to be worn on the nose, but neither of these methods remedy the catarrh. Neither of them eliminate toxemia. Neither of them restore normal nerve energy. Neither of them correct the mode of life. They are only palliative, and as all palliatives encourage an ignoring of cause, they are positive hindrances to recovery.

Fashionable folk are advised to go away to some place where they will not be troubled by dust, pollens, etc. Tilden says:

"By July or August the Schneiderian membrane is so morbidly sensitive that it is irritated by pollen, ragweed, chicken feathers, goose feathers, horse hair, cat fur — any pungent odors or microscopic irritants; and there develops consequently, according to medical science, the very popular disease, hay-fever, which sends thousands scampering to resorts reputed to be free from hay-fever causes. More or less comfort is experienced at these resorts until Jack Frost — that professional 'scab' doctoring without a license — *cures everybody;* and they stay cured until the various causes get to work the next year, and then the hay-fever victims must go hunting cures again. Those who have not the time and wherewithal to fly to dustless, pollenless, ragweedless, catless, horseless, chickenless, gooseless, and senseless resorts, employ doctors who entertain them during the hay-fever season with frequent injections of serums made from all the known and unknown causes; and, if the list is not long enough to last through the season, the resourceful doctor invents enough new remedies to keep the victims busy coming to his lair, hopeful and expectant of cure, until the old quack, Jack Frost, cures them again."

It is true that one may go to the sea or to the mountains and escape the irritating pollens, but this is only another form of palliation. It must be repeated the following year and each year thereafter, for it fails to cure the catarrh that is the essence of hay-fever, and without which the pollens would produce no irritation. Normal membranes are not irritated by pollens — only inflamed membranes are irritated.

Medical treatment does not seek to restore normal condition and function to the mucous membrane. It seeks to get the subject away from the sources of external irritation, or to protect the membranes from contact with irritants by covering them with serates, or by zinc-plating them, or by the use of mechanical filters;

or else it seeks to "immunize" the membranes against the pollens, etc., by the employment of vaccines made of these very substances.

Osler advises ·arsenic, phosphorus and strychnine to improve the stability of the nervous system of hay-fever sufferers. There is nothing like stabilizing the nervous system and there are no stabilizers like strychnine and arsenic!

Occasionally some doctor, or the head of some hay-fever association (the hay-fever sufferers of the country are organized into various associations and hold national conventions) breaks into print with the senseless proposal to destroy all ragweeds or all goldenrods or all male cedar trees, etc. The logically legitimate extension of such a program would convert the whole country into a barren desert. For they would have to destroy not only pollen bearing plants, trees, and grasses, but all suspected animals and even a few sweet-hearts.

Herbert Spencer once remarked that mankind never tries the right remedy until it has exhausted every possible wrong one. So many wrong remedies have been tried for hay-fever that we almost dare to hope that the time is near when we will be forced to try the right one. However, the inventive ingenuity of the human race is almost unlimited and there is still much money to be made out of the commercial exploitation of hay-fever cures that do not cure.

The restoration of sound health and normal function to the membranes of the eyes, nose and throat is so easily and simply accomplished merely by removing the causes of the catarrh and building health by employing the causes of health, that no one need go on suffering from hay fever. The first hay fever sufferer that came under the author's care has been free of hay fever for over twenty years. During the whole of this time the lady could have taken a bath in pollen without producing any discomfort.

Although some cases are a bit stubborn and require a longer time to recover health, my experience has convinced me that fully ninety per cent. of hay fever sufferers can be fully and permanently free of hay fever in five to six weeks. This requires only the elimination of toxemia, restoration of normal nerve energy and correction of the mode of living. Following this the evolution into good health is sure and rapid.

The Ductless Glands

Endocrinology is one of the rackets developed by the medical profession and meat packers during recent years. It followed the discovery of the importance of a group of structures in the body that had formerly been declared to be functionless — relics of man's hypothetical amoeba-worm-fish-r e p t i le-quadruped-primate-pithecanthropus erectus ancestry.

Not so many years ago the adrenal (suprarenal) glands, thymus gland, spleen, thyroid gland, parathyroid glands, pineal and pituitary glands were declared to have no functions. This was all on the well-known scientific principle, recognized by all good physiologists, that ignorance of function is evidence of absence of function; a principle still applied to the tonsils and appendix. Then came the discovery that these small glands do perform functions the importance of which is out of all proportion to their sizes. Indeed, it was found that life is impossible without some of them.

Glandular structures, as they are, they are without ducts (hence, duct-less, glands) and pour their secretions directly into the blood stream (hence, endocrine glands). Other glands — ovaries, testicles, pancreas and perhaps others — though possessing ducts that carry off certain of their secretions, also produce other secretions which are poured directly into the blood. These, too, are classed as endocrine glands.

The internal (endo) secretions of these glands are called *hormones*. Hormone is derived from the Greek and means *agitator*. It is a poor word, for the endocrine secretions are not agitators. They do activate function in some way and do control the nutritive processes of the body. These glands belong to the body's nutritive system.

The discovery of the important offices performed by the hormones in regulating metabolism, activating function and controlling development led enthusiasts and commercialists to declare: *"We are what our glands make us."*

. Unfortunately, as in everything else, instead of trying to understand these glandular functions and instead of searching for the natural conditions upon which normal glandular function depends, the search was directed to finding substitutes for normal functions and means of converting their near-knowledge into cash. I do not think it can be too often emphasized that "modern medicine" is a great big commercial institution or a series of institutions constituting a mighty profit-seeking, dollar-grasping industry. Perhaps the huge army of physicians, nurses, pathologists, bacteriologists, "research" workers, pharmacists (druggists), manufacturing chemists, vaccine and serum producers, glandular products companies, surgical supply houses and all the workers employed by these factories, the medical colleges and their staffs, the thousands of hospitals, sanitariums, clinics, etc., and those who depend on these institutions for their incomes, do not feel that they can afford to have the profitable industry they have built up destroyed by searching for the natural basis of normal function.

The natural outcome of such a deplorable state of affairs is that a gullible public is constantly being deluged with a flood of pseudo-discoveries and pseudo-remedies which are dangled before its eyes by an army of mystery-mongering professionals. Sensation-mongering is the order of the day and the professionals have found that the frequent announcement of a sensational new discovery is very profitable.

Are we what our glands make us? The answer is, no. They are only organs, like the muscles, or the stomach. Glands have no existence, as such, in nature. They exist only in relation to other parts, or rather, in relation to the whole organism. No doubt the whole endocrine system is an organic unit, as is often asserted, but it is no less so than the body and all of its parts. The glandular system is a unit only in relation to the whole body apart from which it has no existence.

Every gland depends upon the cooperation of the others, while the whole organism is dependent, for its well-being, upon a subtle and co-ordinated inter-organic "stimulation" requiring a high degree of subordination of the parts to the common good. "Bear ye one another's burdens," is an admonition that has been obeyed by the organs of the body since the beginning of life. The body functions as an organized unit and not as a mere collection of organs. We cannot separate organs from their reciprocal relations.

All glands of the body, be they ducted or ductless, are under the constitutional or federal government — under the union of the organism (symbiosis). Whatever amount of individual control or individuality the various organs may have, all are bound together by the blood and nervous system. The fact that the sympathetic nervous system regulates the nutrition and functioning of the tissue and the secretion of hormones, makes difficult the understanding of hormones.

The glands have their duties to perform towards "us"; but, we, in turn, owe reciprocal duties to them. Our duties to our glands are usually forgotten. It is not enough to say that these glands are the suppliers of indispensable activators of normal work and leave the matter here. For they require to be supplied by the organism with materials appropriate to the production of their hormones. Every gland depends for its normal function upon the co-operation of other organs (internal control or symbiosis) and, in a wider sense, upon cooperation with biological partners (external control) chiefly through food. We control our metabolism ourselves, the glands being parts of us, take part in the control.

The very use of the term "internal secretion" tends to conceal from us the fact that the vital potencies of the secretions are derived from plants — our symbiotic partners. "Science" investigates everything except the fact that evolution is determined by nutrition.

Glands function efficiently or not depending on their nerve and food supply. If the blood is normal, their supply of food is normal; if the nervous system is normal, they are properly energized. With pure blood and normal nerve force gland function will be normal. These depend upon our conduct — *our mode of living.*

What causes a gland to function? Nerve energy. No doubt inter-glandular reciprocity exists, but over all is a nervous system that furnishes energy for the work. Full nerve energy spells good function. When nerve energy is lowered, functions lag. Glandular function cannot be normal in an enervated body. Glandular mal-functioning is an effect, not a cause. However, "modern medicine" always starts with an established pathology as cause.

The tendency today is to class almost all symptoms as symptoms of endocrine gland disease; to attribute practically all human defects to endocrine disorder. Nowhere is it realized that the endocrine disorder and the defects elsewhere are due to common causes. The commercial program is to ignore causes and treat the glands — stimulate or inhibit them, operate on them, or supply glandular extracts from the glands of animals.

We do not intend to deny that malfunctioning of these glands adds to the pathology. We do insist that the glandular dysfunction is not the primary cause and that any program of care that neglects the primary cause cannot produce satisfactory results. Such a program is merely a system of palliation or patchwork.

The failure of this program is apparent to all except those who are profiting from dispensing the treatments. Sokoloff admits that the diagnosis and treatment of separate glands fail to yield satisfactory results. He adds: "What most frequently takes place is merely further disturbance of the endocrine gland system."

We learn of complications upon complications in the inter-relations of the glands themselves and of the glands and other parts of the body, wherefore, it should be obvious that only a general integrity will avail. To rely upon interference with glands and hormones and their relations is to rely upon things concerning which we have merely fragmentary knowledge. We should rely rather upon preserving (or restoring) intact, our integrity. We must deal with an organism and its ways of life, not merely with theoretically isolated parts of the organism.

Certain, if not all, of the glands are involved in the body's defense against poisons. The supra-renal cortex and the thyroid gland are especially involved in the toxin defense. The glands react to any intoxication by increased functioning.

Chronic irritation, resulting from chronic protein poisoning, will result in chronic hyper-functioning of the glands until exhaustion results in hypo-function. Hyper-functioning may lead to enlargement and consequent change of structure in the glands. Or, a degeneration of the gland's active elements may result, so that often, as a result of "a slight infection of short duration," the organism is permanently thrown out of balance.

The chief cause of intoxication (infection) is protein poisoning, such as that connected with the pernicious habit of meat and egg eating. Man's life and feeding habits are so contrary to the best interests of his body that the ensuing poisoning requires to be specially coped with and provided against by particular glands, the task of which is a very delicate and arduous one, involving frequent fatigue and breakdowns due to overwork, making the task increasingly difficult.

When an organ is overworked enervation follows. Through failing cooperation or reciprocity all the organs are hindered in their functions of assimilation, secretion, and excretion. When an enervated gland fails to function a reasonable remedy would be to find the cause of enervation and remove it. When an over-stimulated (irritated by toxins) gland functions too much, a logical remedy would be to find the cause of the over-stimulation (irritation) and remove it.

No amount of spectacular stimulation or inhibition of the overburdened glands can be depended on to adequately deal with the poisoning. Only a complete revolution of the mode of living can take the intolerable burden of toxins off the glands and permit a return of normal gland function. Treating the adrenal cortex, for instance, with the intent of increasing its toxin-fighting power is ridiculous when we have it in our own hands, by a wise choice of food, or by temporary abstinence from food, to avert poisoning.

Stimulating and inhibiting over-worked glands enervates them still more. No wonder then that, as Sokoloff says, treating separate glands frequently causes "further disturbance of the endocrine gland system."

There is no cure for glandular insufficiency, except to correct the habits of life that are responsible for the enervation which has ended in secretory block. The use of gland extracts in these cases is a failure. The failure of insulin in diabetes is typical of the failure of all other gland extracts. Gland extracts may be used as a crutch by those whose glandular impairment is too great for vital redemption or for compensation. All others should know that these extracts produce their own damages in the body and also that their use leads to an ignoring of cause.

The physiologist, P. G. Styles, says of the adrenal glands: "Their extracts do not successfully compensate for the lack of living cells; the body seems to need a slow uniform delivery of this internal secretion, and periodic dosing does not prove equivalent to the natural condition." There is probably the same need for a slow uniform delivery of all of the internal secretions. At the same time, there is evident an increased or decreased delivery as need occasions. It is impossible to adjust external administration of hormones to the varying needs of the body.

Still another objection to the use of glandular extracts is offered in the fact that after these have been employed for a time, the body seems to learn to destroy them. It seems not to use them. The following item appeared in the *Literary Digest*, September 8, 1934, under the title, "Anti-Hormones End Dream of Remaking Race":

During the last ten years it has been frequently predicted that the human race some day would be remade by endocrine therapy—the use of hormones extracted from or secreted by the still mysterious "ductless glands." It is known that improper functioning of these glands produces giantism and dwarfism, overweight or underweight, and many types of disease. Some physicians have been confident that such conditions readily could be overcome by administering gland substance to make up for that apparently lacking.

But, it now has been pointed out by the *Journal of the American Medical Association*, they have reckoned without the body's resistance to assaults upon its glandular equilibrium. It has been demonstrated by Prof. J. B. Collip and his associates of McGill University that when foreign-gland substances are injected into it, the body manufactures "anti-hormones."

The result is that, after a time, the effect of new injections is neutralized, and the glandular balance of the body becomes about as it was in the beginning.

It is true that powerful endocrine preparations often are administered to patients, and frequently the desired results may be obtained, the editor of the *Journal* pointed out, but physicians have been puzzled by the fact that occasional cases not only fail to improve under such treatment, but become worse. The reason, the *Journal* editor suggested, was that the effect of the treatment had been nullified by the generation of "anti-hormones," with the result that the patient was worse off than before.

How seriously this factor will affect present methods of gland treatment can not be predicted. It probably puts an end to the dream of making giants and dwarfs at will, or of bringing about a medical millennium through glandular therapy.

Who was the wise poet who penned these lines?:

> "And wouldst thou play Creator
> and Ordainer of things,
>
> Be Nature then thy chaos and be
> thou her God."

Removing the glands deprives the body of their functions and, in the case of certain glands, means speedy death. In the case of all of them it means much additional trouble. The evils following the removal of the ovaries are generally known. Whether the whole gland is removed or merely part of it, this does not touch the cause of the trouble. If part of an enlarged thyroid is removed the remaining portion enlarges, due to the persistence of the cause of the original enlargement, and another operation is deemed necessary. Two and three operations upon the thyroid are not uncommon.

None of these methods of treating or mistreating the glands have anything in them to recommend them to an intelligent person. It is unfortunately true, as some philosopher has said, that people would rather die than think. If they could be induced to think they could soon know that we have to put our whole house in order, not by a thousand and one local treatments, but by duly accomodating ourselves to the ordered symbiosis on the grand scale of nature upon which every normal fixture in our body depends. Armed with knowledge they would, when offered, not normalization of the glands, but treatment, or, rather, mistreatment of them, know how to judge of the merits of the measures offered by the professionals.

We forget that the conservation of life-energy is in our own hands and not in the hands of some clever medical profession which will yet discover the right chemicals with which to treat the glands. We ignore, too, the fact that "the crowded foulness of our body" is due to "rioting joys that fringe the sad pathways of Hell." The oft'heard statement, "It's my glands, doctor," is based on the thought that the glands may go wrong without cause, that glandular malfunction is responsible for our troubles, instead of us being responsible for the glandular mal-function. The professionals have fostered this view for professional reasons.

Goitre

Goitre is enlargement of the thyroid gland in the throat. The thyroid gland is one of the body's glands of internal secretion and secretes a substance known as thyroxin which acts as a catalytic agent in the process of oxidation. The human body contains approximately fourteen milligrams of thyroxin, although the amount varies under different conditions. Thyroxin is active in practically all the cells of the body. It quickens the rate of transformation of energy and is a regulator of metabolism. An elevation or depression of one milligram of the thyroxin content of the body results in a corresponding shift of 2.8% in basal metabolism.

Hyperthyroidism is the term applied to the physiologic status that obtains when there is an excess of thyroxin in the body.

Hypothyroidism is the term applied to the condition resulting from deficient function of the thyroid.

Hyperthyroidism can exist without goitre and goitre can exist without hyperthyroidism. This being true it is necessary to carefully weigh the so-called thyroid symptoms to ascertain where they come from.

The secretion of thyroxin seems to depend on an adequate supply of iodine and this has led to the belief that goitre is due to iodine deficiency. As goitre is usually associated with excessive secretion of thyroxin, and as lack of iodine should result in a deficiency of thyroxin, this theory of the cause of goitre would seem to be unsound. Certainly the practice built on this theory of cause has failed; failed both as a preventive and as a cure.

There are several classifications of goitre, but we shall here employ the one which we consider most simple and, therefore, most easily understood by the layman — *simple hypertrophic goitre, cystic or colloidal goitre*, and *exophthalmic goitre*.

The first of these is a simple enlargement of the thyroid gland and may occur without any appreciable disturbance of function. It is frequent in young girls and often disappears at puberty. The voice and swallowing may be affected by pressure exerted by the enlarged gland.

Cystic goitre is a thyroidal cyst containing a fluid or colloid substance within its capsule. It may affect, by pressure, the voice and swallowing.

Exophthalmic goitre receives its name from the manner in which the eyes protrude from their sockets — *exophthalmia*. There is an increased pulse rate, frequently running up to 140 and even 160 a minute, often violent palpitation, increased metabolism, nervous and mental symptoms, loss of weight and energy and, often, there is sugar in the urine.

The thyroid gland is very closely linked with the sex glands. Apparently there is a more fundamental relationship between the female sex organism and the thyroid than between it and the male sex organism. At least disturbances of the sex functions in females have a more profoundly disturbing effect upon the thyroid than do disturbances of the male sex functions.

Medical science (?) would have us believe that all the disagreeable symptoms peculiar to exophthalmic goitre are due to systemic poisoning from excess secretion. That this is not true is obvious from the fact that many of these symptoms precede the hyperthyroidism. The goitre is merely a link in a chain.

Hyperthyroidism (goitre) results from toxemia, the essential and ever-present first cause of over activity of the thyroid. To us, all goitres are toxic goitres. Supersaturation of the body with toxins from checked elimination, excessive eating of proteins, starches, pies, puddings, etc., and neglect of raw vegetables and fruits, and from various poison habits and the pyramiding of the effects of bad habits, is the cause of goitre.

It has been shown experimentally that the thyroid gland may be stimulated into activity by sympathetic impulses and Cannon and others say that a continuation of such impulses over a considerable period of time produces a condition in animals like exophthalmic goitre in man. Clinical observations indicate that in men and women this condition may result from prolonged nervous strain or even that it may follow a single violent emotional disturbance.

Domestic and social discord, worry, irritation, etc., may easily produce enough sympathetic stimulation of the thyroid to result in exophthalmic goitre. Overwork, the various poison habits — coffee, tea, tobacco, alcohol, etc., habits — too frequent childbearing or other drains upon the organism and the various indulgencies common to modern living are factors in the production of goitre. We consider it very significant that among animals in captivity only carnivores suffer from goitre. Vegetarian and fruitarian animals are not so affected.

The sex factor in the development of goitre has not received sufficient consideration. Dr. Weger says that in practically all female goitre patients who have reached maturity and also frequently in girls who have just past puberty there is an intimate association and pathological involvement of the ovaries or uterus or both. "In the majority of cases there exists a small uterine fibroid. * * * In many cases the uterine tissues are themselves in a state of fibrous enduration and enlargement. Almost invariably there is found a complicating chronic endometritis or endocervicitis with retained secretions."

Tilden says, "thyroid enlargement is secondary to uterine and ovarian perversion in the female, and gonadal perversion in the male, and the perversion of these reproductive functions is super-induced by over-indulged appetite and passion, for the most part by suppressed lasciviousness and salaciousness." Again: "I have never seen a case of goitre in women who have not been troubled with toxemia, and who have not been suffering with gastro-intestinal catarrh and a catarrhal state of the womb. I have found drainage from the womb invariably imperfect."

"The thyroid and mammary glands are auxiliary to the, reproductive system and anything that perverts the functions of the reproductive organs causes abnormalities of the thyroid and breasts." "Lumps in the breasts," so generally scare-headed into cancer, are invariably associated with the same kind of pelvic derangements as is goitre.

In goitre, the breasts of the female are often enlarged and the glands hard and sensitive. The womb is often enlarged and sensitive with catarrh and even ulceration of the membrane of the neck and body of the womb. The breast and thyroid troubles are reflex affections due to womb sepsis. The imperfectly drained (retained) secretions of the womb undergo decomposition and are highly toxic.

Sexual repression is especially common in females and many of these repressed women are as lascivious as any libertine. If married, they enter the sexual relation without responding, consciously or subconsciously (usually the latter) repressing themselves, and thus helping to pervert the functions of the thyroid.

To remove the thyroid, or to give gland extracts, or to treat the gland, or to give iodine, has no effect whatsoever on the cause of goitre. Removal of part of the gland is followed by subsequent enlargement of the remaining portion for the cause has not been removed. Two and three such operations are sometimes performed before the patient finally dies.

Goitre rests upon a physical derangement of enervation, toxemia, intestinal putresence and uterine sepsis and to ignore this derangement and treat the goitre *per se* cannot but fail.

Dr. Weger says "most hypertrophic goitres can be made to absorb. Absorption of a cystic goitre is a very rare occurrence." Dr. Tilden says: "exophthalmic goitre can be cured just as easily as a fibroid tumor of the uterus can be cured. Indeed, these diseases can be cured even after many of the heads of the surgical profession of our leading cities declare that they cannot be cured without an operation."

Complete and ultimately successful recovery can occur only, as Dr. Weger says, if "the patient is put to bed in an environment that will insure absolute physical and mental rest — away from friends and even relatives. The reasons for this are only obvious to those who have had experience in getting nervous patients under control. Outside influence and interference are sometimes insurmountable obstacles and always decided handicaps."

We have emphasized above the office of nervous irritation, domestic difficulties, etc., in overstimulating the thyroid. It should be obvious to anyone how necessary it is to get away from the sources of these disturbing factors. Proper rest of the nervous system is not possible so long as they exist. Physical and mental rest are vitally important in goitre cases.

Toxin elimination is best secured by fasting — *physiological rest*. This will also hasten the absorption of the enlargement. Indeed it often results in a rapid reduction and disappearance of the thyroid enlargement and of the sensitiveness, enlargement and hardening in the breasts. and womb or ovaries.

Dr. Weger adds: "Physiological rest can best be obtained by a complete fast. All foods must be withheld and nothing but water given until the pulse is normal and all active symptoms have subsided "

Uterine drainage is essential and if this is not re-established, success need hardly be anticipated. Inflammation and ulceration will not heal or will heal slowly if the constitutional toxemia is not eliminated.

The diet after the fast is vitally important, not merely immediately but for a long time thereafter. A low-carbohydrate tolerance, lasting even for months, is usually present and sugar in any form is forbidden. Fruits and green vegetables are the most important food needs.

A return to the old living habits — tobacco, alcohol, coffee, domestic discord, repression of lasciviousness, over-eating, wrong eating, etc., — will quickly rebuild the trouble. Goitre may be prevented in the first place by right living; right living alone can prevent a recurrence after recovery.

Colitis

Colitis is inflammation of the colon or large bowel. It is necessary to re-emphasize that the suffix, *itis*, means inflammation and when joined to the end of the name of an organ or part, it indicates inflammation of that organ or part. Thus, rhinitis is inflammation of the nasal mucous membrane; iritis is inflammation of the iris; conjunctivitis is inflammation of the mucous membrane of the eye, or conjunctiva; laryngitis is inflammation of the larynx; pharyngitis is inflammation of the pharynx; otitis is inflammation of the ear; stomatitis is inflammation of the mouth; odontitis is inflammation of a tooth; cholangitis is inflammation of the bile duct; orchitis is inflammation of the testicle; ovaritis is inflammation of the ovary; nephritis is inflammation of the kidney; duodenitis is inflammation of the duodenum; proctitis is inflammation of the rectum; endoappendicitis is inflammation of the mucous membrane lining the appendix; endocranitis is inflammation of the endocranium, or dura mater; osteitis is inflammation of a bone; arthritis is inflammation of a joint; neuritis is inflammation of a nerve; — and, thus, we might run on indefinitely naming the *many* "diseases" and find them to be not names of different *diseases*, but of the same *disease* in different locations.

The multiplication of *diseases* has gone even further than this would indicate. Every fraction of an inch of anatomy calls for a different name and the inflammation therein becomes a *different disease*. Inflammation in different parts of the same organ is named as different *diseases*. Although inflammation is everywhere the same process; it is denominated a different disease in every location in which it may be necessary and, as the tendency is to name inflammation in each tissue of an organ, and in each quarter inch of the same tissue differently, there seems to be no conceivable end to the number of *diseases* man may develop.

Examples of the manner in which inflammation of different parts of the same organ receive different names are carditis, inflammation of the heart; myocarditis, inflammation of the heart muscle (myocardium); endocarditis, inflammation of the lining membrane of the heart (endocardium); pericarditis, inflammation of the investing membrane of the heart (pericardium); endopericarditis is combined endocarditis and pericarditis; while endoperimyocarditis is inflammation of all the layers of the heart; metritis, inflammation of the womb; endometritis, inflammation of the lining of the womb; (endometrium), perimetritis is inflammation around the womb; cervicitis, inflammation of the neck of the womb (cervix uteri); endocervicitis, inflammation of the lining membrane of the cervix, or neck of the womb; phlebitis is inflammation of a vein; endophlebitis is inflammation of the inner coat of a vein; periphlebitis is inflammation of the outer coat of a vein — and thus we could fill pages of these minute distinctions between inflammation in the various organs and tissues of the body. It is all as foolish as considering a stye on the upper eye lid as *one disease* and a stye on the lower eye lid as *another disease;* it is as absurd as to consider acne on one check *one disease,* and acne on the other check another *disease*.

Simple colitis is a catarrhal inflammation of the colon. It does not differ from catarrh of the nose (rhinitis) and throat (laryngitis), or of the vagina (leucorrhea), or catarrh anywhere else in the body. Catarrh of the colon is no more mysterious than catarrh of the nose and throat. It is not a *different disease* from catarrh of the nose and throat; it is the same condition or process in a different location. When this fact is realized the whole matter becomes simple. The ordinary layman may comprehend the essential facts of pathology and its development once the mystery-veil, woven out of thousands of Greek and Latin terms, has been drawn back.

Colitis is one of the most common "diseases" with which civilized man suffers. It might be appropriately described as a chronic "cold" of the colon. During the course of chronic colitis, the more intense inflammation may be localized in one or more circumscribed areas of the colon. This more acute phase of the inflammation is usually named after the section of the colon in which it is located. Hence, if it is in the sigmoid flexure it is called sigmoiditis; if it is in the rectum it is denominated proctitis. The line of demarkation between sigmoiditis and proctitis is only an imaginary one. Such distinctions are very misleading.

Colitis may be very mild and somewhat obscure for a long time. The abdominal distress of which the sufferer is conscious, may be attributed to gas and constipation. Colitis may not be suspected until considerable mucus appears in the stools. There may be mucus masses of jelly-like consistency, or suspicious-looking ropy shreds, like casts of the bowels, or the feces may be coated with mucus, and it is sometimes streaked with blood.

Constipation, almost always of the spastic kind, is the most outstanding symptom. Indeed there is almost always some colitis in all cases of chronic constipation. In colitis accompanying inflammation of the ileum, or small bowel (ilieitis) or in ulcerative colitis, there may be diarrhea, or diarrhea alternating with constipation.

Colonic spasm is almost invariably present in colitis and there is almost always a sagging of the colon — *enteroptosis*. There may be enteroptosis without mucus and there may be mucus without enteroptosis, but, usually, they co-exist. Spastic constipation seems to be an unfailing accompaniment of either or both these conditions. The medical opinion that the spastic constipation causes the colitis is as ridiculous as would be the opposite opinion — that is, that the colitis causes the spastic constipation. They are merely two parts of the same condition and both depend upon the same underlying cause.

One of the most prominent features of advanced colitis is the negative or depressive psychosis — the *colon complex*. This *complex*, seen in chronic cases, usually involves the emotions. The depressed mentality seen in these cases is likely to be dismissed as *neurasthenia* by the average physician, because he does not understand the connection that almost invariably exists between colitis and the mental and emotional depression.

Dr. Weger gave it as his opinion that a chronically diseased colonic mucous membrane forms the basis of more mental and physical derangements than any other single functional abnormality. All of the thoughts of such a sufferer become introverted and center around his digestive tract and his constipation. No matter how hard he tries he cannot divert his thoughts from their center of interest.

Some try bravely to repress their feelings, while others no longer attempt to conceal their constant state of apathy. They are irritable, grouchy, nervous, excitable and sometimes they border on melancholia or actually become hysterical. As Dr. Weger expresses it: "Few diseases can compete with colitis in developing obsessions."

The subjective symptoms presented by the sufferer from colitis are uniformly consistent. Certain feelings are more marked in some than in others — in one person the digestive disturbances seem paramount; in another nervous symptoms predominate.

Constipation, usually measured in years, is almost always present. The purgatives, laxatives, teas, oils, enemas, diets, etc., that have been used, have seemed to give temporary relief in some cases and have aggravated the condition in others.

All of the sufferers complain of gastric and intestinal indigestion, with gas and rumbling in the intestine, and there is more or less pain, sometimes of a colicy nature. Nausea and uneasiness are common and there is often a sense of fullness. Dull and constant or sharp and recurrent headache is usually complained of. There may be a feeling of stiffness and tension in the muscles of the neck. A sub-occipital pain or drawing sensation is quite common. There is a feeling of extreme exhaustion, and a lack of ambition and initiative.

Objectively these cases are likely to be thin and undernourished, though colitis may be seen in overweight individuals. Most cases appear anemic and dysemic. There is usually a coated tongue, offensive breath and an unpleasant taste. The nausea experienced immediately preceding the expulsion of a large accumulation of mucus is followed by a feeling of great relief. Misery and dejection are written all over the face of the sufferer and this is frequently combined with anxiety.

I quote the following resume of the many objective and subjective symptoms that color the picture of chronic colitis, from Dr. Weger; "insomnia, nervousness, shortness of breath, premonitions of impending evil, disturbing and fearsome dreams, bloating, fullness, gas, reverse peristalsis, loss of appetite, bilious spells with occasional nausea, headache, weakness, cutaneous hyperesthesia, mouth cankers, bad breath, backache, pain and weakness in the legs, varying aspects of malnutrition, pessimism, irritability, and an unwillingness to think or talk of anything but the ever-present misery — intensified, of course, by the never-ending hypercritical speculation and the habit of inspecting the stools. The most trivial intestinal movement or unrest is often seized upon as an excuse for complaining.

Pains in the arms, legs, shoulders and chest, even pseudoanginal seizures, often occur in the nervous and hypersensitive type, especially during those periods when large quantities of mucus form."

The reader will understand that all of these symptoms are never present in any one individual and that many of them are present only in advanced or long standing cases. Many cases are mild and often require years to reach the advanced stage seen in the worst cases.

No case of long-standing or advanced colitis exists without the coexistance of many "other diseases" in the same individual. In all such cases, there will be catarrh of the nose and throat, perhaps polyps in the nose, catarrh of the stomach (gastritis), intestine (endoenteritis), and of other parts. Sinusitis is a frequent concomitant. Hay fever and asthma are frequent. In women leucorrhea is almost invariably present, while cystitis is common in both sexes. The catarrh is likely to extend up the gall duct to the gall bladder, or up the pancreatic duct to the pancreas. Often the eyes and ears are involved. Metritis and painful menstruation are seen in women while not a few such sufferers have had operations for the removal of tonsils, appendix, gall bladder or other organ. In women the sagging colon may force the womb out of position.

A long-standing catarrhal condition in the nose (rhinitis) may culminate in ulceration of the nose; a long-standing catarrhal condition of the stomach (gastritis) may end in gastric ulcer; a chronic catarrhal condition of the colon (colitis) may result in ulceration of the colon — *ulcerative colitis*. Cancer is the next and final stage in this process of pathological evolution.

Colitis sufferers become habituated to the use of drugs. They try every stomach and bowel "remedy" that is advertised. They exhaust the list of cathartics, laxatives, digestants and tonics.

They use enemas, colonic irrigations, cascades and try different systems of dieting. They go from doctor to doctor and from one system of treatment to another, "studying their symptoms and confusing their feelings."

There are many theories of the cause of colitis; there are thousands of treatments. But we find colitis considered incurable and daily we see individuals who have suffered with colitis for years, meanwhile trying all the treatments and growing steadily worse. However, the condition is not as hopeless as this makes it appear.

Colitis (catarrh of the colon) is an outgrowth of toxemia — of retention of toxic waste in the blood and lymphatic system. Toxemia is a development out of enervation and this results from a mode of living that uses up nerve force in excess.

There is no treatment for colitis. It gets well when its cause is removed; it will not get well until this is done. What is its cause? A wrong mode of living and the enervation and toxemia that rest thereon. How, then, may cause be removed? Restore nerve energy to normal, eliminate the toxemia and correct the mode of living.

Rest — physical, physiological, mental and sensory — is the great need in these cases. After rest has eliminated the toxemia and restored nerve energy to normal, proper food, exercise, sun baths and a general health-building program will do the rest. Feeding is often a problem in these cases as no two sufferers can be fed alike. Special exercises are often required to restore the fallen organs to their normal positions.

Peptic Ulcer

Peptic ulcer is the name given to ulcers in the stomach and duodenum, this latter being the upper end of the small intestine. Such ulcers rarely develop in the jejunum or middle section of the small intestine. They are confined almost wholly to those areas of the digestive tract that are subjected to the pepsin and hydrochloric acid of the gastric juice. It is estimated that at least ten per cent of the population develop peptic ulcer, more than ninety per cent of these occurring in the stomach.

Ulcers of the stomach and intestine develop more in middle life rather than in advanced age. This is especially true of their development in women. The disease seems to be more common in men than in women, although this is not universally so. In Germany, for instance, peptic ulcers are about equally divided between the sexes.

Going through the literature on the subject one is struck with the decided lack of dependable knowledge about the condition. Why or how ulcers develop is unknown. There is no agreement about what causes them and no harmony about what is the best form of treatment. There is a great maze of confusion and much uncertainty.

The fact stands out on every page of the literature that the cause of peptic ulcer is still unknown. Efforts to account for their occurrence are usually mere attempts to fix the blame on disease elsewhere in the body. Bad teeth and tonsils, sinus infection, appendicitis, gall-bladder "infection," and similar troubles are usually blamed. Chemical and mechanical causes are sometimes invoked, while heredity and nervous derangement occasionally come in for a share of the blame.

For the most part the authorities are studying the preceding and concomitant states of disease in other organs of the body and, instead of seeing in these, evidence of a general deterioration of the body, from which they all, including the gastric or duodenal ulcer, stem, they hold that "one disease" causes the "other disease."

Peptic ulcers can be produced experimentally in animals by a great variety of methods. But, so far, this has not thrown any light on the cause of ulcers in man and there is grave doubts that such experimental production of ulcers will ever aid in discovering the cause. In the first place experimental ulcers are produced by a variety of methods, some, at least, of which, we can rule out entirely as causes of ulcers in man. Experimental ulcers are seldom or never like those in man and do not act the same. Again, they are not characterized by the tendency to persist, as in man.

We of the Hygienic School hold that peptic ulcer is not a local disease of the stomach or duodenum, or, rarely, of the esophagus; but that it is merely a local manifestation of a general or systemic derangement. This is the meaning of all the other "diseases" and symptoms that precede and accompany peptic ulcer. They are all outgrowths of a common cause.

The ulcer is an endpoint in a chain of causes and effects which reaches back into the life of the patient for several years. A typical case gives a history of recurring "attacks" of indigestion, pain and distress in the stomach region after meals, a sense of fullness, chronic gastritis, constipation, frequent colds, and other minor ailments. Finally the teeth begin to decay, abscesses form in them, sinus troubles develop, chronic enlargement of the tonsils occurs, the gall bladder may be affected and, lastly, an ulcer or several ulcers develop in the stomach or duodenum.

None of these preceding affections cause the peptic ulcer. They represent merely so many successive stages or steps in the gradual deterioration of the body. The ulcer is the outgrowth of the same causes that produce these precedent troubles. They all stem from a common cause and are not causes of one another.

Ulcers are never found in those parts of the body that are bathed in an alkaline medium. Acidity is essential for their development. In peptic ulcer there is always hyperacidity of the stomach. Some authorities believe acidity to be the most essential factor in the causation of ulcers. It is obvious, however, that the abnormal acidity of the gastric juice is itself the effect of other causes. There must not only be the acidity and its causes, there must also be lowered resistance to the action of acids, for these structures possess a high degree of immunity to gastric acidity.

It therefore becomes necessary to account for the lost immunity and for the excessive acidity. Hyperacidity of the stomach is an expression of "acidosis" — of a lessened alkalinity of the body generally. Acidosis is a condition characterized by a deficiency of fixed alkalis in the body, which leads to an increased production of ammonia in the urine and a high urinary acidity. The decline in blood alkalinity may be due to one or more of many factors such as the excessive intake of fat, the free use of acetic acid in vinegar, acid fermentation in the digestive tract, etc. The most common cause is a diet of denatured foods—one that is preponderantly acid-forming — and wrong combinations of food.

Lost immunity is also to a great extent an outgrowth of this same lack of alkaline minerals. The man or woman who has peptic ulcers has a mild form of scurvy. There is calcium deficiency and vitamin deficiency.

Hyperacidity and lost immunity may exist without producing peptic ulcer. Other factors are essential. First there is enervation and toxemia due to wrong living. Neurotic, emotional, worrisome and hard working people are most likely to develop peptic ulcer. Due to emotional interference with digestion and to overwork, digestion is impaired. Fermentation and putrefaction result.

Poisons and gases resulting from decomposition of food set up irritation and cause inflammation. The indigestion becomes chronic so that the irritation is persistent. This results in induration or hardening in the stomach and intestine. The hardening goes on until ulceration results.

Any influence that lowers constitutional vigor and lessens resistance favors the development of an ulcer. Alcohol and tobacco using, general malnutrition, lowered vitality, with its consequent checking of elimination and impairing of digestion, must be included among the antecedents of gastric ulcers. The use of drugs that derange digestion and directly injure the walls of the stomach and intestine is often a direct cause of ulceration.

Chronic provocation prevents the ulcer from healing. Perforation of the stomach or intestine occurs and the patient dies of peritonitis.

Every step in the development of this condition is built on the preceding one. Enervation, indigestion, irritation, inflammation, induration, ulceration, perforation, peritonitis, death — these are all evolutions out of uncorrected causes that lie in the eating habits and general living habits of the patient. The indigestion and the ulcer are not separate and distinct diseases, but separate links in a syndrome of causes and effects extending from childhood to death.

Not all ulcers produce perforation. Many of them heal. Some of them heal without the individual ever knowing of their existence. In many cases there are only occasional spells of indigestion, the person thinking he is all right between spells.

Ulcers sometimes evolve into cancer. Approximately twenty per cent of gastric ulcers become malignant. The chronic irritation and hyperacidity favor cancerous growth. Perhaps in all cases where the ulcer does not heal cancer would develop did not death occur first.

The diagnosis of peptic ulcer is very difficult, even for the X-ray specialist. Other conditions such as "irritable bowel" and inflammation of the bile-duct, or of the gall bladder are frequently mistaken for peptic ulcer.

Hyperacidity, pain in the stomach sometimes (two or three hours) after meals, relief of pain by eating or by taking alkalis, and periodical "attacks" of discomfort are the usual symptoms of a simple case. Vomiting and hemorrhage sometimes complicate these cases. The actual location of the ulcer can be determined only by the X-ray expert and he finds this difficult.

Many cases presenting most of the above symptoms are diagnosed peptic ulcer when their trouble is not that at all. One case which came under my own care will illustrate this. The case had been studied for some time and careful tests made. Every thing seemed to point to gastric ulcer and the diagnosis was so made. An operation was advised and refused. Three days of fasting brought relief from discomfort, after which the patient was fed foods that would have caused much pain and distress had he had an ulcer. There was no recurrence of symptoms and he returned to good health.

It is extremely unfortunate that the feeding and care of patients with peptic ulcer is designed simply to relieve pain. Frequent small feedings of soft, bland, well-cooked, non-irritating foods is the practice. Food is taken every two hours or five meals a day are advised. The stomach is never allowed to be completely empty. Belladonna and alkalis, such as magnesia, are prescribed.

The alkalis neutralize acidity but prevent digestion.

The diet is preponderantly acid forming and
cannot possibly remedy the already existing "acidosis." All raw fruits and vegetables are prohibited. Denatured carbohydrates and acid forming
proteins constitute the bulk of the diet.

Any change of diet which removes the immediate irritation of the conventional diet will
afford relief from pain and will permit healing in
a certain percentage of cases. But the diets
usually employed are of a character to perpetuate
the unstable body chemistry present in all such
cases and this assures the persistence of the
hyperacidity and toxemia.

The failure of the usual methods of treatment is apparent from the advice of a leading
American surgeon that operation should be advised after the patient has been cured nine
times. Treatment directed at the relief of local
conditions and which ignores the constitutional
state must fail.

In spite of such a diet, a certain percentage
of ulcers heal, but recur later for the reason
that the systemic condition that was back of
them and the mode of living that caused them
are not corrected. Most cases, "after a fair
trial" of the above methods, are operated upon.
Patients are led to believe that after the operation is performed they may return to their previous manner of eating and living. Recurrences
are therefore quite common.

Opposed to this ceaseless puttering with palliatives, we offer a method of radical correction
of the causes of peptic ulcer and a resulting return to vigorous health. With intelligent living
thereafter there will be no recurrence of the
ulcer.

Our method is not directed at the control of
symptoms, but at the removal and correction of
causes. Instead of lopping off a few branches,
we apply our axe to the root of the trouble and

the results are a thousand fold more satisfactory than those that flow from the conventional methods of caring for such cases.

Complete rest in bed is necessary. Cases may recover without this, but never in so short a time as with rest. Mental and physical rest should form an integral part of the care of each case.

Physiological rest, particularly of the stomach, is even more important. This means fasting. Fasting will usually increase the patient's discomfort for the first two to four days. The frequent feeding commonly resorted to is designed to use up the excess of acid thrown into the stomach by the over active gastric glands. During the first part of the fast the excess acid will continue to be thrown into the stomach and will produce the usual pain that accompanies an empty stomach in these cases.

Fasting, however, soon ends the secretion of gastric juice. In two to four days the secretion ceases, the pain abates and the patient is comfortable. This effect of fasting is the opposite of the feeding methods in vogue, which stimulate the production of gastric juice and add to the "acidosis" that is back of hyperacidity of the stomach.

Fasting accelerates elimination from the body of the excess of toxins and succeeds in increasing the percentage of lime in the body. By thus overcoming lime deficiency the mild scurvy from which such patients suffer is remedied. The fast is demonstrably the quickest means of remedying systemic "acidity" and restoring normal body alkalinity.

The fast should be sufficiently prolonged to allow complete healing of the ulcer and a thorough cleansing of the body. When to break the fast is best determined by the doctor in charge of the case. Such a doctor should have full knowledge of fasting and should have had much experience in conducting fasts.

The fast must not be ended until all reactions indicate that the renovation of the body is complete. For, if it is broken too soon, dependable healing will not occur. Permanent and satisfactory healing follows upon the elimination of excess "acid" and toxins, and not until then.

Feeding after the fast is important. In most particulars it should be exactly opposite to the feeding methods commonly employed in cases of ulcer. An alkaline diet is essential. Fruits and green vegetables and these raw, should make up the bulk of the diet. If at first there is sensitiveness to the roughage in these foods, raw fruit and vegetable juices may be employed. Purees and strained vegetable soups may be used but are not as valuable as the raw juices. Cooked fruits are never to be used.

As soon as possible whole fruits and whole vegetables should be added to the diet. A week after the fast is broken carbohydrates and proteins may be employed and these gradually increased in amount until a normal amount of each is being taken. Baked potatoes will prove the best source of carbohydrates and cottage cheese will serve best as a source of protein until digestion is restored to normal vigor.

Sun baths will be found invaluable both during and after the fast. The office of the sun in rejuvenating the blood will hasten the healing process and improve nutrition in general.

As soon, after the fast is broken as the patient can stand it, mild exercise should be instituted. As strength increases, the amount and vigor of the exercise should be increased. At first it is well to take the exercise while lying in bed. Later walking and other forms of exercise may be added.

At the beginning all tobacco, alcohol, tea, coffee, cocoa, chocolate and drugs should be discontinued. No alkalis, no magnesia or baking soda, etc., should be employed. Nor should any of the above named poison habits be returned to subsequent to recovery.

Patients of a worrisome disposition should be taught not to worry. The greatest part of any truly remedial program is that of educating the patient out of his bad mental and physical habits. For, outside of correction of cause, there is no cure.

The inebriate who sobers up will get drunk again if he returns to drink. The sick man who gets well, will get sick again if he returns to the habits of living that made him sick before. The ulcer patient who gets "well" under the prevailing plan of care and who leaves the hospital as ignorant of right living as when he went there, is certain to have a recurrence of the ulcer.

Obviously the earlier the above ·plan is adopted the earlier will recovery occur. The victim of peptic ulcer should not wait until after he has had several hemorrhages and his digestive tract is a mass of irremediable changes before he adopts rational methods of care. Natural methods should be employed first and not last, as is so often the case. Don't wait until the ulcer becomes cancer or until perforation has occurred before these methods are employed. Natural methods cannot remove the scar tissue that forms and narrows the passage, cannot enlarge the pyloric valve that has been narrowed by the formation of a scar; cannot overcome stricture of the duodenum from the same cause. These conditions should be avoided by resorting to natural methods before they develop.

Surgeons advise the removal of possible "foci of infection" — teeth, tonsils, gall-gladder, appendix, etc., — in treating these cases. The above described methods will care for these troubles and enable the patient to retain his organs. Health is not restored by cutting out important organs of the body.

There is a great army of sufferers from

digestive derangements who are going from one doctor to another vainly hoping to find a cure for their trouble without due attention to diet. Many of them are, indeed, on diets of various kinds, but a glance at such diets reveals a pathetic ignorance of the first principles of dietetics. Failure and recurrence is certain under such conditions.

Patients who have been operated on one or more times for peptic ulcer can usually paint a dark and uninviting picture of the after effects — of subsequent operations for adhesions or the removal of other organs. They are disillusioned by the return of symptoms and subsequent development of another ulcer. Often the symptoms return in an aggravated form leaving the patient bitter and wrecking his faith in medicine and surgery.

To such as these Hygienic methods offer a measure of hope. Even where important organs have been removed and the continuity of structure has been broken by the surgeon and where strictures and adhesions give trouble, comfort may still be restored and compensatory adaptation to the abnormal conditions established. A measure of health and comfort may be built up and maintained if the sufferer can be educated into a new way of living and induced to continue it.

Diabetes Mellitus

This is the name given to a group of symptoms that center around an impairment of carbohydrate metabolism. Commonly we are told that it is a disease of the pancreas, but it is coming to be realized that it is a disturbance of the metabolic processes involving the entire organism and not strictly localized in any one organ. It is, in other words, a manifestation of a systemic derangement and, however important the pathology in the pancreas may be, this is secondary to the systemic derangement which has resulted in the disease of the pancreas.

The *Islands of Langerhans* may be described as little organs within the pancreas or sweetbread. These structures produce an internal secretion commonly known as *insulin* which is essential to the oxidation of sugar. When they fail to secrete sufficient *insulin* an excess of sugar accumulates in the blood and is eliminated by the kidneys in the urine. Hence sugar in the urine (*glycosuria*) is the principal symptom of what the layman calls *sugar diabetes*. But it is a subordinate symptom and is valuable chiefly as a criterion of the progress of the condition.

The condition of the pancreas of diabetics has been thoroughly studied after death and the destructive changes therein found have been carefully described and catalogued. But the patient may have had diabetes ten or more years before death and the pathologist, studying the end-point of the pathological process after death, gives us a false picture of the condition of the pancreas in any save the terminal stages of the disease. Thus the hopeless view of diabetes taken by medical men.

There is no destruction in the pancreas when the disease first begins and the destructive changes take place slowly against the weakened resistance of the body. Enervation (fatigue) of the *Islands of Langerhans* is the probable beginning of diabetes. It is toxemia that produces the pathology (the destruction) in the pancreas. Toxemia produces first a mild, chronic pancreatitis which may persist for a long time before marked damage to the pancreas occurs.

Under causes of diabetes, Dayton's *Practice of Medicine* gives: "Heredity, male sex, adult life, Jewish race, obesity, cerebral or spinal disease or injury, infectious diseases, overwork and nervous strain predispose. Actual cause is unknown. Pancreatic disease is probably important."

Heredity! Male sex! Adult life! Jewish race! These are not causes of anything. If adult life predisposes to diabetes then it is certainly dangerous to grow up. If male sex and Jewish race predispose then it is dangerous to be a man and a Jew. We ought all to be females, and "gentiles" and should all die young.

If adults have more diabetes than children it is because more years of wrong living have produced more pathology in them. If men have more diabetes than women, it is because their mode of living is worse. If Jews have more diabetes than heathen it is because something in their mode of living produces the diabetes.

Perhaps pancreatic disease is important, but it certainly is not self-originating and self-evolving. It must be the outgrowth of causes antecedent thereto; must be secondary to other causes and conditions. Healthy men and women, Jews or heathens, do not develop diabetes.

Heredity! Is there such a thing? It is true that there are many cases of diabetes in children and youth and it is quite possible that there is marked larval endocrine deficiency in all such children. It may even be a lesser degree of larval endocrine deficiency that establishes the tendency to diabetes in adults. The time of life at which carbohydrate tolerance breaks down may be considered an index to the larval endocrine imbalance in the individual. But we must not overlook the fact that of two individuals with the same degree of larval endocrine deficiency, the one that subjects his body to the most enervating influence and consumes the greatest amount of carbohydrates will break down his carbohydrate tolerance first.

In those cases developing after the thirty-fifth or fortieth year we think the larval deficiency may be considered negligible and think that the cause is a decidedly over-crowded general nutrition in which carbohydrate consumption has been excessive throughout life. The *Islands of Langerhans* have merely been overworked through the years.

Worry, anxiety, grief, shock — fright, accidents, surgical shock — will so impair the function of the pancreas that sugar shows up in the urine immediately. In many cases of diabetes, emotional stress is the chief cause, but it is never the sole cause. Every so-called disease is a complex effect of a number of correlated antecedents.

Diet and drink, sex and sleep, work and play, and many other factors enter the cause of every so-called disease. *Any form of over-stimulation — mental, emotional, sensory, physical, chemical, thermal, electrical — may give rise, first to functional, and, finally, to organic, disease.* Diabetes is a functional disturbance at its beginning.

Diabetes is more markedly on the increase in those countries in which sugar consumption has mounted to such high figures during the past fifty years — France, Germany, Britain and the United States. Every fat person is a potential diabetic. The overfeeding which is responsible for the fat overworks the pancreas and as overwork of any organ results in impairment of the function of the organ, pancreatic failure results. If its causes are not corrected, functional impairment gradually passes into organic disease.

Carbohydrate excess places a strong stress on the pancreas and when this gland is over-worked by too great an intake of starches and sugars, there will be first, irritation and inflammation, then enlargement, followed by degeneration (de-secretion); after which the body loses control of sugar metabolism and of the excess acidity caused by too much starch and sugar.

But it should not be thought that overeating of carbohydrates alone impairs the pancreas. Anything that produces *enervation* — tobacco, tea, coffee, chocolate, cocoa, alcohol, soda fountain slops, sexual excesses, loss of sleep, overwork, general overeating, emotionalism, etc. — impairs organic function in general including pancreatic function.

Sedentary habits added to overeating increase the tendency to diabetes, as they do to all other so-called *degenerative diseases of later life.*

Let us glance briefly at the symptoms of diabetes. The urine is frequently voided, is pale and of high specific gravity unless there is inflammation of the kidneys in which case specific gravity is not usually so high. The urine contains varying amounts of sugar and certain acids that are absent from the urine of healthy subjects.

There is great thirst and a ravenous appetite with, commonly, loss of weight. Headache, depression and constipation are common. The breath is sweet, though unlike that of the healthy person. The mouth and skin are dry, even parched, the tongue is red and glazed, and when the disease is advanced the teeth usually decay and become loosened. There is a tendency to pyorrhea and bleeding of the gums. Loss of sex power is common, while Bright's disease may develop as a "complication." Impairment or loss of vision may occur. Boils and eczema are also frequent. The disease progresses more rapidly in young patients than in older ones and it is thought by some *Hygienists* that children rarely if ever make a complete recovery.

Recovery — the medical dictum is "once a diabetic, always a diabetic" — depends upon the amount of functioning tissue left in the pancreas. Fortunately, the pancreas, like all other organs of the body, possesses a great excess of functioning power over that needed for the ordinary activities of life, so that even after part of the *Islands of Langerhans* have been destroyed the remainder will be able to function sufficiently to meet the regular needs of life provided the impairing causes are removed and they are given opportunity to return to a state of health.

When organs are not destroyed beyond repair, rest, poise, self-control, and a restricted, proper diet will restore normal functioning. In diabetes, rest and proper food, with diet restricted to the patient's digestive capacity, and full cooperation will result in dependable health in a few years. Failure is for all those who are not willing to carry out instructions.

All enervating influences and habits must be corrected or removed. Sufficient rest for restoration of nerve energy is imperative. A fast, not merely to give the pancreas a rest, but of sufficient duration to free the body of its load of toxins, must be followed by a diet that is designed to produce all possible regeneration in the pancreatic gland. Feeding that is designed merely to cause the disappearance of sugar from the urine may speedily kill the patient. After health is restored the patient must be taught to live within his compensating capacity.

Arthritis - Rheumatism - Gout

These are merely three terms for the same condition — inflammation of the joints. Gout is usually used only with reference to inflammation of the joints of the toes. Rheumatism may also be used with reference to muscular inflammation. Lumbago is a term applied to rheumatism in the small of the back, while pleurodynia is applied to rheumatism of the intercostal muscles. Rheumatoid arthritis and arthritis deformans is rheumatism of the joints with deformity.

These conditions may be acute, sub-acute, or chronic. The acute form is usually very severe and accompanied by fever. The sub-acute form of rheumatism or arthritis is the same as the acute form in all respects, except in the fact that its symptoms are not nearly so severe. Acute and sub-acute rheumatic illness may recur from time to time and gradually become chronic. Chronic gout and chronic arthritis tend to spread from joint to joint and in time the joint structures may be destroyed and the ends of the bones unite — ankylose.

These conditions are said to be due to germs and are traced to colds, tonsilitis and other troubles. Instead of colds in the head, scarlet fever, tonsilitis, measles and other acute "diseases," which often precede rheumatism, being the cause of acute or chronic rheumatism, they are but crises of a constitutional derangement on which the rheumatism, or arthritis, depends.

Acute rheumatism, simple chronic rheumatism, arthritis deformans, chronic osteo-arthritis, and simple arthritis are merely so many crises in a general constitutional derangement, consisting first of a rheumatic diathesis (the so-called *gouty* or *arthritic*, or *lithic* or *uric acid* diathesis), or tendency, and secondly, of a combined enervation and toxemia caused by errors in the habits of living and errors in diet.

Rheumatic arthritis is perverted nutrition in those of the "gouty diathesis." It is related to stone in the gall-bladder and kidneys, hardening in the arteries, lime deposits in the valves of the heart, and all those forms of "rheumatism" called gout. It belongs to the "deficiency diseases."

Rheumatism and "rheumatic heart trouble" are brought on from auto-infection, and anything that enervates and weakens the digestive power; then, if those who are weakened persist in eating beyond their digestive capacity, they will develop intestinal fermentation; this fermentation alters the alkalinity of the blood, and places those who are predisposed to rheumatism and heart disease in a condition for the development of these diseases.

Although chronic gastro-intestinal symptoms are common in chronic arthritis, it is doubtful if the average person can realize that the majority of people who have rheumatism get it from overeating and from improper food combinations.

The rheumatic individual represents one who has "lived well" but not wisely. He liked "good food" and lots of it and, as a rule, he has overeaten on starches and sugars. This he continued until he broke down his capacity to handle food.

Too much starch, or too much starch and sugar combined, is a greater factor in producing rheumatism in any of its forms than is meat; the old-fashioned jelly-bread, or preserves with bread, and bread with sugar, or syrup or molasses with bread or hot cakes, and cereals with sugar, have played a greater part in producing rheumatism-arthritis-gout than any other foods or combinations of foods. Bread with meat, eggs with bread, bread with fruit, bread three times a day, bread every time you eat, even between meals, bread in addition to cereals, potatoes, cakes, etc., plays a big share in the production of rheumatism.

In chronic articular rheumatism there is, as a rule, more or less stiffness of the joints. This is usually worse after eating and in the morning after a night's sleep.

Where there is rheumatism of the heart little beads of fibrin are deposited along the valves of the heart, which by contracting, prevent normal closing of the valves, so that valvular heart defect results. It is not correct, however, to say that arthritis of the knee, for instance, causes heart trouble. It is more true to say that the heart is damaged by the toxins that are causing the arthritis — that the heart defect is also due to auto-infection, superadded to a primary or metabolic toxemia.

Heart disease has another and perhaps more common cause in rheumatic conditions. Over sixty years ago Sir Lauder Brunton pointed out that salicylates, while relieving the pain of rheumatism, are likely to add heart disease to the original complaint. Today doctors persist in employing salicylates in rheumatism and frequently discuss the great prevalence of heart disease following rheumatism. At the same time they are searching for the "guilty microbe."

Dr. Richard C. Cabot says in his *Handbook of Medicine*, while dealing with rheumatism; "The group of drugs called the salicylates, or aspirin, which is a first cousin, give us great relief of pain in this disease. They do not cure it; they do not shorten the duration of illness; they do not protect the heart; they do nothing except check pain; but this is a good deal. They have been a great blessing to us, making it unnecessary to use morphine and such drugs, as was formerly the custom."

It is not true that "they do nothing except check the pain." They "check pain" by sandbagging the nerves into insensibility and this cannot be done without damage both to the nerves in particular and to the body in general. Any standard work on materia medica will reveal their damaging effects.

Why submit to their damaging effects if they do not cure, do not shorten the illness and do not protect the heart? In what way can such poisons and their evil effects be truly said to have been a great blessing? Only in the way that they have been substituted for more damaging drugs, such as morphine, and are thus the lesser of two evils.

The present popular manner of handling these cases is by removal of teeth, tonsils, gall-bladder, appendix, ovaries, etc. The cleaning up of these so-called "foci of infection" is essential, not because these cause arthritis, but because they represent part of the general pathology. Pent-up secretions must be drained, but organs need not be removed. They may be restored to good health.

Why submit to an operation for the removal of the appendix and gall bladder to cure rheumatism, when the cause of rheumatism, appendicitis and cholecystitis is the same? Since all of these conditions rest on one cause, toxemia, can any intelligent person expect to cure one of the three by cutting out the other two? The physician's promise to relieve gout, arthritis, rheumatism by removing an inflamed appendix or gall-bladder — these latter conditions resulting from the same cause that produced the former — is as absurd as would be the promise to relieve a corn on the big toe by trimming an ingrowing nail on the little toe.

Even when the heart is involved, rheumatism usually ends in recovery, though sometimes the heart may be permanently damaged, and, though "rheumatic inflammation" of the heart does sometimes end in death. But recovery from an acute rheumatic inflammation of the toes (gout), joints (arthritis), or muscles (muscular rheumatism), does not mean recovery of health. One crisis passes and a few days or a few weeks later another develops. Crises come and go, but the underlying toxemia, metabolic perversion and wrong mode of life continue.

Need we wonder that arthritic cases find it difficult to return to health? They are all extremely enervated, heavily toxemic, and often on their last leg — which is usually a cane, or crutches, or wheel chair by the time they reach us. They have a markedly perverted metabolism and they very much dislike to surrender their bad habits and clean house. They are easily discouraged, a thing for which previous disappointing experiences with treatment is largely responsible. Many would not follow instructions if the severity of their symptoms did not drive them to it.

Sufferers from gout and arthritis we have received at the *Health School* have been treated by the conventional forms of care — drugs, vaccinal, surgical, physiotherapeutic, chiropractic, osteopathic, hydrotherapeutic, dietetic, and even with Christian Science — with little or no apparent beneficial results, or with only temporary apparent benefit. My place seems to be the place of last resort.

Considering the uniform failure of the curing methods and the remarkably high percentage of recoveries we have with Hygienic or health building methods, it is difficult to understand why our institution is looked upon as a last resort. Why do they say: *"We can go to Shelton after everything else has failed us"?* Is it because they know that at Shelton's they will be required to cease producing their gout and arthritis, whereas the treating plan permits them to continue their pet disease-producing habits and tries to cure them in spite of cause.

By strict elimination of all the habits of life which bring about enervation and produce a poison-absorption from the gastro-intestinal tract, "attacks" of rheumatism-gout-arthritis may be avoided, even though a tendency to it may have been acquired. On the contrary, given a tendency or a diathesis to a disease, whether the disease is called gout, arthritis, tuberculosis, neurasthenia, Bright's disease; or, by any other name, and add to it the enervation and toxemia that are in keeping with the habits of the individual, and it will not be long before a real crisis in the patient's life is developed.

Often we hear of medical institutions that are treating arthritics dietetically. If this is so, why are they not getting the results that we are getting in our own institution? First, because they are ignoring enervation and toxemia and the mode of living upon which these depend. Second, because with their drugging habits, they employ foods as drugs; that is, they are trying to cure with diet without removing the cause of arthritis.

Arthritics do not handle sugars and starches well, due to metabolic disturbance. However, best results are obtained, not by a mere reduction of carbohydrates, but by a general reduction of the diet, for the carbohydrates are not alone to blame. The toxemia present is the result of long abuse with a redundancy of foods of all kinds and in wrong combinations.

Not a mere reduction of foods, but abstinence from all food, will most rapidly remedy the gastro-intestinal catarrh which represents the starting-point of all cases of rheumatoid arthritis. But to this must be added a correction of the whole mode of living and sufficient rest for the restoration of full nerve force.

High Blood Pressure

High blood pressure is a symptom that is present in many so-called diseases. It is one of many endings of a series of crises in toxemia, the first of which was a so-called cold—a catarrhal fever. The cold, according to Hygienic philosophy, is the earliest symptom of an initial pathology, which, if its cause is not removed, leads on and on through many crises, to an ending that may be high blood pressure or any one of the many chronic so-called organic diseases—diabetes, Bright's disease, tuberculosis, diseases of the heart and arteries, paralysis, insanity, cancer, etc.

Until the many so-called organic diseases, from which people die, are recognized as end-points in a progressive pathological evolution, starting in early life and punctuated by frequent crises (acute diseases) along the way, sanity in the care of the sick can never exist. When these so-called diseases are recognized as merely different end-points in one and the same pathological evolution, and not separate and specific diseases, that giant system of delusion that proudly styles itself Modern Medical Science will cease to murder its victims by the tens of thousands.

When the principle of evolution is admitted into the realm of pathology, doctors of all schools will recognize the folly of directing their prophylactic and therapeutic treatments at the end-points of the pathological process and will remove the cause of the pathological evolution long before the end-point has been reached.

Doctors know little or nothing about the causes of high blood pressure. Instruments of precision can tell when patients have high blood pressure and how high the pressure runs, but what is this worth? The instrument cannot tell the cause. It certainly does not benefit the patient. Nor does it do the patient any good to examine him at intervals and tell him how high his pressure is. The only one who benefits by these examinations is the doctor who gets the fee.

Without a knowledge of cause doctors merely attempt to force blood pressure down in spite of cause. Drugs to depress the heart, or to relax the arteries are popular. Removal of the thyroid gland has also been resorted to and about a year ago Dr. Crile advocated removal of the solar plexus. None of these things even remotely affect cause. They only cripple the patient.

Nerve irritation always precedes high blood pressure. Nervous irritation causes the blood vessels to contract and the small capillary vessels are almost shut off from any circulation of blood. This fact seems to have been behind Dr. Crile's proposal to remove the solar plexus — perhaps on the theory that it is easier to remove the irritated nervous structure than to remove the source of the irritation.

Almost any chronic or frequently repeated irritation of the sympathetic nervous system will sooner or later result in high blood pressure. Irritation of the nervous system from pressure by an enlarged prostate may cause high blood pressure.

If removal of the prostate gland is followed by a lowering of blood pressure, does this justify the doctor or surgeon in declaring that enlargement of the gland causes high blood pressure and that all such cases should be operated upon? Of course not. Yet this is medical reasoning at the present time.

A true cure will remove, not the enlarged prostate, but the cause of the enlargement. If the gland is removed and the cause ignored, this cause will evolve another source of nervous irritation and the patient will have to be "cured" all over again.

"Progressive" physicians and surgeons, like Crile, are now advancing the idea of removing the nerves that carry sympathetic impulses. Men who reason in this manner should be hod carriers.

Remove the causes, of which there are many, to remedy high blood pressure. To destroy or cripple the nerves that carry impulses is senseless. Nature will take care of the nerve reflexes if we remove the causes of the trouble. Functional and reflex irritations will all disappear when cause is removed.

Hard arteries produce high blood pressure. What do hard arteries mean to the average physician? Nothing, beyond the mere recognition of their presence. What leads up to the hardening, when it has its actual beginning and how it may be overcome — these form a closed book to him.

Irritation causes the arteries to feel hard, at times almost like whip cord, and no doubt, if it were possible to feel or see the hair-like capillary vessels, we would find them hard and stiff. The irritation is of toxic and emotional origins. The toxic irritation grows largely, if not wholly, out of excesses and poison habits.

"The people troubled with high blood pressure," says Tilden, "are those who are going at top-speed to a premature end, enjoying as much as they can, the pleasures of life — the luxuries of high life such as money buys, and the luxuries of low life common to all. The poor have luxuries that belong to sensualism and there is nothing that can be accomplished so easily as partaking of the tree of knowledge prematurely. Sex-lust stands at the head, but there is also a lustful spirit — an indomitable lust for any or all of the things that people desire."

Plethory, an abnormal fullness of the blood vessels — is a general hyperemia. It means that there is an excess of blood. This is not an ideal state. Hypertension — excess tension in the circulatory system; high blood pressure — due to plethory increases toxin poisoning.

Plethory is due to excess in eating and drinking. It is an over saturation of the body with food and fluid. Excessive drinking of non-stimulating beverages, even water and fruit juices, may in time produce high blood pressure. Excess fluid is one of the causes of obesity, and obesity always raises blood pressure.

High blood pressure may mean an excessive amount of blood and lymph (plethory), or it may also mean the opposite. For, high blood pressure may sometimes be seen in anemia.

High blood pressure may be a symptom of the influence of tobacco on the organism. It may be a symptom of the influence of alcohol, or of tea or coffee, or of other poison habits. No one who is addicted to any of civilization's many poison vices is safe from high blood pressure. Salt, pepper and other spices and condiments produce enough nerve irritation to bring on high blood pressure.

Perhaps the greatest single cause of high blood pressure is toxemia resulting from checked elimination. Secondary toxemia, such as that seen in nephritis (Bright's disease), and intestinal autointoxication arising out of gastro-intestinal fermentation and putrefaction, all produce enough nerve irritation to cause high blood pressure. A high protein diet gives rise to a particularly virulent irritation when it putrefies in the digestive tract.

Any form of excess — over eating, overwork. excessive venery, over enjoying, and over indulgence in anything — taxes the nervous system and brings on enervation, which checks secretion and excretion. Checked secretion produces indigestion with its consequent intestinal autointoxication; checked excretion produces toxemia. Learning one's limitations in expending nerve energy and then respecting these limitations will prevent enervation, guarantee good digestion and efficient elimination, and thus insure health and long life.

High blood pressure may result from losing one's temper every day. Suppressing anger or hate may build high blood pressure. Men and women may have high blood pressure, not from carrying an excessive amount of blood, but from too much anxiety, excessive introspection, worry, anguish, trouble, etc. The banker or other business man who is expecting to have his business closed on him at any time is very likely to have high blood pressure. The gambler who is in a constant state of tension, the thief who is afraid of being caught, the liar who is never in a state of poise, the gossip who is always under apprehension — these people are likely to develop high blood pressure.

Besides the immediate nervous tension produced by trouble, threatened loss, lying, gambling, stealing, and all forms of dishonor and dishonesty, these things all produce enervation, and enervation always produces toxemia.

Few things can be so easily, quickly and permanently remedied as hyper-tension — high blood pressure. A world of irritation is removed when the subject goes to bed, refrains from eating, and certainly from worrying, and discontinues his or her poison habits. How foolish to take drugs to remedy a condition brought on by the causes described above and do nothing about the causes!

Rest and fasting do not cure high blood pressure. They remove a load of toxins and irritations and blood pressure falls rapidly. But the real cure is to teach these subjects poise of mind and body; to train them in healthful physical, dietetic, emotional and sexual habits. The real cure is a healthful mode of living. For, to go to bed and fast and reduce blood pressure, and then return to the former mode of living — the former excesses and indulgences, to the poison vices and emotional habits, to the prior sexual excesses and to dishonesty, gambling, etc. — is to rapidly rebuild the pathological state that produced the high blood pressure.

To see blood pressure fall consequent upon a reduction of weight and then to regain the weight is to see it rise again. If there is excess fluid intake the obesity cannot be cured until the over consumption of fluid is discontinued. It is always necessary to remove cause.

Paradoxical as it may seem at first sight, the same mode of living that causes high blood pressure may also produce the pathology that is back of low blood pressure; and the same correction of cause that reduces blood pressure in the one instance will increase blood pressure in the other. Normal blood pressure depends upon normal living.

Acne

Acne is an inflammation of the oil glands of the skin and of the follicles of the fuzz-like hairs attached to the oil-glands. It manifests as small and large pimples, often containing pus, which detract greatly from the appearance of the sufferer.

I am not sure that I am right, but it seems to me that there is far more acne now than there was twenty-five years ago. Sure I am that it is very common today and that it is the source of much anxiety and mental discomfort in those who have this affection. More than one otherwise beautiful young girl has consulted us who was on the verge of suicide, so much were they concerned over their appearance and over the persistent failure of their efforts to remedy their skin trouble.

Various qualifying terms have been added to the term acne to distinguish its most important features. Thus we have:

Acne Simplex, or simple acne, which is the most common form, hence the term *Acne vulgaris.*

Acne Indurata, which differs from the simple form chiefly in the degree and extent of its symptoms and the hardening (*induration*) *which* is present.

Malnutritional Acne, called, also scrofulous acne, or, acne scrofulosum, and acne cachecitcorum, occurs in undernourished or scrofulous or emaciated individuals. It develops chiefly on the trunk and lower limbs, though, occasionally the arms and face are affected.

Artificial Acne, or acne artificialis, is papules produced by the internal use of such drugs as the bromides and the iodides, and the external application of tar, chrysarobin, etc.

Atrophic Acne, or acne atrophica, is simple acne in which the lesions are followed by scars or small pits.

Papular Acne, or *acne papulosa,* is simple acne in which papular eruptions (solid raised spots on or in the skin) predominate.

Pustular Acne, or *acne pustulosa,* is acute acne simplex with papules developing into pustules.

Overgrowth acne, or *hypertrophic acne,* is applied to acne followed by thickening of the skin from an overgrowth of connective tissue.

Scurvy Acne, or *acne scorbutis,* is a papular acne with hemorrhages into the skin.

Acne Rosacea is acne plus *rosacea,* or a chronic congestion of the nose and parts of the face.

Acne Varioliformis is a form of acne the pustules of which resemble those of variola (smallpox). It develops chiefly on the forehead, along the hair margin, also the scalp, face and neck and, sometimes, the shoulders and breastbone.

No effort will be made to describe each of these forms of acne. Suffice is to say that, except artificial acne, these forms are all the outgrowth of toxins. Since they are merely variations of simple acne and all yield to the same care let us confine our remarks chiefly to this form.

This form is seen more often in women and girls than in men and boys. It develops chiefly on the forehead, cheeks, lower jaw and chin and sometimes on the chest, shoulders, upper arms and even down the back and thighs. It develops chiefly during the adolescent years and tends to disappear upon the attainment of maturity, although it may persist long after thirty is passed. It is often aggravated before and during menstruation.

Blackheads usually constitute the center or nucleus for the beginning of the inflammation. A papule develops around this center, and later becomes a pustule. However, acne may develop without blackheads, and blackheads may exist without acne developing.

A crust forms on the pustule then falls off, leaving a redness which lasts a few days, or a depression or scar may be left. In many cases no pustules develop, the condition remaining in the papule stage, in which cases, the papules are absorbed after a few days.

On the same face, or other portion of the body, and without any semblance of regularity, there may be seen all stages — blackheads, papules, pustules, crusts, redness, pittings and scars. I frequently see faces that have been so badly pitted their owners look like they have had smallpox. Few things can so completely spoil the beauty of the face as acne.

The scars may be permanent, or they may gradually smooth out. In some cases no scars are left. The stain that often remains tends to fade out eventually.

If the papule of acne is opened or squeezed, blood, pus and fatty substance and, if present at the beginning of the papule, the blackhead, are found. Healing is usually rapid after evacuation of the contents, though squeezing usually tends to aggravate the local lesion. If the pustule is not molested spontaneous evacuation takes place.

In *acne indurata* the areas of hardening vary from the size of a pea to as large as a hazel nut. They begin deep below the epidermis, are usually deep red or purplish, often involve several adjacent glands, thus giving the appearance of boils and may contain much pus. The lesions often fail to rupture spontaneously. When opened and evacuated artificially, they tend to refill rather than to heal. Scar formation is often very pronounced especially where there has been much squeezing or direct pressure. Fibroid changes in the scars may cause them to resemble fibroid tumors.

There are no general symptoms of acne and the sufferer is inclined to regard himself or herself as otherwise healthy. Observing that their friends who do not have acne (but who often have much worse troubles) eat and drink as they do, they are not easily convinced that their mode of living is in any way responsible for their trouble.

The skin is the largest organ of the body, but because it is on the outside we tend to forget that it is helped or hurt by the same internal conditions that help or hurt the other organs of the body. We do not sufficiently recognize its dependence upon the blood.

"Diseases" of the skin occur as the direct or indirect result of a large number of constitutional and visceral failures. Functional weakness and actual pathology of the stomach, intestine, liver, kidneys, nervous system, etc., frequently lead to eliminative efforts through the skin. These are also seen in rheumatism, gout, diabetes, etc.

Carbuncles, furuncles and other skin eruptions seen in diabetic cases are explained by the saturation of the skin with sugar and, even if we grant the claim of bacteriologists, that these things represent staphylococcal infection, the sugar saturation is necessary to provide a favorable nidus for the growth of the microbes.

Pruritis and eczema occurring in a patient suffering from chronic interstitial nephritis is due to the failure of elimination through the defective kidneys. There is also an intimate relationship between gastro-intestinal disorders and skin "diseases" — eczema, pruritis, urticaria, acne, etc., are frequently observed in association with and to be influenced by digestive disturbances which involve decomposition of food and partial digestion.

Pruritis is often observed in connection with pathology of the liver, especially when jaundice exists; xanthoma and chronic jaundice are often associated. Eczema and gout are so common together that they have both been classed as belonging to the "gouty diathesis," while there is also a close connection between psoriasis and chronic arthritis.

It is often difficult to trace the relationship between eruptions and other skin symptoms and the internal failings and "pathologies" with which they are associated; but we may be sure that faulty digestion, incomplete metabolism, and deficient excretion, these growing out of faulty dietary habits and other evil practices, are the underlying causes for these skin troubles.

Acne in particular is definitely related to toxemic states and nutritional impairments. The large amounts of sweets consumed during adolescence tends to saturate the skin with sugar and lay the foundation for this and other troubles.

The first principle in the care of skin diseases is to deal with the internal conditions with which they are associated, by removing or correcting the causes of these. Locally, the only care necessary is cleanliness.

Functional impairments, — faulty elimination, digestive derangements, glandular defects, etc. — growing out of enervation and toxemia, must be overcome by removing or correcting the causes of enervation and toxemia.

For parents to permit their sons and daughters to suffer with acne until their faces are a mass of scars is inexcusable. In all cases the condition may be quickly remedied by fasting, improved diet and general hygiene.

The local application of salves, ointments, lotions, etc., is of no value. Some of these preparations will suppress the condition for a time, but the minute their use is discontinued the acne reappears. Often the acne reappears while their use is continued. The only time they appear to produce a lasting "cure" is when they are used coincident with spontaneous disappearance of the trouble. It should be remembered that in most cases the acne disappears without any treatment or change in the mode of living, after adolescence.

It is never wise to wait upon the spontaneous termination of acne at the end of the adolescent period; for, by that time, the face may have become a mass of scars and its owner the victim of an inferiority complex that makes life miserable.

Goodbye to Neuralgia

Neuralgia is a term applied to paroxysms of severe pain occurring along the line of the sensory nerve-trunk, without inflammation or obvious anatomical changes in the nerve itself. In this particular, neuralgia differs from neuritis which denotes a pathologic change in the nerve itself or in its sheath.

Neuralgia is characterized by sudden, sharp, darting, and arresting pains. The pain is relieved by pressure; but there are tender spots, so-called *points douloureax*, where the nerve emerges from bony canals or muscular coverings. The condition is more or less chronic and the pain is often intense.

Neuralgia may occur in almost any part of the body. Neuralgia of the right abdomen over the appendix region has been the occasion for thousands of operations for chronic appendicitis. Neuralgia, a little lower in women has furnished the excuse for removing many healthy ovaries. Neuralgia in the lower back has caused much needless anxiety about the kidneys; neuralgia over the heart is frequently mistaken by sufferers as a symptom of heart disease; while neuralgia in the gall-bladder region has resulted in the removal of many gall-bladders.

The most frequent and most important neuralgias, named according to the location of the pain and the special nerves involved, are discussed below:

Trifacial Neuralgia, or Neuralgia of the fifth nerve, the trifacial nerve, is known as *Tic Douloureaux* and *Prosopalgia*. It is characterized by pain in one or more branches of the trifacial nerve with tender points both above and below the eyes, extending well down the cheek and centering in some cases at a point immediately above the teeth of the upper jaw. Reflex spasms of the muscles, muscular twitchings, are common. In old chronic cases the hair on the affected side may become coarse and bleached.

The real sufferer from tic douloureaux presents a pathetic picture of abject misery and suffering. In the chronic form this trouble often persists for years and may utterly incapacitate the sufferer. Despair and mental apathy are common depressive mental concomitants and, when the disease has become a fixture, the two form an almost indissoluble union.

Cervico-Occipital Neuralgia, which involves the upper cervical nerves, is characterized by paroxysmal pain extending down one or both sides of the neck as far as the collar bone and upward to the check. A spot of tenderness may be found midway between the mastoid process and the upper cervical vertebrae. Cramps in the muscles, sensitive skin, and, sometimes a surface eruption of vesicles, may accompany this form of neuralgia. Frequently a cracking at the nape of the neck proves very annoying. This form of neuralgia may also accompany tuberculosis of the spine.

Cervico-Brachial Neuralgia, involving the lower cervical nerves, presents paroxysmal pain with numbness and weakness radiating down the arm to the hand, across the shoulder to the scapula, and sometimes by a surface eruption of vesicles. Swelling or edema of the arm and later atrophy of certain muscles with pale, dry, harsh, and glossy skin are often seen in long standing cases.

Dorso-Intercostal Neuralgia, following the course of the intercostal nerves, is characterized by paroxysmal pain that is usually confined to the fifth and sixth intercostal spaces. This means that the pains are felt between the ribs. It is frequently associated with an eruption of herpes zoster — shingles. Spots of tenderness may be found near the spinal column, in the axilla and near the sternum.

Lumbo-Abdominal Neuralgia presents paroxysmal pain along the courses of the iliohypogastric and the ilioinguinal nerves radiating from the hip to the groin and inner side of the thigh.

Sciatica, though usually a neuritis, may also sometimes be a neuralgia, the pain radiating down the inner side of the thigh and leg.

The chief symptom of neuralgia is intense pain of a sharp, stabbing character. The pains last from a few minutes to many hours and its subsiding may be accompanied by the passage of a large quantity of pale urine. The interval between paroxysms varies in different individuals; sometimes being several weeks or even months long. The "attacks" often tend to recur at regular intervals. The pain is often relieved by pressure.

The area supplied by the affected nerve is usually very sensitive and palpation (exploration with the hands) may locate spots of extreme tenderness at points of exit of the nerve. Inspection of the part usually reveals nothing abnormal although a slight swelling may be seen in some cases. Herpes, or shingles, occasionally precedes or follows an "attack." In some cases reflex spasms of the muscles attend the pain.

Neuralgia is seen almost wholly in adults. It is more common in women than in men. Exposure to cold and wet may act as an exciting cause in "susceptible" individuals.

Medical works list heredity as an important cause of this disease. This is a fallacy that will soon be outgrown. Hereditary disease belongs to the days of our grandparents. Modern biology admits of no such thing.

The disease is no doubt of toxic origin. It is frequently seen in cases of chronic lead poisoning. Malaria and gout are often accompanied with neuralgia. Eye-strain and cavities of the teeth are listed as reflex irritants that may cause trifacial neuralgia. At most they can act only as secondary contributing causes. Neuralgia often accompanies anemia, but whether as a result of deficiency or as an expression of toxemia is undetermined.

Organic disease of the nerve-centers often produces neuralgia. Degeneration or tumor of the gasserian ganglion is sometimes a cause of trifacial neuralgia.

Anemia, dental caries, nervous degeneration, nerve tumor, malaria, gout and other conditions listed as causes of neuralgia are all outgrowths of toxemia: It is safe to say that practically all cases of neuralgia are due primarily to toxemia. Dr. Tilden thinks some cases are due to pressure on the nerves.

One standard medical author, in outlining the treatment for neuralgia, says: "If the disease is associated with anemia, iron and arsenic are indicated. If there is any suspicion of syphilis, mercury and iodides should be tried. If a malarial element is present, quinine may effect a cure. In gouty subjects much may be expected from regulation of diet, systematic exercise, and the administration of alkalis. In chronic lead-poisoning, iodides are serviceable."

In giving measures to "improve the general nutrition, which is almost always disturbed," he includes "the use of such tonics as iron, arsenic, codliver oil and hypophosphites."

Ordinary palliative measures and drugs have little or no effect during a paroxysm of neuralgia and it is not uncommon for these patients to become addicted to the use of morphine or similar drugs.

Morphine and other pain-killing (or had we not better say "patient-killing") drugs are given to patients for neuralgia. Soon a morphine disease, morphinism, is produced; the drug disease supplants the neuralgia and the "cure" proves to be a hundred times worse than the "disease" for which it was given.

A barbarous practice becoming popular with the medical profession is that of removing the nerves of painful parts. Dr. Edward Podolsky tells us in his book, *Medicine Marches On*, that they remove the nerves in "painful affections of the legs which no drug on earth could heal," in painful menstruation, painful constipation, cancer, angina pectoris, spastic paralysis, Raynaud's disease, and trifacial neuralgia.

The whole plan of treatment is destructive—poisoning; poisons to improve nutrition, poisons to relieve pain, surgery to destroy the nerves — is there any wonder that "for permanent cure" the prognosis "must be guarded?" Such "cures" only produce worse trouble.

It is true that this medical author does mention the necessity for removing the cause of neuralgia, but he does not mean the same thing we do when he talks of cause and its removal. He says that in "the interval" between "attacks" "careful search should be made for an exciting cause, which, if found, must be removed. The teeth, eyes, nose, gastro-intestinal tract, urine, and blood should be carefully examined." It is here that he looks for causes and his conception of removing cause is that of pulling teeth, fitting the eyes with glasses, removing tonsils, appendix and gall bladder, giving arsenic for anemia, mercury for syphilis, quinine for malaria, alkalis for gout, iodides for lead poisoning, and arsenic to improve nutrition. He mentions "proper food," but the expression is meaningless.

The late Dr. Weger well sums up the hygienic care of neuralgia when he says of trifacial neuralgia:

"All but one of the few cases we have been privileged to treat have made permanent and satisfactory recoveries by persistently following the most rigid dietetic regime for many months. Some cases require a year or two to overcome the toxic cause and the vicious pain habit that frequently persists after the cause is removed. The psychic aspect of some cases that have had as many as fifteen ganglion injections without relief, is a factor that is often underestimated. The power of the will must be enlisted and utilized to overcome, to endure, to ignore, and to minimize the pain consciousness. We have found a rather protracted fast or even several fasts at intervals of a few months absolutely necessary to accomplish a cure. All carbohydrate food must be withheld for several months. Sweets, condiments, and stimulants of all kinds must be absolutely avoided. The diet must be non-irritating in order to avoid reflex excitation from a sensitive gastric or intestinal mucous membrane. Food containing all of the necessary basic cell salts and vitamins should be given in proper combination. The physical and mental morale must be raised and the patient carefully guided and encouraged. The only failure we have to record was in a patient near the seventieth year who was not capable of understanding or carrying out specific instructions."

Dr. Weger has here outlined the care of long standing chronic cases of trifacial neuralgia which have had weeks, months and years of medical abuse before coming under hygienic care. The reader will readily understand that milder cases, cases of not so long standing, and cases that have not been medically abused or that have been abused but slightly, do not require such long periods for recovery.

All "forms" of neuralgia are to be cared for alike. The location of the pain makes no difference in the care.

It is essential to correct the life of the patient. Excessive eating and all stimulants must be given up. Sexual abuse or excess, the tobacco and alcohol habits, the coffee and tea habits and all other injurious habits must be discontinued. The emotional life will have to be adjusted. A prolonged rest for recuperation is essential. Daily exercise and daily sun bathing are necessary.

When all of the causes of impaired health
have been removed, nervous recuperation secured
and toxins eliminated from the body, a health
building program including all the natural hygienic agencies, will build a high degree of health
and the neuralgia will presently end.

Neuritis

The term neuritis signifies inflammation of a nerve and, since nerves ramify all parts of the body, neuritis may develop in any part of the organism. The condition is almost wholly confined to the peripheral nerves. As it is often difficult to distinguish between neuritis and neuralgia, thousands who have the latter condition imagine they have neuritis.

In this article we shall discuss *simple neuritis*, as distinguished from *multiple neuritis*. Simple neuritis is characterized by inflammation of the nerve trunks accompanied by pain, impaired sensation and motion, and atrophy.

Three sets of symptoms are commonly described for *acute neuritis*, as follow:

Sensory Symptoms: These are severe pain following the course of the inflamed nerve, which is tender upon being touched. The pain is often associated with burning, tingling, numbness, etc. At first the affected part is likely to be very sensitive but later may lose sensation.

Motor Symptoms: These are impairment of muscular power, diminished or lost reflexes and tremors.

Trophic Symptoms: Herpes eruptions sometimes develop along the course of the affected nerve. The skin may become glossy, and the nails lusterless and brittle. In advanced cases the muscles undergo atrophy.

Chronic Neuritis is characterized by pain, loss of sensation, paresis, wasting and contraction of the muscles, glossy skin, and thickening and brittleness of the nails.

Optic Neuritis is inflammation of the optic nerve and involves chiefly the intra-ocular end of the nerve.

Sciatica is inflammation of the sciatic nerve (sciatic neuritis) and is characterized by sharp shooting pains running down the back of the thigh. Movement of the leg increases the pain.

The pain may be evenly distributed along the course of the nerve, or there may be local spots where it is more intense. Tingling and numbness are often present. The nerve may be extremely sensitive to touch. The symptoms tend to be worse at night and upon the approach of cold or stormy weather. In long standing cases there is likely to be much wasting of the muscles and impairment of locomotion.

Medical works list such "causes" of neuritis as "exposure to cold," "trauma," "infectious diseases" ("diphtheria, influenza, measles, etc."), "chronic intoxication" ("gout, alcoholism, diabetes"), "pressure of a tumor," "relaxation or chronic inflammation of the sacro-iliac joint" (in sciatica), "rheumatism," "lead, arsenic, carbon-monoxide, sulphonal, etc., poisoning," "malnutrition," and "advanced arteriosclerosis." Optic neuritis is said to be due to "tumor of the brain," "cerebral meningitis," "syphilis," "toxic agents" (lead and alcohol), "infectious fevers," "anemia," and "Bright's disease." Sciatica numbers among its causes "uterine fibroid" in women and "carcinoma of the prostate" in men. Dr. Richard C. Cabot says most cases of neuritis are due to alcohol.

Pressure Neuritis is due to pressure upon the nerve by tumors, misplaced parts, or by outside forces. One form of this, called "Saturday night paralysis" is seen in the drunk who sleeps all night on a bench in the park with his arm over the back of the settee and his head on his arm. The alcoholic stupor prevents him from changing positions and relieving the pressure when it becomes uncomfortable, so that when he awakes next morning his arm is paralyzed.

Neuritis resulting from injury — wounds, blows, crushes of the arm or leg, operations — and from great strain upon the arm is quite common. Operations are a frequent cause of neuritis. Indeed, such cases are more common than the public is aware of.

Many of the "causes" given in medical works are not causes at all and many of the others are only complicating causes. If injury (trauma) is the cause of neuritis, this disease should follow every severe injury to a nerve. If "infectious diseases" cause neuritis, all cases of such "diseases" should be followed by neuritis. If alcohol causes neuritis, all drinkers should have neuritis. A cause that needs an ally is not a cause. A cause that causes an effect once in a hundred times is not a cause.

The primary, the basic cause of neuritis is toxemia. This is the *constant* that is needed to prepare the groundwork for neuritis and to perpetuate it once it has developed.

But not all toxemic subjects develop neuritis. Not all toxemic subjects who are injured or who use alcohol develop neuritis. Only those develop neuritis whose nerves are lacking in resistance. Cause is a composite of many factors.

Checked elimination brought on by enervation produces toxemia. Impaired secretion, resulting from enervation, permits gastro-intestinal fermentation and putrefaction, and produces chronic auto-intoxication.

When to toxemia and auto-intoxication there are added drugs, alcohol, injury, etc., those parts of the body that offer least resistance become diseased.

If the inflammation is in the kidneys, the so-called disease is named nephritis (Bright's disease); if it is in the liver, the disease is called hepatitis; if it is in the lungs, it is called pneumonia; if it is in the nerves, it is called neuritis.

Injuries to the nerves — wounds, blows, pressure, etc. — are speedily recovered from if the blood is normal. If toxemia is great, instead of recovery, the inflammation produced by the injury becomes chronic. Chronic inflammation may result in so much degeneration of the nerve that paralysis follows. This means loss of sensation, or motion, or both.

It is necessary not to make the mistake of believing that people have neuritis merely because they have pains in the arm, or shoulder, or thigh. Neuritis is really not as common as is generally thought. Pain is produced by many things and to mistake all acute or chronic pains in the limbs for neuritis is to make a great mistake.

Dr. Cabot says: "The great thing about neuritis is that it gets well and that it is rare and that treatment has very little to do with it." By this statement Dr. Cabot means for us to understand that the treatment has very little to do with the recovery. It does not follow from this, however, that it has very little to do with failure to recover; for, the treatment employed often prolongs and intensifies the disease.

Drugs such as sedative lotions (lead-water and laudanum), blisters, salicylates, phenacetin, morphine, acetanilid and codeine, produce more enervation and by thus putting an added check upon elimination, increase the toxemic state while, at the same time, lowering nerve tone — *resistance*.

Hot and cold applications, massage, electricity, baking, and hypodermic injections of strychnin, all employed after the acute symptoms have subsided, to "promote nutrition," are as injurious as the above listed drugs and positively do not promote nutrition. Massage and heat and cold are particularly likely to aggravate the affected nerve.

Medical works tell us to remove the cause, where possible. By this, they mean remove tumors, pull teeth, cut out tonsils, excise the womb or prostate gland or cut out the use of alcohol. Basic causes are not touched and not recognized.

It is, of course, necessary to discontinue the use of alcohol and other drugs (and this covers all drugs) that enervate and impair. Nothing will be gained by substituting strychnin or opium for alcohol. It is just as essential to discontinue tobacco and coffee as to drop alcohol. All enervating indulgencies must be corrected.

Absolute rest is essential until the acute symptoms subside. Cause must be removed and since the factor of toxic irritation must be reckoned with, toxemia must be eliminated. The elimination of toxemia by fasting produces speedy results. In chronic cases rest and fasting are equally valuable.

After the symptoms have subsided, exercise — passive where necessary, active when and as soon as possible — plus proper food and sun bathing will promote nutrition in a manner that massage, heat, electricity and strychnin can never do.

Sun bathing is of value during the painful stage, but care must be exercised not to overdo sunbathing, as this increases the pain and suffering.

Infantile Paralysis

At the end of every summer, when the regular orgy of vaccinating school children is completed, we have epidemics of *poliomyelitis*, or as it is commonly called, infantile paralysis. An instance of this nature is supplied us by the recent experience of Iowa.

Following the Fall round-up of the children of that state and their forcible infection with cow-pox pus, there developed an epidemic of infantile paralysis. Several cases were reported in Des Moines, Ft. Dodge, Waterloo, Boone, West Point, Otumwa, Brooklyn, Centerville, Leon and other cities and many country districts of Iowa, all reported many cases.

That the medical authorities are aware of the connection between vaccination and infantile paralysis, is shown by the fact that while there was an epidemic of infantile paralysis in New York City, in 1931, the health authorities of that city temporarily suspended the requirement of vaccination as a precedent to school attendance.

The *New York American*, Sept. 23, 1931, carried an item in which are the following words:

"Dr. John Oberwager, Department of Health expert, told superintendents to permit children to enter school without being vaccinated during the period of the epidemic. He said it was wise for parents to defer vaccination, removal of tonsils and other minor operations during the danger period."

The New York *Sun*, Sept. 25th, 1931 carried the following words:

"On the advice of Health Commissioner Shirley W. Wynne, Superintendent of Schools, O'Shea has temporarily suspended the requirement that pupils newly enrolled must present vaccination certificates. • • •

"The temporary waiver of the requirement, Dr. O'Shea explained, was a concession to parents who feared that the resistance of their children to infantile paralysis might be weakened if they were vaccinated at this time. So far as is known, the vaccination rule has never before been waived in the schools."

Unfortunately human welfare means nothing when it runs up against the desire for profits. Iowa learned nothing from its recent experience. Even before the infantile paralysis epidemic had ended, county health nurses were making surveys in the schools of that state — *immunization survey* — and of the people to determine who had not been "immunized." The great god, *Profit*, must be served when the medical gang are in control.

Known also as acute anterior poliomyelitis and acute infantile spinal paralysis, or infantile paralysis, this condition develops chiefly in young children, rarely in adults. Anatomically it is characterized by inflammation of the gray matter of the spinal cord with destruction of the nerve cells in the anterior horns, and clinically by fever and rapid atrophic paralysis of various muscles.

It begins with slight fever (101° – 103° F), restlessness, headache, pain in the back and limbs, and muscular soreness. In a few cases there is vomiting or diarrhea, and occasionally convulsions. In the course of a day or two a flaccid paralysis develops. The legs are especially likely to be involved, but all four limbs, the trunk, the lower limbs, one limb only, a group of muscles, or the respiratory muscles may be involved. The paralysis reaches its maximum in a few hours or days, then begins to improve, in many cases very little paralysis remaining at the end of a few weeks or months, in other cases much paralysis remaining. Complete recovery is more frequent than is generally known. Where paralysis persists permanently, deformity often ensues from the failure of growth in the paralyzed parts and the over contraction of the unantagonized muscles.

The paralysis may be due to changes in the brain or in the spinal cord. Several forms are described, but these relate to location and not to the actual cause or causes of the affection. In addition to the spinal form there are (1) abortive cases, in which the constitutional symptoms are unattended by paralysis and complete recovery occurs in a few days; (2) meningitic cases, in which the early symptoms closely simulate those of epidemic cerebrospinal meningitis; (3) bulbar cases, in which the nuclear centers in the medulla oblongata are involved; and (4) polyneuritic cases, in which pain in the limbs and general hyperesthesia are for a few days the most outstanding symptoms.

Unless the initial symptoms are very severe, or the respiratory muscles are affected, the prognosis as regards life is good. The death rate under regular care ranges from 5 to 30 per cent. In all cases that live, much of the paralysis disappears and occasionally the improvement is so marked that the usefulness of the affected parts is not seriously impaired. Undoubtedly many cases of death and permanent disability are due to the drugs and serums used in treating the patient in its early or acute stages. I have never seen paralysis develop in a case under drugless treatment of whatever nature.

Those demanding a unitary specific cause say poliomyelitis is due to a "minute anaerobic organism," but care based on this premise is often worse than the so-called disease itself.

Infantile paralysis is divided into intra-uterine and post-natal classes. Tilden says: "the anti-birth causes are not hereditary; for an influence to cause paralysis to be hereditary would prevent conception; or, in other words, sterilty prevents such calamities." Cases developing before birth are due to injuries and poisons. Doubtless most of these cases are due to injuries received at birth. Cases developing after birth result from infection, either from gastro-intestinal decomposition or from vaccination. Epidemics of poliomyelitis develop at the end of each summer when children are vaccinated for school. A plethoric state, due to over-eating, is described by medical men as a "well-nourished" state. They say that acute epidemic poliomyelitis "appears in children previously well nourished." Such "well-nourished" states are commonly occompanied by intestinal sepsis.

While we have stressed the office of intestinal sepsis and vaccination in producing infantile paralysis, it is necessary to add that these can produce the disease only in enervated and toxemic subjects. The child of full resistance will throw off both forms of sepsis (vaccine is septic matter) and no serious disease will develop.

Overfed and overweight children, children that are stuffed on cookies, candies, eggs, and meat, and children that are enervated from the many causes that lower nerve energy will develop enough toxemia along with the intestinal sepsis to develop any so-called disease.

Drugging, coffee using, too much excitement and lack of rest and sleep produce enervation in children. Whipping, scolding and the deliberate frightening of children, indulged in by many parents, are great enervating factors. Fear is especially destructive to nervous integrity.

Vaccination is a form of poisoning — septic poisoning or septic infection. Vaccine is either septic, or else it is inert. If it is inert, it does not "take." If it "takes," it means disease. This infection is, itself, a severe shock to the nervous system.

Even should none of the vaccinal matter ever reach the spinal cord, it so shocks the nervous system that it lowers its resistance, inhibits excretion and impairs the digestive functions.

Finally, let us emphasize the fact that the symptoms of poliomyelitis are those of a virulent sepsis, such as can evolve only from high protein foods. Meat and eggs are high toxic potentials and evolve virulent poisons when, due to over consumption .or to impaired digestion, they putrefy in the digestive tract. Vegetarian children should not have infantile paralysis.

Rest in bed, with plenty of fresh air in the room are essential. Stop all food until all convulsions, twitchings, spasmodic movements, spastic contractions, fever, etc., are gone. After this feed the child a fruit diet for a week, then feed it normally. Cases that are left with muscular and nervous incoordination require muscular and nervous re-education in the form of educational gymnastics, for which see Volume IV of *The Hygienic System*.

The "iron lung" has received an undue amount of publicity during the past few years. It has much of the element of the spectacular in it and medicine is nothing if not one spectacular stunt after another.

The "iron lung" is no lung at all, but merely an expensive piece of machinery designed to keep up artificial respiration in the patient whose respiratory center has been destroyed. It succeeds in keeping this type of patient alive for a few days to a few weeks, in one or two cases, for a year or two, but they all eventually die, for there is no way of restoring the destroyed nerves.

It is necessary to say that paralysis does not develop in all cases, even under medical abuse. We doubt the wisdom of the braces that are employed in those cases in which paralysis does develop. These braces prevent the reestablishment of muscular and nervous coordination.

Fasting for Children

"Daddy I feel bad," said a little fellow to his father the other day. "Come over here son and let us see what is ailing you," said the father. The little boy walked over to his "daddy," who took him in his arms and immediately detected that he had a slight fever. "Where do you hurt, son: do you have a headache?" he asked. The little fellow replied "No," "Does your stomach hurt," asked the father. Again the boy replied, "No." "Where do you hurt, then," asked daddy. "I don't hurt any where," replied the boy, "just feel rotten."

Then followed a few questions about what the boy had been eating, what he had eaten the day before, where he had been, what he had done, etc., and then the father said: "You go into your room and go to bed and don't eat anything until your fever is gone and you will soon be all right." Protesting that he did not want to do without food, the little fellow went to bed and in the course of a few hours was all right again.

Pain, fever, and inflammation suspend the digestive secretions, stop the rhythmic contractions (miscalled hunger contractions) of the stomach and cut off the desire for food. All of the necessary physiological conditions of digestion are absent when child or adult is acutely ill.

The dry mouth and tongue seen in fever are matched by a similar dryness of the stomach. The coated tongue and bad taste in the mouth prevent any relish of food.

In even a mild gastritis (catarrhal inflammation of the stomach) large quantities of mucus are poured into the stomach. The reader may get a picture of this if he will imagine all the mucus that pours from the membranes of the nose and throat in a cold pouring into the stomach from the membrane lining the stomach.

In severe gastritis the amount of mucus poured out is even greater. In typhoid fever the condition of the stomach and intestine is worse than that of the stomach in gastritis.

In all acute disease — measles, scarlet fever, whooping cough, diphtheria, etc., — there is more or less gastritis and in all of them digestion is suspended. Pneumonia suspends the digestive function as surely as does typhoid fever.

With these facts in mind, how foolish becomes the popular advice to the sick to eat "plenty of good nourishing food to keep up strength." Instead of feeding and nourishing the body and keeping up the strength it does just the opposite. Indeed, it is an everyday occurrence to see a mild feverishness, that would end in a day or two, persist and grow worse due to feeding. All "fevers" require fasting.

Fasting shortens the course of the illness; feeding prolongs it. Feeding increases the pain and discomfort and causes the temperature to rise. It increases restlessness and thus prevents rest. The sick child that is fed cries much, sleeps little or none at all and keeps the whole household awake at night.

The sick child that is not fed rests peacefully and sleeps most of the time. Parents do not realize how much unnecessary suffering they cause their feverish children and how much avoidable anxiety they cause themselves by feeding their sick children.

Complications result almost wholly from feeding and drugging. They almost never develop in cases that are not fed and not drugged. If fasting is instituted at the very outset of whooping cough the child may never whoop. Vomiting does not occur in whooping cough when no food is given. Scarlet fever ends in four to five days and no complications develop. Measles, pneumonia, diphtheria, smallpox, etc., soon end if no food is given.

Fasting in Heart Disease

Recently a business executive came to the *Health School* for care. Repeatedly during the preceding two years he had been refused life insurance because of the condition of his heart. Here at the *Health School* he had a fast of forty two days, during most of which time he took light exercise for a few minutes each day. One month after the fast was broken he was given ten thousand dollars life insurance. The life-insurance examiner found his heart to be in excellent condition.

In 1924 I cared for a young man from New York City who suffered with a heart affection that his physicians had declared was incurable. This young man had a fast of thirty days with complete recovery. When I last saw him, two years ago, twelve years after his fast, his heart was still in excellent condition and he was in splendid general health.

This young man had been warned against exercise. Each day when I made my rounds he reported that he had taken his exercise. On the fifteenth day of his fast, I examined his heart. After examining him at rest, I asked him to do ten deep-knee bends. He looked frightened and asked: "won't it hurt me?" I assured him it would not and with fear and trembling, his mouth wide open, and fear plainly registered on his face, he gradually lowered his body to squatting position. He then raised up to an erect position and looked relieved that he was not dead. He finished his exercise and I again examined his heart. It was good.

He then exclaimed: "I am going to do my exercise every day hereafter!" To my question, "have you not been exercising daily, as you reported?" he replied: "No, I lied to you. I was afraid to exercise and I knew that if I told you I had not exercised you would have me do it."

He did his exercise faithfully through the remainder of his fast.

Only a few years ago the medical profession dogmatically declared that if one goes six days without food, his heart will collapse and he will die. Since the above young man had his fast of thirty days that resulted in recovery from an "incurable" heart affection, one of my patients, who had just gone on a fast, was gravely warned by her former physician that if she went without food for six days her heart would collapse and she would die.

Although many patients with various forms of heart disease have fasted under my care for greater or lesser periods, none of them have suffered heart collapse and death. On the contrary, most of them completely recovered from their heart trouble.

Everyday people die of "heart attack" or "heart failure" who are eating three square meals a day and extra food between meals. Often these deaths follow immediately upon the heels of a hearty meal, or occur even while the meal is on. If "plenty of good nourishing food" will prevent heart collapse these people should not die.

The simple truth is that very few sufferers from heart disease, be they doctor or layman, fail to note from experience that their comforts depend to a great extent upon what and how much they eat. Heart "attacks," from simple acceleration and palpitation to the severe anginas, are in the great majority of instances, due to overloading, fermentation, distention, and indigestion of the stomach.

Eating places a load upon the heart; overeating but needlessly increases the burden. Fasting relieves the heart of the excess load it is carrying and provides an opportunity for rest.

The heart that is pulsating at the rate of 80 times a minute, -pulsates 115,200 times in twenty-four hours. Shortly after the fast is instituted the heart rate decreases and, while it may temporarily go much below 60 pulsations a minute, it ultimately settles at 60 beats a minute and remains there for the duration of the fast. This is 86,400 pulsations in twenty-four hours, or 28,800 fewer pulsations each day than it was doing before the fast.

This represents a decrease of twenty-five percent in the amount of work the heart performs. The saving in work is seen not merely in the reduction of the number of pulsations but also in the vigor of the pulsations. It all sums up to a real vacation — a rest — for the heart. During this rest the heart repairs its damaged structures and replenishes its tissues.

But fasting does more than give the heart a rest. It supplies the body with the needed opportunity to free itself of accumulated toxins. With toxemia eliminated, tissue repair is more rapid and more ideal. Toxic irritation of the heart ends and it makes a "come back" that is often more than surprising.

What we have said above applies to most cases of heart trouble. But there are occasional exceptions. Rarely we see a case in which heart action becomes depressed and erratic while fasting, necessitating breaking the fast. In such cases there may be real danger in continuing the fast.

All cases of heart trouble who undergo a fast should do so under the direct and personal supervision of one experienced in conducting fasts. No unnecessary chances should be taken in these conditions.

Hunger Pains

The *Times Herald*, Dallas, Texas, November 15, 1940, carried the following bit of news: **KANSAS FARMER ON 45TH DAY OF FAST FOR AILMENT**

Inman, Kan., Nov. 15 (INS).—J. I. Friesen, 42-year-old farmer, today was on the forty-fifth day of a fast, according to relatives.

Undertaken to relieve gall bladder and liver trouble, the fast has accomplished its purpose and, incidentally, dropped Friesen's weight from 210 pounds to 162.

He has drunk normal amounts of water during the forty-five days.

Strong hunger pains that assailed him on the seventh, fourteenth and twenty-first days did not manifest themselves during recent weeks, it was said, and Friesen will wait until he gets normally hungry again before he breaks the long fast with orange juice.

It is the medical, as well as the popular, view that hunger is a painful sensation; indeed that it may often be a very painful experience. "Strong hunger pains that assailed him on the seventh, fourteenth and twenty-first days did not manifest themselves during recent weeks." It will be difficult to explain how this faster was "hungry" only at intervals of seven days; how his "hunger" was intermittent, even though he did not take food; how his "hunger" ceased to manifest after more than twenty days without food.

So careful an investigator as Dr. Walter B. Cannon makes this same mistake. In his *Bodily Changes in Pain, Hunger, Fear and Rage*, he says:

"The sensation of hunger is difficult to describe, but almost everyone from childhood has felt at times that dull ache or gnawing pain referred to the lower mid-chest and the epigastrium, which may take imperious control of human action. As Sternberg has pointed out, hunger may be sufficiently insistent to force the taking of food which is so distasteful that it not only fails to arouse appetite, but may even produce nausea.

The hungry being gulps his food with a rush. The pleasures of appetite are not for him — he wants quantity rather than quality, and he wants it at once.

* * *

Hunger may be described as having a central core and certain more or less variable accessories. The peculiar dull ache of hungriness, referred to the epigastrium, is usually the organism's first strong demand for food; and when the initial order is not obeyed, the sensation is likely to grow into a highly uncomfortable pang or gnawing, less definitely localized as it becomes more intense. This may be regarded as the essential feature of hunger. Besides the dull ache, however, lassitude and drowsiness may appear, or faintness, or violent headache, or irritability and restlessness such that continuous effort in ordinary affairs becomes increasingly difficult. That these states differ much with individuals — headache in one and faintness in another, for example — indicates that they do not constitute the central fact of hunger, but are more or less inconstant accompaniments. The 'feeling of emptiness', which has been mentioned as an important element of the experience, is an inference rather than a distinct datum of consciousness, and can likewise be eliminated from further consideration. The dull pressing sensation is left, therefore, as the constant characteristic, the central fact, to be examined in detail."

Any man of experience, reading the above will recognize at once that Professor Cannon has never seen a hungry man and has mistaken the morbid sensations of a food-drunkard for the normal expressions of life.

Real hunger, rather than producing "lassitude and drowsiness," "or faintness," produces alertness and activity in the search for food.

Dull ache in the epigastrium, violent headache, irritability, restlessness, lassitude, drowsiness, faintness and a decreasing capacity for continuous effort — how like the effects that follow the missing of the accustomed cigar, pipe, cup of coffee, or tea, glass of whiskey, or dose of morphine are these symptoms! How did Dr. Cannon miss their true significance?

The "feeling of emptiness," and the gnawing that he describes, are not accompaniments of hunger. Neither is the "dull pressing sensation" which he has left as the "central fact" of hunger, any part of the physiological demand for food, which we call hunger. These are both morbid sensations.

Let us arrive at an understanding of hunger by seeing what it is not. Headache is not hunger. Pain in the abdomen is not hunger. Gnawing in the stomach is not hunger. Lassitude is not hunger. Drowsiness is not hunger. Irritability is not hunger. Weakness is not hunger. Faintness is not hunger. A "feeling of emptiness" is not hunger. A "dull pressing sensation" is not hunger. Restlessness is not hunger.

Think of thirst. Is it a pain? Is it a headache? Is it irritability? Is it faintness? Is it drowsiness? Is it any of the sensations described by Dr. Cannon as belonging to hunger?

It is none of these things. Thirst is felt in the mouth and throat and there is a distinct and conscious desire for water. One does not mistake headache for thirst. The sensation of thirst is too well known.

Genuine hunger, too, is felt in the mouth and throat. In real hunger there is a distinct and conscious desire for food. The condition is one of comfort, not of discomfort and suffering. There is a "watering" of the mouth (flow of saliva) and often a distinct desire for a particular food. Hunger is a localized sensation and is not in the stomach. The healthy person is not conscious of any sensations in or about the stomach when hungry.

To return, then, to the "strong hunger pains" Mr. Friesen is said to have suffered on the "seventh, fourteenth and twenty-first days" of his fast: What were they? They were not "hunger pains," for the reason that there are no such things.

Such pains are seen in certain fasting subjects — dyspeptics, nervous persons, so-called gall-bladder cases and those individuals who are inclined to worry, fear, apprehension, etc. Where they are not due to actual pathology, as in gastric and duodenal ulcer, gall-stones, etc., they are due to spastic contractions of the stomach and intestine resulting from psychic or emotional disturbances of the sympathetic control of the stomach and intestine.

In more than twenty years of experience during which time I have conducted more than ten thousand fasts ranging in duration from three days to fifty-five days I have yet to see a single case in which pain, headache, drowsiness, a "feeling of emptiness" etc., accompanied the development of real hunger.

Nor does the really hungry person gulp his food, or seek for quantity rather than quality. Dr. Cannon has carried on his researches with a group of neurotics, dyspeptics, and food drunkards and none of them have ever gone without food long enough for full adjustment to follow.

Gluttony a Neurosis

Habits fasten themselves upon us slowly and insidiously. To smoke one cigarette, or to take one drink of alcohol, or one cup of coffee does not constitute the tobacco, alcohol, or coffee habit. Eating one huge meal does not constitute gluttony. One masturbation does not constitute auto-eroticism. If these are practiced until they become established habits — *addictions* — changes occur in the nervous system resulting in neuroses — *habit neuroses* — that grow upon the habits that produced them. Once a practice becomes ingrained in the nervous system it continues to cry for expression. The individual now finds that his habits are master, he is slave.

Over-eating and frequent eating tend to develop a gastric neurosis which is commonly called gluttony. Once gluttony has become a fixed habit, it tends to grow upon the glutton until he finds himself eating many times as much as his body needs.

We have seen many individuals who ate three big meals a day and ate frequently between meals and at night. We have seen them get up out of bed at all hours of the night to eat. Although they were constantly eating, they complained of always being hungry.

If they did not eat they were uncomfortable. They were, of course, food-poisoned. Their discomforts were identical with those of the coffee, tea, tobacco, alcohol or drug addict who is deprived of his poison.

Some of these neurotics suffered both before and after taking food. Though they knew that eating would cause discomfort, they were driven by their neurosis to eat, anyway.

The worst types of gastric neuroses are called *bulimia*. This is a voracious appetite. In such a state the sufferer often eats all the time and eats all manners of substances. Indeed cases have been reported of individuals who would gnaw their own flesh if food was not present. This condition is usually accompanied with vomiting and diarrhea.

Craving for food becomes irresistable and leads often to eating substances that have no food value, or to eating all manners of disgusting substances.

The worst feature of these cases is that they cannot be made to realize that what they mistake for hunger is not hunger. They believe they are hungry and insist on eating. "My body demands food," they will say, when told that their supposed hunger is a *perversion* or *neurosis*.

In many cases the *neurosis* tends to become a *psychosis*. It "goes to the head," to use a popular expression. They get so they think and talk of nothing but food.

Meet one of these men on the street and he will say: "What did you have for breakfast? I had —" and so on through a recital of each item of his breakfast and the amount of each item consumed. Finishing with this recital. he will begin with a detailed story of what he plans to have at his next meal. He may even go over his whole eating program of the day before.

Eating at all hours of the day and night, drinking juices of all kinds, trying new foods and food concentrates, experimenting with different diet programs, talking all the time about food and suffering always from excess, these poor victims of their own follies fail to find the relief they seek — whether they seek relief in drug or drugless palliation — because they never cease their gluttonous indulgence.

They have lost all control of themselves, they have become slaves to a morbid change in their nervous system and, since they fail to recognize that they do not need and cannot possibly use the amounts of food they habitually burden their digestive and excretory systems with, they continue to eat and suffer. Eating causes them to suffer and suffering causes them to eat. The morbid chain of affinities binds them and holds them until an early death releases them from the slavery they have built for themselves.

It should be understood that the neurotic who demands repeatedly to experience the desired thrill or sense of pleasure, is not only profoundly enervated, but that each repetition of his indulgence increases his enervation. Hence the ever growing demand for newer, stronger, more frequent excitement, every repetition of which fastens the habit more firmly upon him. Many become so bound by the fetters of habit that they are unable to free themselves. They need, and must have, the aid, even the control, of others.

To teach these people that they are over-eating and that over-eating is causing their troubles; that over-eating originally produced their neurosis and over-eating perpetuates it, is futile. Even if they can be made to understand these things, they still cannot control their morbid cravings. They will not eat until it kills them and cram food into the mouth with their last gasp.

Fasting and the Teeth

A letter comes to the editor from a lady in New York, who writes:

"I went to a Dr. — , who is supposed to be a Naturopath, Dentist, Osteopath and what have you and he suggested pulling a tooth rather than removing the nerve. He said he cleaned your teeth once, and thought you had a mighty fine set of them, but as for your methods he thought they were too harsh.

"He remarked that one of your patients who was on a long fast came to him with most of his teeth in an awful state, as a result of this long fast. But I notice that people lose their teeth without fasting, as has been true in my case."

This dentist is mistaken about having cleaned my teeth. It's true I have a good set of teeth, it is also true that no dentist has ever examined them. The dentist who thinks he once cleaned my teeth has never seen my teeth beyond what he could see as we talked to each other on many occasions. My teeth do not need cleaning.

Are "my" methods too harsh? Who is to judge: those who have been cared for at the *Health School,* or a man who has never been in the *Health School* and knows very little about what is done here?. I challenge anybody anywhere to find an institution in America (hospital, sanitarium, health home, health resort, health school, or by whatever name it is called) that uses milder methods than we use at *Dr. Shelton's Health School.*

A dentist who jumps at conclusions will often land in a hole. No doubt some of those who have fasted under our care have gone to this man with their tooth troubles. So far as we know, no one ever claimed that fasting would restore soundness to teeth that are decayed. We get many patients whose teeth are practically worthless, not because they have fasted but because they have not been properly nourished.

It behooves the dentist to ascertain, when such patients come to him, what the condition of the teeth was before the fast. To conclude that the condition of the teeth, as he finds it, is due to fasting, when they probably began to decay ten to twenty years before the fast was undergone, does not evince a desire to get at the truth about the matter.

Such jumping at conclusions may be the result of mental shortcomings, educational inadequacies, prejudice, commercialism, or fear of breaking away from the beaten path. Let us turn to some very orthodox scientific testimony, which, while orthodox, does come from a man who has taken the trouble to investigate the matter thoroughly before expressing himself.

In his monumental work, *Inanition and Malnutrition*, C. M. Jackson, M. S., M. D., LL. D., Professor and Director of the Department of Anatomy, University of Minnesota, says:

"Like the skeleton, the teeth appear very resistant to inanition, * * * In total inanition, or on water alone, the teeth in adults show no appreciable change in weight or structure * * *"

In *total inanition* the experimental animal is deprived of all food and water. It is obvious that the animal will not live as long when deprived of water as when receiving water. But the reader will note that no changes occur in the teeth in animals that are given water only until they starve to death.

In certain animals, exceptions to this are found. This is especially true of rabbits in which the teeth grow continuously. The teeth are not damaged, but a temporary lessening of the organic materials of the teeth is produced. A similar thing might probably occur in the teeth of very young children if they were forced to undergo a very prolonged fast, but such children never have to undergo such fasts.

Jackson points out that the teeth are "especially susceptible to rickets and scurvy" and that in both animal and man:

"There are slight changes in chemical composition, especially in chronic (incomplete) inanition. In the young, such inanition may delay the process of dentition, but persistent growth and development of the teeth (as of the skeleton) occur in young rabbits held at a constant body weight by underfeeding.

"The effects of partial inanition have been studied in rickets and in scurvy. In both human and animal rickets there is delayed and abnormal dentition. Both enamel and dentine may be defective and imperfectly calcified."

Without additional quotations about the effects of deficient diets (partial inanition) upon the teeth in rickets and in scurvy, let us point out that dentists who have studied the effects of inadequate and deficient diets upon the teeth and who do not know that fasting does not produce the same results as such diets, are likely to conclude that fasting injures the teeth. Indeed there is a tendency in all who study the effects of dietary inadequacies and deficiencies to run away from fasting, for, they reason, if a defective diet produces such undesirable results, no food at all should produce much worse results. They are blissfully unaware that fasting not only does not produce any of the so-called deficiency diseases, but that it is actually beneficial in everyone of them.

Dr. Jackson says that:

"In scurvy, the gums are markedly congested and swollen in about 80 per cent of adult human cases, * * * The alveolar bone and peridental membrane undergo necrosis, with consequent loosening of the teeth, and ulcerations or pyorrhea may occur."

In the pyorrhea that "four out of five" are said to have, we see inflammation and ulceration of the gums, pus formation, loosening of the teeth, necrosis of the jaw, and even falling out of the teeth. In numerous cases of pyorrhea that we have cared for, the gum inflammation has subsided, the ulcers have healed, pus formation has ceased and the loosened teeth have become firmly fixed in their sockets, and all of this has occurred while the patient was fasting. The effects of fasting must not be confused with the effects of a white - flour - lard - pie - pasteurized - milk-mashed-potato diet.

The lady who wrote the letter mentioned at the head of this article, asks: "do you approve of the dentists' methods of treating gums with different drugs, scraping, electricity, injections and other methods?"

We do not approve of anybody's methods of treating anything. We do not believe in treatments.

If the drugs of the dentist are beneficial in *disease* of the gums, then why not use the drugs of the physician in *disease* of other tissues of the body? If electricity is beneficial in *disease* of the gums, why not beneficial in treating *disease* of the liver, or kidneys, or brain, or heart? If injections are beneficial in *disease* of the gums why would they not be beneficial in treating *disease* of the stomach, or pancreas, or spleen?

Dentistry is a medical specialty. Dentists are trained in and accept the absurd theories of the "regular" medical profession. They believe gum troubles and tooth troubles are due to germs. They believe in immunization, in antiseptics, in drugs, serums, vaccines, operations, radium and X-ray treatment, etc. Dentists helped to popularize the obvious fallacy that "a clean tooth never decays," they helped to popularize the vulgar habit of brushing the teeth and that of using tooth powders and tooth pastes. They have taught the public almost as many fallacies as the pill peddlers.

Dentists became as enthused as the mixers of dope (M.D.) over the pulling of teeth to cure rheumatism, neuritis, heart disease, anemia, epilepsy, etc. Indeed some of them got to the point where they refused to fill a tooth. As they did all the pulling, they pulled car loads of sound teeth, knowing they were sound, because they are indissolubly linked with the medical profession and because the dental profession is as highly commercialized as the medical profession.

They have preferred to pull and plug teeth to preserving them in a sound state. Only within recent years have a few of them, stung to the quick by the lashings of Hygienists, begun to look to means of preserving the structural integrity of the teeth. Even these have not been able to throw off the stultification of their medical training, so they are seeking to preserve teeth by diet. Every day I see people's teeth decay who are on diets that are said to preserve the teeth.

Until these men learn that it is no more possible to maintain healthy teeth with diet alone than it is to maintain health of any other part of the body by diet alone, their work will not become successful. It must be recognized that nutrition is a composite resultant of many factors.

When, several years ago, the editor offered the slogan, *a well nourished tooth never decays,* as a substitute for the old threadbare fallacy, *"a clean tooth never decays,"* he recognized that teeth can not be well nourished, no matter what the diet, if nutrition is perverted or deranged from any cause.

Fictional Objections to Fasting

Mr. Frederick Hoelzel, of Chicago, has published a brochure on *Fasting, Water and Salt*, in which, though approving of fasting, he puts forth the claim that it always produces a condition of "hidden edema." Hidden edema is a term used to designate a slight excess of salt and water in the tissues.

Hoelzel says: "I have not known of any case of fasting, even when for only five days, where some post-fasting edema was not present. I have also noted edema developing in rats after fasting or protein restriction. A wet diet (with plenty of water), in my opinion only seems to produce edema more easily in rats than a dry diet because rats eat more freely of a wet diet (made up largely of vegetables) and thus obtain more salts, etc. There seems to be no exception to the rule that edema will develop after starvation or sufficient protein restriction in humans or rats, excepting that there naturally are expected differences in time and degree of edema production."

I have seen several cases of edema of the feet and ankles following prolonged fasting, but these are rare occurrences. However, Mr. Hoelzel discusses "hidden edema" for which there is no accurate test and of the existence of which we cannot always be sure. The "pitting test," whereby the skin on the legs over the skin-bone is depressed by the finger, can reveal edema only after it is no longer hidden. The intra-dermal salt solution (called the McClure-Aldrich test), which consists of injecting a little salt water into the skin and noting how long it takes for the blister to disappear, is claimed to be an improvement over the pitting test, but even this fails to reveal slight edema.

Hoelzel thinks that a more accurate and more valuable test of hidden edema than the pitting test and McClure-Aldrich test is the presence of the following symptoms: "Swollen feet and enlarged ankles; a puffy or bloated face; hypersensitiveness to drafts or to shaving; skin that cuts, chaps or bruises easily; a shiny skin, including a shiny nose; frequent colds; some types of headache; a continuous sense of fatigue and lack of ambition; mental depression; abnormal blushing and coyness; cases of obesity in which the fat is not firm; and some troubles associated with menstruation and pregnancy," or what have you?

Hoelzel says that "fasting is not even necessary to predispose one to the development of edema as it develops after simple protein restriction, when this has been sufficiently prolonged. Moreover, table-salt is not necessary as many natural and unsalted foods (some vegetables and some types of meat) contain enough natural or mineral salts or unoxidizable crystals to produce edema after sufficient protein restriction. It is known that carbohydrates can contribute to edema, apparently by being retained as glucose instead of being changed to glycogen."

One certainly does not get an excess of salts nor of carbohydrates while fasting, nor is an excess of water consumed if the demands of instinct rather than of theory are obeyed. It is the rule that the sodium-chloride produced edema is eliminated during the fast. As the protein restriction during the fast is no greater than the restriction of other substances (except water and air) the body succeeds in establishing and maintaining a balance.

Mr. Hoelzel's experience with fasting has been extremely limited and his method is not one of which we can approve. He became technician in gross anatomy at the College of Medicine of the University of Illinois in 1916, but carried on most of his experiments with fasting in the Department of Physiology in the University of Chicago, where he was granted the courtesy of the use of the laboratory from time to time by

Professor A. J. Carlson, to carry on his independent experimentation.

He tells of fasting fifteen days in the University of Chicago in 1917 and following this with six days of fasting during which he took cotton fibre soaked in lemon juice to which common salt was added. He used about one-third of an ounce of salt a day. With this as "food" he gained over two pounds a day in weight, storing fifteen pounds or more of salt water in the six days of "fasting." He says, "I stopped after six days because the edema had become obvious in my legs and I was becoming sluggish generally." He recounts another gain of twelve pounds in twenty-four hours after eating two moderate sized meals which contained salt food (ham and cabbage), and a weight increase of two pounds daily after a nine day's fast when only salt (ten grams daily) was taken in addition to sufficient water to satisfy thirst.

This is not an objection to fasting, nor does it prove that fasting produces hidden edema. It is an objection to salt-using and excess water-drinking. The use of salt and salted foods and the consequent drinking of lots of fluid water-logs the tissues of all who practice it — fasting or feeding. I know of no one (except Ghandi) who advises the use of salt while fasting. Without salt-using and excess water-drinking no gains in weight, such as Mr. Hoelzel describes, ever take place. Excess water drinking in the absence of salt never registers more than slight temporary gains.

The rapid post-fasting gains he describes do not occur in properly fed cases. The most rapid gains I have seen have been produced by the milk diet, but here again it was a mere water-logging of the tissues from excess fluid intake. Even in these cases I have not seen any apparent edema. Cases fed on fruits, vegetables, and moderate quantities of proteins and carbohydrates do not present the difficulties he describes, nor do their tissues fill with excess water. On the other hand, additional protein alone is not always enough to overcome malnutritional edema. It may even aggravate the condition. Simple fasting, of whatever duration, is not open to any of the objections raised by Mr. Hoelzel. On the contrary, it is the most rapid means of removing the accumulated fluid in edema.

Exercise and the Heart

Every one of man's organs is supplied with a reserve of functional power and ability, in excess of the needs of ordinary life, to be used in meeting emergencies or unusual demands. A considerable portion of the liver may be removed without its possessor appreciably missing it; about two-fifths of it may be removed, but if three-fifths are removed he begins to feel it. We have much more liver than we really need for the preservation of life. This same is true of all the other organs of man's body, the heart included.

The capacity of the heart muscle for work is thirteen times as great as the amount of work it is ordinarily called upon to do. This most wonderful organ is one of the strongest and most resistant in the body. It is capable of outlasting any other organ of the body except the brain. Instead of work or heavy exercise injuring the heart, the muscles of the body become too tired to go on before the normal heart feels any strain.

The heart is a muscular organ — it is almost all muscle — and like all other muscles of the body, is strengthened by use. A heart that is never called upon to do vigorous work does not grow vigorous and strong. If it always does light work it tends to become soft and flabby. It needs periods of vigorous work to build up and maintain its maximum strength and ability.

Running is the best exercise known for the heart. Running is the one universal exercise among the higher animals. Whether running merely for play, as one may observe dogs, cats and horses doing, or running away from an enemy or after prey, as one often observes in the wilds, running is frequently indulged in by life all around us.

Children run in play as naturally as do young kittens and calves, puppies and cubs. Running is the most natural form of exercise and has long been known to be the finest "conditioner" that athletes can employ in their training. "Road work" (running) is employed by the boxer to build up that condition of the heart and lungs that spells staying power when he comes into the ring for the fight.

Stop being afraid of your heart. What does it matter that some nit-wit has advised you not to attempt to climb even three steps? They have been killing those who take this advice seriously, for a long time. The best way to weaken your heart — to let it grow flabby like the muscles of your arm — is to never give it any vigorous work to do.

Stair climbing, started moderately and increased prudently, will result in recovery in many cases of supposed bad heart weakness. The late President Harding restored his heart to soundness by stair climbing after years of petting and pampering under the directions of his favorite pill roller had failed to help.

Any form of exercise — running, dumb-bell exercise, Indian club swinging, swimming, etc., — started moderately and increased prudently, will produce heart and lung development and lead to the establishment of robust health. Of all forms of exercise, running, as pointed out above, is perhaps best for the heart.

Although "regular medicine" never tires of telling us how many heart defects and other defects are susceptible of prompt eradication by proper measures, they seem never to be able to find the proper measures. Their program of inactivity and drugging certainly does not remedy heart defects and every day we see heart cases grow from bad to worse under this program of care.

The most difficult task in heart cases is that of ridding the patient of fear implanted by physicians. Yet the elimination of fear is one of our most important tasks. Fear paralyzes action and prevents the patient from carrying out the necessary exercise program. Fear cripples the heart itself. It impairs digestion and checks elimination and tends to prevent recovery.

In 1911 Clarence DeMar entered his name for a 26 mile Boston Marathon. His heart was examined by a doctor who told him to drop out if he got tired and advised him to give up running thereafter. DeMar won the race in record time. Since then DeMar's record in 66 marathons, including three at the Olympic Games in 1912, 1924, and 1928, is 20 first, 12 seconds, 9 thirds, and he is still a keen marathon runner. Had he allowed the advice of the physician to frighten him and had he ceased running as advised, the name of DeMar would not stand so high in the athletic world.

Fear is man's greatest enemy. Fear is the greatest nerve annihiliator known. It not only paralyzes action, it deranges digestion, impairs glandular action and checks elimination. Enervation, perverted metabolism, and toxemia are the results. Cases have come under my observation in which fear of activity (both conscious and sub-conscious) was so great, that the victims of fear were weak and always tired. Slight exertion exhausted them and made them feel bad. Those patients had been frightened by doctors and parents about their hearts and thus their hearts, being denied the one thing that could make and keep them vigorous, had grown weaker and weaker.

Only exercise can strengthen and rebuild such hearts and their fear of exercise prevents them from employing it. Fear paralyzes effort and denies their hearts the one thing essential to its recovery of vigor.

There are times and conditions in which the heart needs rest and nothing else will take the place of rest; but perpetual rest becomes rust. After rest has done its work, exercise is needed and nothing will take the place of exercise. After a period of preliminary preparation, vigorous exercise should be indulged.

There are still many physicians who warn us of the grave dangers to the heart and other parts of our body that exist in athletics. Nobody ever warns the dog running after the hare, or the wolf chasing a deer, that running is bad for the heart. Only man seems to be built so poorly that he cannot indulge in the strenuous activities of life.

Physicians like to tell their heart cases that their heart troubles have been brought on by strenuous play, like tennis, foot ball, handball, swimming, running, jumping, etc., because any trouble so caused is supposed to be hard to *cure* and physicians find that patients have more patience with them when they fail to "cure" in a reasonable time, if they believe their troubles were caused by athletics.

Actually, this is one of the chief reasons why these patients are never restored to health. So long as physicians are mistaken about cause, so long as they fail to find the real cause, they cannot care for the patient in a manner that will restore health. Wrong care must always flow from an erroneous cause.

Mixing Acids with Proteins

Among those who have some knowledge of correct food combining and who give some attention to this feature of proper eating, there are many who advise mixing acid foods — tomatoes, lemons, limes, oranges, grapefruit, pineapple, etc, — with proteins. The practice goes back many years and is based on the thought that acids help to digest proteins. Indeed, we have heard it asserted that "acids digest proteins."

All of this is based on ignorance of physiology, or else, on a failure to understand the facts of digestive chemistry. Acids do not digest proteins, and acids, except that secreted by the stomach itself, do not help to digest proteins. Indeed, as we shall see, acids retard the digestion of proteins.

All of this has reference to gastric (stomach) digestion, for there is no protein digestion in the mouth, while all the digestive processes in the intestine take place in an alkaline medium.

The active work of splitting up (digesting) complex protein substances into simpler substances, which takes place in the stomach and which forms the first step in the digestion of proteins, is accomplished by an enzyme, or digestive ferment known as *pepsin*.

Pepsin acts only in an acid medium; its action is stopped by alkali. The gastric juice ranges all the way from nearly neutral to strongly acid, depending upon what kind of food is put into the stomach. When proteins are eaten the gastric juice is acid, for it must furnish a favorable medium for the action of *pepsin*.

The normal stomach secretes all the acid required by *pepsin* in digesting a reasonable quantity of protein. An abnormal stomach may secrete too much acid (hyperacidity) or an insufficient amount (hypoacidity). In either case, taking acids with proteins does not aid digestion.

While *pepsin* is not active except in the presence of hydrochloric acid (I can find no evidence that other acids activate this enzyme), excessive gastric acidity prevents its action. Excess acid destroys the *pepsin*.

Drug acids and fruit acids demoralize gastric digestion, either by destroying the *pepsin*, or by inhibiting its secretion. Gastric juice is not poured out in the presence of acid in the mouth and stomach.

The renowned Russian physiologist, Pavlov, positively demonstrated the demoralizing influence of acids upon digestion — both fruit acids and the acid end-results of fermentation. Acid fruits by inhibiting the flow of gastric juice — an unhampered flow of which is imperatively demanded by protein digestion — seriously handicaps protein digestion and results in putrefaction.

Nuts and cheese containing, as they do, considerable oil and fat (cream), are about the only exceptions to the rule that *when acids are taken with protein, putrefaction occurs*. These foods do not decompose as quickly as other protein foods when they are not immediately digested.

Furthermore, acids do not delay the digestion of nuts and cheese; because these foods contain enough fat to inhibit gastric secretion for a longer time than acids do.

Fat depresses the action of the gastric glands and inhibits the outpouring of gastric juice. It lowers the amount of *pepsin* and hydrochloric acid and lowers the entire digestive tone fifty per cent. This is the reason cheese, nuts, and fat meats require a longer time to digest than other proteins.

The inhibiting effect of fat upon gastric secretion may be counteracted by consuming a plentiful supply of green vegetables, especially raw, at the same meal. For this reason, it were better to consume green vegetables with cheese and nuts than to consume acid fruits with them, even though, this latter is not particularly objectionable.

When we consider the actual process of protein digestion in the stomach and the positive inhibiting effects of acids upon gastric secretion, we realize at once the fallacy of consuming pineapple juice or grapefruit juice or tomato juice with meat, as advocated by certain so-called dietitians, and the fallacy of beating-up eggs in orange juice to make the so-called "pep-cocktail," advocated by other pseudo-dietitians.

Lemon juice, vinegar or other acid used on salads, or added to salad dressing, and eaten with a protein meal, serve as a severe check to hydrochloric secretion and thus interfere with protein digestion.

Since acid fruits do not undergo any digestion in the mouth and stomach and do not normally remain in the stomach more than a few minutes and, since their presence in the stomach interferes with both protein and starch digestion, they should not be eaten at a regular meal. Nor should they be taken a half hour or an hour after meals. The habit of drinking quantities of fruit juices — lemon juice, lime juice, orange juice, grapefruit juice, grape juice, tomato juice, papaya juice — between meals is responsible for a large amount of indigestion in those who think they are eating healthfully. This practice, revived during the last few years, was quite the vogue in *Hygienic* circles forty to sixty years ago, and the digestive and other evils that flowed from it caused many to abandon the reform diet and return to the flesh pots. Let me quote Dr. Robert Walter's experience with the juice drinking fad, as he records it in his *Exact Science of Health*.

He says that in consequence of the treatments he had undergone in his efforts to recover health (first medical and then hydropathic), he had a "ravenous appetite for food" and as a consequence of the irritation of his stomach he had developed into a "gourmand which no amount of food could satisfy." He adds:

"My sufferings from thirst were always great, but I did not like water, and having been taught the superior qualities of fruits, I could never get enough of the cooling juices, which fermented in my stomach, creating and perpetuating the very fever they temporarily relieved, all of which * * * kept me in a fever of nervous hunger which no suffering in other respects ever equalled."

This experience caused the doctor to renounce vegetarianism and return to meat eating. Eating at all hours of the day (for drinking juice is eating), he developed a neurosis which he mistook for hunger. Trying to satisfy a neurosis is like trying to put out a fire with gasoline.

Those who mistake gastric irritation for hunger and who continue to "appease" their "hunger" with the use of the cause of the irritation must grow from bad to worse. Turning from vegetarianism saved Dr. Walter, not because vegetarianism is wrong, but because he began to eat but one meal a day and ceased to imbibe fruit juices between meals.

No diet is so good but that it will be spoiled by the juice drinking practice and no diet is so bad but that this practice will make it worse. And this is true, not because the juices are bad, for they are excellent, but because their use in the ways condemned above disorganize digestion.

Many mistakes that are now being made by so-called dietitians could be avoided if they were acquainted with the history of diet reform. All of their "discoveries" were made and tried long ago, and some of those that are just now enjoying a heyday of popularity, were found evil and abandoned.

For instance, nearly fifty years ago, Dr. Salisbury, popularized the exclusive meat diet in tuberculosis, arthritis and other diseases. For several years physicians in both Europe and America swore by this diet and reported their cures. However, like all the cures that do not cure, it passed into oblivion. Shortly after the end of the war to end war this diet was revived and all the old mistakes are being repeated.

Nearly forty years ago a physician conceived the idea of separating the alkaline minerals from fruits and vegetables and giving these to the sick to alkalinize their bodies — that is, to neutralize excess acids. At first, he used juices as a substitute for fasting. Later he put up the first food pills made of fruit and vegetable minerals in concentrated form. For several years his mineral concentrates enjoyed a wide vogue among both medical men and drugless men. But it, too, passed. Since the world was made safe for democracy this man's ideas have been plagarized and his pills have been imitated by every Tom, Dick and Harry in the field of commercialized "dietetics" and the public is being fed a dietetic pharmacopia that bids fair to equal in size and in number of remedies, that of the medical profession.

Since the inventive ingenuity of the human mind seems to be infinite, there is no remedy for this evil, except that of enlightenment. So long as the people do not know, there will be those who will take advantage of their ignorance to exploit it.

Autolysing Tumors

The word autolysis is derived from the Greek and means, literally, self-loosing. It is used in physiology to designate the process of digestion or disintegration of tissue by ferments (enzymes) generated in the cells themselves. It is a process of self-digestion.

Enzymes exist throughout nature. All organic processes are accomplished by their aid. Seeds sprout by the aid of enzymes. Every tissue has its own enzyme.

It is now common knowledge that the processes of digestion that take place in the mouth, stomach and intestine are made possible by active agents or ferments known as enzymes. For instance, starch is converted into sugar by digestive enzymes that are said to be starch splitting, or amylolytic; proteins are converted into amino-acids by protein-splitting, or proteolytic, enzymes. The digestive enzymes digest only "dead" substances and therefore, do not digest the stomach and intestine.

Acids and alkalies do not accomplish the work of digestion. They only supply favorable mediums for the work of the digestive enzymes. The enzyme, ptyalin, of the saliva acts only in an alkaline medium and is destroyed by a mild acid; the enzyme, pepsin, of the gastric juice works only in an acid medium and is prevented from working by an alkali.

It should be equally well known that the chemical changes that take place in the cells and tissues are instigated by enzymes, of which there are a number in every living thing. Simple sugar (monosaccharide) is absorbed from the intestine and carried to the liver where it is converted, by an enzyme, into glycogen (animal starch) and stored until used. When the body needs sugar the glycogen is reconverted into sugar, again by enzymic action. It is now general knowledge that insulin secreted by the pancreas is necessary to the metabolization (oxidation) of sugar and that when the pancreas fails to turn out sufficient insulin, unoxidized sugar is excreted in the urine.

A number of autolytic enzymes are known and are included under the general terms, *oxidases* and *peroxidases*. Physiologists know that proteolytic (protein digesting) enzymes are formed within many, if not in all, living tissues.

These various intra-cellular enzymes play a conspicious part in the metabolism of food substances; that is, in the normal or regular function of nutrition or metabolism. A few familiar examples of autolysis will prepare the reader for what is to follow about tumors.

When a bone is broken, a bone-ring support is built around the fractured section, extending each way from the point of fracture. After the bone is reunited and knitting or healing is completed, and the circulatory channels are re-established, the bone-ring support is softened and absorbed, except about a quarter of an inch about the point of fracture.

If planaria, or flat worms, are cut into small pieces and placed where they can absorb nourishment, each piece will grow into a small worm. If they cannot get nourishment, they cannot grow. Each piece, therefore, completely re-arranges its materials and becomes a perfect, but very minute worm. The piece that contains the pharynx, finding this too large for its diminished size, will dissolve it and make a new one that fits its new size.

The manner in which an abscess "points" on the surface of the body and drains its septic contents on the outside is well known to everyone of my readers. What is not generally known, is that this "pointing" on the surface is possible only because the flesh between the abscess and the surface is digested by enzymes; that is, it is autolyzed and removed.

Certain animals have specialized stores in which they store up a reserve of nutrition to feed them during periods of scarcity or during hibernation. These physiological store-houses are analogous to the "water tank" possessed by the camel. Examples of this are the big-tailed sheep of Persia, the gila monster of our Western plains and the Russian bear. Other animals, including man, possess only the generalized reserves found in the bone-marrow, liver, blood, fatty tissue, etc., and the private reserve possessed by each cell in the body.

Both types of animals may draw upon these reserves for supplies with which to nourish their vital tissues, if raw materials from without are not to be had; or, if, due to sickness, they cannot be digested.

These tissues (fatty tissue, bone marrow, etc.) and food substances (glycogen) are not fit to enter the blood stream before they are acted upon by enzymes. Indeed human fat, or human muscle is no more fitted to enter the circulation without first being digested, than is fat or muscle from the cow or sheep. Glycogen (animal starch), stored in the liver, must be converted into a simple sugar before it can be released into the blood stream. This conversion is accomplished by enzymic action.

Many more examples of autolysis could be given, but enough have been presented to convince the reader that it is a common fact of everyday life. It remains now to show that the body possesses control over this process, just as it does over all the other processes of life: that the process is not a blind, undirected bull-in-a-china-shop affair.

A remarkable example of this control is afforded by the piece of diced plenarium that contains the pharynx. Here is manifest the ability to tear down a part and shift its constituent materials. The same thing is seen in the softening and absorption of the bone-ring support around a point of fracture. Only part of the bone-ring is digested, the remainder is allowed to remain to reinforce the weakened structure.

The phenomena of fasting supply many examples of the control the body exercises over its autolytic processes. For instance, tissues are lost in the inverse order of their usefulness — fat and morbid growths first, and then the other tissues. In all animals, from worms to man, the various organs and tissues differ very greatly in their rates of loss while fasting. Usually the liver loses more in weight relative to the rest of the body than the other organs, especially in the earlier stages, due to the loss of glycogen and fat. The lungs lose almost nothing and the brain and nervous system still less.

The vital tissues are fed on the stored reserves and the less vital tissues, so that abstinence from food can produce damage only after the body's reserves have been exhausted.

The body possesses the ability to shift its chemicals and fasting furnishes many remarkable instances of this. The digestion and reorganization of parts seen in worms and other animals, when deprived of food, the digestion and redistribution of reserves and surpluses and non-vital tissues, as seen in all animals, when forced to go without food, constitute, for the writer, some of the most marvelous phenomena in the whole realm of biology.

The body is not only able to build tissue; it can also destroy tissue. It can not only distribute its nutritive supplies; it can also re-distribute them. Autolysis makes redistribution possible.

I propose now to show the reader that this process of autolysis can be put to great practical use and be made to serve us in getting rid of tumors and other growths in the body. This fact is not exactly new for it has been known for a long time. Over a hundred years ago, Sylvester Graham wrote that when more food is used by the body than is daily supplied "it is a general law of the vital economy" that "the decomposing absorbents (the old term for the process of autolysis) always first lay hold of and remove those substances which are of least use to the economy; and hence, all morbid accumulations, such as wens, tumors, abscesses, etc., are rapidly diminished and often wholly removed under severe and protracted abstinence and fasting."

To fully understand this, it is necessary for the reader to know that tumors are made up of flesh and blood and bone. There are many names for the different kinds of tumors, but the names all indicate the kind of tissue of which the tumor is composed. For instance, an osteoma is made up of bone tissue; a myoma is composed of muscular tissue; a neuroma is constituted of nerve tissue; a lipoma consists of fatty tissue, etc.

Tumors being composed of tissues, the same kinds of tissues as the other structures of the body, are susceptible of autolytic disintegration, the same as normal tissue, and do, as a matter of experience, undergo dissolution and absorption under a variety of circumstances, but especially during a fast. The reader who can understand how fasting reduces the amount of fat on the body and how it reduces the size of the muscles, can also understand how it will reduce the size of a tumor, or cause it to disappear altogether. He needs, then, only to realize that the process of dis-integrating (autolyzing) the tumor takes place much more rapidly than it does in the normal tissues.

In his *Notes on Tumors*, a work for students of pathology, Francis Carter Wood says: "In a very small proportion of human malignant tumors spontaneous disappearance for longer or shorter periods has been noted. The greatest number of such disappearances has followed incomplete surgical removal of the tumor; they have occurred next in order of frequency during some acute febrile process, and less frequently in connection with some profound alteration of the metabolic processes of the organism, such as extreme cachexia, artificial menopause, or the puerperium."

No more profound change in metabolism is possible than that produced by fasting and the change is of a character best suited to bring about the autolysis of a tumor, malignant or otherwise.

The conditions Dr. Wood mentions as causing spontaneous disappearance of tumors are, for the most part, "accidents" and are not within the range of voluntary control. Fasting, on the other hand, may be instituted and carried on under control and at any time desired. It is the rule that operations are followed by increased growth in the tumor. Spontaneous disappearance following incomplete removal is rare. The same may be said for extreme cachexia and artificial menopause. In' fevers we have rapid autolysis in many tissues of the body and much curative work going on, but we cannot develop a fever at will. Pregnancy and childbirth occasion many profound changes in the body, but they are certainly not to be recommended to sick women as cures for their tumors. Even if this were desirable, it would be a hit-or-miss remedy. The effects of fasting are certain. There is nothing hit-or-miss about the process. It works always in the same general direction.

Fever is a curative process and does help to remove the cause of the tumor. None of Dr. Wood's other causes of spontaneous disappearance assist in removing the cause of tumors. Fasting does assist greatly in the removal of such cause.

During a fast the accumulations of superfluous tissues are overhauled and analyzed; the available component parts are turned over to the department of nutrition to be utilized in nourishing the essential tissues; the refuse is thoroughly and permanently removed.

I could quote numerous men of wide experience with fasting to corroborate what I am going to say about autolysing tumors, but I do not desire to weary my reader with quotations. I will content myself with one quotation. Mr. Macfadden says: "My experience of fasting has shown me beyond all possible doubt that a foreign growth of any kind can be absorbed into the circulation by simply compelling the body to use every unnecessary element contained within it for food. When a' foreign growth has become hardened sometimes one long fast will not accomplish the result, but where they are soft, the fast will usually cause them to be absorbed."

Due to a variety of circumstances, some known, others unknown, the rate of absorption of tumors in fasting individuals varies. Let me cite two extreme cases to show the wide range of variation in this process.

A woman, under forty, had a uterine fibroid about the size of an average grapefruit. It was completely absorbed in twenty-eight days of total abstinence from all food but water. This was an unusually rapid rate of absorption.

Another case is that of a similar tumor in a woman of about the same age. In this case the growth was about the size of a goose egg. One fast of twenty-one days reduced the tumor to the size of an English walnut. The fast was broken due to the return of hunger. Another fast a few weeks subsequent, of seventeen days, was required to complete the absorption of the tumor. This was an unusually slow rate of tumor-absorption.

Tumor-like lumps in female breasts ranging from the size of a pea to that of a goose egg will disappear in from three days to as many weeks. Here is a remarkable case of this kind that will prove both interesting and instructive to the reader.

A young lady, age 21, had a large hard lump — a little smaller than a billiard ball — in her right breast. For four months it had caused her considerable pain. Finally she consulted a physician who diagnosed the condition, cancer, and urged immediate removal. She went to another, and another and still another physician, and each made the same diagnosis (an unusual thing) and each urged immediate removal.

Instead of resorting to surgery the young lady resorted to fasting and in exactly three days without food, the "cancer" and all its attendant pain were gone.

There has been no recurrence in thirteen years and I feel that we are justified in considering the condition cured.

Hundreds of such occurrences under fasting have convinced us that many "tumors" and "cancers" are removed by surgeons that are not tumors or cancers. They cause us to be very skeptical of the statistics issued to show that early operation prevents or cures cancer.

The removal of tumors by autolysis has several advantages over their surgical removal. Surgery is always dangerous; autolysis is a physiological process and carries no danger. Surgery always lowers vitality and thus adds to the metabolic pervertion that is back of the tumor. Fasting, by which autolysis of tumors is accelerated, normalizes nutrition and permits the elimination of accumulated toxin, thus helping to remove the cause of the tumor. After surgical removal tumors tend to recur. After their autolytic removal, there is little tendency to recurrence. Tumors often recur in malignant form after their operative removal. The tendency to malignancy is removal by fasting.

In Europe and America literally thousands of tumors have been autolyzed during the past fifty years, and the effectiveness of the method is beyond doubt. The present writer can give no definite information about bone tumors and nerve

tumors; but, since these are subject to the same
laws of nutrition as all other tumors, he is dis-
posed to think they may be autolyzed as effectual-
ly as other tumors. These things are certain —
the process has its limitations and tumors that
have been allowed to grow to enormous sizes will
only be reduced in size; while, not all cysts will
be thus absorbed. It is advisable, therefore,
to undergo the needed fast or fasts while the
tumor or cyst is comparatively small.

One other limitation must be noted; namely,
tumors that are so situated that they dam-up the
lymph stream will continue to grow (feeding
upon the accumulated excess of lymph behind
them) despite fasting.

In cases where complete absorption is not
obtained, the tumor is sufficiently reduced in size
not to constitute a menace. Thereafter proper
living will prevent added growth. Indeed, we
have seen a number of cases where a further decrease in size followed right living subsequent
to fasting.

Index

CHAPTER   PAGE

Introduction 5
Orthopathy — Physiological Lawfulness 8
Disease a Vital Process 10
Organic Unity — Its Relation to Cure ... 14
Toxemia 19
Foci of Infection 27
Health First 33
Half-Way Houses of Science 37
Allergy 40
The Fallacy of Diagnosis 47
Rational Care of the Sick 54
Reform vs Cure 60
Avoiding and Remedying Colds 63
What Caused the Quints' Tonsillar Troubles? 71
Bronchitis 81
Sinusitis 86
Bronchial Asthma 92
Hay Fever 99
The Ductless Glands 105
Goitre 114
Colitis 120
Peptic Ulcer 127
Diabetes Mellitus 137
Arthritis — Rheumatism — Gout 142
High Blood Pressure 148
Acne 154
Goodbye to Neuralgia 160
Neuritis 167
Infantile Paralysis 172
Fasting for Children 177
Fasting in Heart Disease 179
Hunger Pains 182
Gluttony a Neurosis 186
Fasting and the Teeth 189
Fictional Objections to Fasting 194
Exercise and the Heart 198
Mixing Acids with Proteins 202
Autolyzing Tumors 207

FOOD and FEEDING

—BY—

HERBERT M. SHELTON, D.P., N.D., D.N.T.

—AUTHOR OF—

Fundamentals of Nature Cure
Principles and Practices of Orthopathy
Living Life to Live it Longer
Author of "Living To Live."—N. Y. Eve. Graphic

Editor of How To Live

Professor of Naturopathy,
American School of Naturopathy
New York City.

Published by How To Live Pub. Co.,
Hugo, Oklahoma.
1926

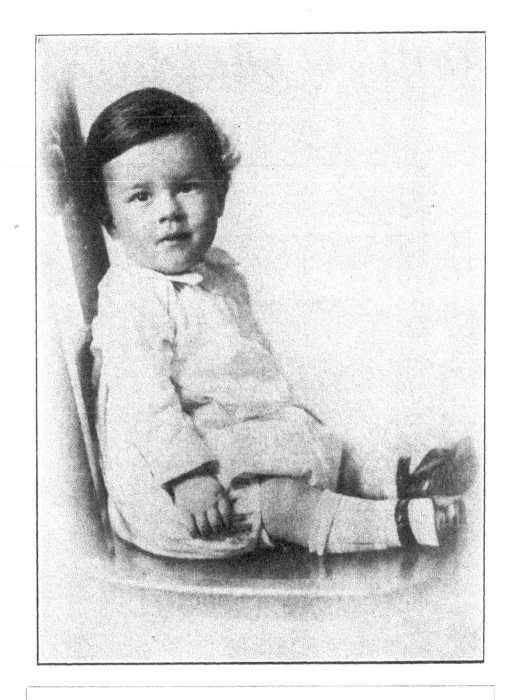

TO MY SON, BERNARR HERBERT SHELTON, WHOSE SUPERB
HEALTH, UNUSUAL STRENGTH AND SUNNY DISPOSITION
IS DUE TO THE PRINCIPLES PRESENTED IN THESE PAGES,
THIS BOOK IS LOVINGLY DEDICATED, BY THE AUTHOR.

HERBERT M. SHELTON.

Introduction

There are so many books on diet now that it would seem a work of supreme egotism to write another. However, this book is intended to be different and in being different, it is intended to fill a place that is filled by no other book on this subject.

Most worthwhile books on diet are written by specialists who have become obscured by the subject of their specialty and have allowed themselves to become more or less one-sided. Often they are unable to see the other side of a question. Many diet specialists are simply laboratory workers who work with test-tubes, rats, chickens, etc., and announce their discoveries, perhaps prematurely, to a credulous world. These men go on day after day, seemingly unaware that their theories fail in practice. Then, there is another class of books that are written by those who are neither laboratory men nor physicians. I know of one work on diet written by a man who is advertised as an authority on diet. This man is only a journalist.

In writing this book I had in mind giving my readers a working knowledge of dietetics as it has been so far worked out in the laboratory and in practical experience. I have studied all the various systems of diet and tried them out. I am familiar with their successes and failures, their shortcomings and defects. While teaching dietetics in the American School of Naturopathy, I was handicapped by the lack of a reliable and complete text-book on the subject. No such book exists. We were forced to draw upon a variety of sources and, more than ever before, I was struck by the differences of opinion and claims presented by the various writers on diet. Often my own bewilderment was about as great as that of the students. I often asked myself: ''If I become so bewildered in these studies, what must be the state of mind produced in the layman by all these conflicting claims?'' I set myself the task of unraveling the problem and I am convinced that I have presented the true solution in the final chapter of this book. Although the principles laid down in that chapter run through all the other chapters of the book, I have thought it well to lay special emphasis upon these in this final chapter. It is chiefly these principles that make this book different and reveal why a diet works or appears to at one time and fails at another.

In the final chapter of this book I have tried to impress upon the reader the fact that every case must be handled individually. The practice of dietetics as I have set it forth in these pages might be summed up in three propositions, viz.,—

1. Feed such foods as will supply to the body all the necessary food elements in an assimilable form.

2. Feed such combinations and under such conditions as will insure perfect digestion and avoid gastro-intestinal fermentation and putrefaction. The chief purpose of careful eating is to avoid decomposition.

3. Make all the corrections in the patients manner of living that are necessary to insure normal function of all the organs of the body to the end that nutrition and drainage may be normal.

I believe that if these three aims are kept in mind and purpose, the problems of dietetics will soon clarify themselves.

I have not deemed it worthwhile to give the reader a long table of the analyses of various foods. Such tables would be understood only if you have a knowledge of Organic and Physiological Chemistry and would be of little value to you even then. My object has been to teach you how to eat. I trust I have accomplished this.

CHAPTER 1
Diet As a Factor in Health

Among the useful things in regaining and maintaining health, strength, youth and beauty, diet holds a chief seat. Its value is coming to be recognized more and more by both the laity and the medical profession. Nature Curists have given dietetics a prominent place in their practice from the very beginning. Indeed, it can truthfully be said that until recently about all the knowledge about diet that was of any advantage was confined to the ranks of Nature Cure.

There is and has been such a multiplicity of conflicting plans and theories about diet, every one of which, were claimed by their proponents, to be the one true system that the student has been more inclined to decide that they are all wrong, and give up in despair and disgust, than to continue with his studies. However, most of the plans and systems of diet have a grain of truth in them, which, if separated from the chaff, will be found very useful. Dietetics is really not a complex subject and is not hard to understand and apply when properly presented. In these chapters we shall attempt to present the most important of these principles and explain them in a way that will enable the reader to apply them to himself and the members of his household in an intelligent manner.

Dietetics is the science and art of correct eating and involves a knowledge of the proper selection, proportion, combination and quantity of foods and their use, in different climates, and seasons; in the different stages of life and the varying conditions of life and labor; together with a knowledge of how and when to eat. This may all seem complicated at first glance but we assure you that before you have completed these chapters you will begin to see how simple and easy it all is. You will realize too how natural and sensible the whole plan is and will wonder why these things were not found earlier in history. For this knowledge will save health, life and expense.

During life two simultaneous processes are in continual progress—a building up and breaking down process. The two processes taken together are called metabolism. The constructive process is known as anabolism; the breaking down process as katabolism. In the healthy organism during childhood and youth and well into maturity the constructive process exceeds the destructive process. During sickness and in old age the destructive process exceeds the building up.

It is to supply material with which to carry on the building up and replace that which is broken down; in other words, to supply material for growth and repair; that we eat. At least this is one of the purposes served by food. It serves other purposes also.

Other processes besides those of growth and repair are continually going on in the body. For instance, there is the work of preparing food for use by the body. This work is known as digestion and is accomplished largely by the action of certain juices or secretions which act upon the food chemically. These juices have to be manufactured by the body for its own use. Food furnishes the necessary material for the production of these and the many other secretions of the body.

The broken down products of the cells are acid in character and are highly irritating and poisonous. If permitted to remain in the body unchanged they would soon destroy life. Therefore, they are not only eliminated, but are changed chemically by being combined with certain alkaline mineral elements, thus rendering them less irritating and harmful and also preparing them for elimination. The mineral elements with which this detoxifying change is made are supplied by our food.

Foods are also burned in the body to supply heat and energy.

The normal alkilinity and normal specific gravity of the blood is maintained by food.

These uses of food may be summed up in a few words

by saying: Food is any substance which, when taken into the body can be used by it for the replenishment of tissue (growth and repair) and for the performance of organic function. This definition can be made to include the oxygen of the air, however, oxygen is not usually classed as a food. Such substances if they are to be classed as true foods must be without deleterious effects. Many things that are eaten by man have deleterious effects although they do possess food value. Obviously, such foods should be abstained from as long as other foods are to be had.

To accomplish the many purposes served by food only a few elements are required. Of the eighty or ninety elements which chemical science has so far recognized some sixteen are essential constituents of the human body. These are:

Iron	Potassium	Silicon
Calcium	Magnesium	Nitrogen
Phosphorus	Manganise	Oxygen
Sulphur	Carbon	Chlorine
Sodium	Hydrogen	Iodine
		Florine

Other elements have been found but as yet their function in the system is not understood. In fact, it has not been determined whether they are normal constituents of the body or are foreign substances that have been taken into the body.

These 16 elements are used in the structure and functions of man's body. They must be supplied from the outside by food. It by no means follows, however, that any substance containing one or more of the elements can be used as food. Crude rock phosphorous as it comes from the mines is a powerful poison. Its use in the manufacture of matches has been prohibited by law because of its poisonous character. It is often administered as a medicine, but its continued use, even in small doses causes emanciation and anemia.

Man cannot supply his body with sulphur by eating it in its crude mineral form.

The same is true of iron. Iron is essential to health

and life. But it cannot be supplied by eating saw filings or railroad rails. This too is often administered in drug form. If long continued it upsets digestion producing gastric distress, causes headache and constipation.

Calcium (lime) cannot be supplied the organism by eating crude lime rock, or chalk. Lime in this form is an irritant and if in the "unslacked" condition is extremely destructive of the soft tissues, while in the slacked state is still destructive of these. The attempt to supply the body with lime in this way would prove disastrous.

The same is true of the other elements of the body. A handful of soil contains all sixteen of the needed elements but we cannot beat the high cost of living by consuming dirt. These elements, to be useful to the body and not harmful must be in the organic form—that is, they must be supplied to the system in the form in which they are found in fruits and vegetables.

The power to assimilate crude inorganic matter as it is found in the soil and convert it into living protoplasm and other organic substances or to use such substances in performing physiological function does not belong to the animal organism. It is the office of plant life or vegetation to convert the primary elements from their crude inorganic state into the organic state. This conversion cannot be accomplished by any synthetic process known to the laboratory.

After the plant has raised the crude inorganic matter of the soil into plant protoplasm the animal may take these and raise them to a still higher plane—that of animal protoplasm. But the animal cannot do the work of the plant. He must get his food either directly or indirectly from the plant kingdom. That is, the animal must either eat the plant or its fruits (as in the case of vegetarian and fruitarian animals) or (as in the case of the carniverous animals) he must eat the animal that has eaten the plant. Food must be in the organic form. Air and water form the only exception to this rule.

Food substances as they come from the plant and animal contain:

(1) Nutritive matter,

(2) Water,

(3) Refuse—or waste.

The different articles of food are placed into different classes according to the food elements that predominate. Thus, there are:

1. PROTEIN FOODS: These are rich in protied which contains nitrogen as a distinguishing element. It also contains carbon, hydrogen and oxygen. Most proteins contain sulphur and some other elements. Chief among the protein foods are:

Lean meats of all kinds—including fish, poultry, etc.

Eggs—all varieties.

Legumes—beans, peas, lentils, peanuts.

Nuts—all kinds except chestnuts.

Olives.

Grains—all kinds.

2. CARBOHYDRATE FOODS: which are rich in carbohydrates (starches and sugars) which are composed of carbon, hydrogen and oxygen with hydrogen and oxygen in proportion to form water H_2O. Chief among the carbohydrate foods are:

Cereals and cereal products of all kinds.

Tubers—potatoes, sweet potatoes, carrots, artichokes, parsnips, etc.

Nuts—a few varieties—acorns, chestnuts and cocoanuts.

Fruits—bananas, all sweet fruits, hubbard squash, etc.

3. HYDROCARBONS: which are rich in hydrocarbons (fats and oils) which contains carbon, hydrogen and oxygen. Fats and oils (hydrocarbons) are manufactured in the body from carbohydrates and proteins. Chief among the hydrocarbons are:

Dairy products—cream, butter and some cheese.

Flesh of dead animals, especially pork, mutton and beef that has been fattened.

Fat fish—herring, shad, salmon, trout.

Legumes—peanuts, soy beans.

Nuts—almost all varieties.

Fruits—olives.

4. ORGANIC MINERALS (ash): These are essential to health and growth and cannot be substituted by inorganic elements. They are found in varying quantities in all food substances but are present in more abundant quantities in the succulent vegetables and juicy fruits. Chief among these are:

(1)   Succulent vegetables:

Tubers—asparagus, beet, carrot, turnip, radish, onion, cone artichoke, rutabaga, garlic.

Leafy vegetables—celery, lettuce, kohlrabi, cabbage, spinach, dandelion, endive, turnip tops, mustard, parsley, cauliflower, brussel sprouts, kale, chard, lotus, cress, field lettuce, romaine, chicory, rhubarb, beet tops, radish tops, etc.

Fruiting plants—okra (gumbo) cucumber, summer squash, pumpkin, string beans, green peas, corn "in milk" (fresh), oyster plant, etc.

(2)   Juicy Fruits:

Acid: Orange, (sour), lemon, lime, sour apple, grape fruit, pineapple, peach, sour plum, apricot, cranberry, gooseberry, loganberry, pomegranate, strawberry.

Sub-acid: sweet apple, sweet orange, pear, blackberry, mild grape, tomato, fresh prune, raspberry (red and black), avocado, cherry, currant (fresh), nectarine, plum.

Non-acid: Melons—water-melon, musk-melon, cantaloupe, casaba, honey dew, etc.—sweet grape, huckleberry, fresh fig, etc.

Many other foods are used both in America and other parts of the world but all may be placed in some one or the other of the above classes. Some foods such as nuts, grains and legumes may be placed in two classes.

The bountiful hand of mother nature has supplied us with an abundant and pleasing variety of foods. This wonderful variety of foods which are designed to please the senses of sight, taste and smell as well as supply the needs of the body are all made of but a few simple elements of the soil—"the dust of the earth."

Food forms the raw material from which the tissue elements used in repairing and reconstructing the body are taken. The process of cell renewal is constantly going on. These processes of cell destruction and cell renewal are much more rapid than the earlier physiologists thought. Some modern physiologists claim that the body is completely renewed in every part as often as once in every twelve months. This is probably not true in the case of the harder structures such as teeth and bones, although some claim this to be so, even in these.

From this it would appear to be true as one often hears stated: "Man is what he eats." This is, however, not true. What man eats plays a very important role in the human economy, but it is not the only important factor. It cannot even be said that a man is what he assimilates.

Every thought and action of an individual helps to make one what he or she is. What one eats, breathes, drinks, thinks, says and does, these with other factors such as exercise, sun and air, elimination and drainage, one's associates, etc., all have a part in making one. Yet, even these do not make man what he is. Heredity plays a very important part. If we feed a negro child and an English child on the same food, give them the same air to breathe and water to drink, rear them in the same environment, the one would grow up a negro, the other an Englishman. Heredity does this. Man is a product of heredity and environment plus his individual reaction to these. Food is only one of the factors making up man's environment.

Dr. Richard C. Cabot says: "Almost nothing is known about diet. There are numerous books on the subject which are useful for pressing leaves, but not for much that they contain."—A Layman's Handbook of Medicine.

From this one may see that Dr. Cabot who is one of the greatest living medical men, does not think much of medical and popular works on diet. We think, however, that the doctor is in error when he says: "Almost nothing is known about diet." In Nature Cure literature and Nature Cure schools is to be found a profound knowledge of the fundamentals of diet together with a thorough knowledge of the proper application of these principles. It shall be our endeavor in these chapters to present the reader with this knowledge in such a way that he or she shall be able to apply it in daily life.

Diet more, perhaps, than any other one factor is of vital importance in health and disease. More errors in eating are made by the average individual than in any other department of living. Present day eating might well be called a comedy of errors were its consequences not so serious. Haphazard eating is the rule and the person who maintains health by such eating does so only by chance. He is but one in a million. We should live by knowledge not by chance. The Bible says: "My children are killed for want of knowledge." If you want health, strength, youth, beauty and a long, useful life you must learn how to live to attain and preserve these. Learn how to eat, what to eat, etc.

CHAPTER 2
Nature's Food Refinery

Foods as we receive them from the bountiful hand of Nature are not fitted for entrance into the blood and lymph or for use by the cells. They must undergo a disorganizing and refining process by which the structure of the food is broken down and the useful is separated from the useless in food. This process is called digestion.

The process by which apples, corn, beans, celery, etc., are transformed into blood, bones, nerves, muscles, skin, hair, nails, etc., is intensely interesting and is worthy of the attention of every one. Digestion, the first step in this wonderful process, is the process by which food is prepared (in the mouth, stomach and intestines) for absorption into the blood and lymph to be used by the body. Digestion is carried on partly by mechanical, partly by chemical means. Mind, too, has an important role in this affair.

Before considering the processes of digestion let us get some idea of the work accomplished by these. First, it is a refining process breaking down the structure of the food and separating the nutritive portions from the waste or useless parts. Second; it splits up the large and complex molecules of food into smaller, less complex ones, in this way adding to the diffusibility of the food. Diffusibility is the capability of spreading and enables substances to pass through ordinary membrane. Lastly; it standardizes our food. By this we mean it obliterates many of the characteristics of the various foods consumed and gives us, finally, practically the same set of products whatever the meal eaten. From the many strange and foreign compounds that are taken into the mouth, as food, are formed a few acceptable compounds. From this it may be readily seen that digestion is both a complicated and interesting process.

The chemical part of digestion is performed by a series of digestive juices, alternating between alkalies and acids. The active principals in these juices or fluids are ferments known as enzymes. All true digestive juices contain enzymes. These are substances which possess the power of instigating chemical reactions, without themselves being transformed or destroyed in course of the process. Digestive enzymes bring about chemical changes in the food eaten. They are known as protein-splitting or proteolytic, fat-splitting or lipolytic, and starch-splitting or amylolytic, according to the type of food-stuff upon which they act. They are specific in their action, by which is meant, they are not capable of inciting several different reactions but each enzyme acts upon but one class of food. If a digestive juice affects two distinct types of food it is considered to contain two enzymes. They are destroyed by heat short of boiling and are prevented from acting by cold, although as a rule this does not prevent them from resuming their activity upon being warmed.

If they are compared with other chemicals a very striking peculiarity is disclosed. That is, enzymes are not used up in proportion to the work they do. If one is pouring hydrochloric acid upon iron to make hydrogen gas he is forced to continue pouring the acid if he is to continue evolving the gas. But if starch is being converted into sugar by ptyalin the amount of sugar formed depends less upon the amount of saliva present than upon the time. A small amount of digestive juice, containing a much smaller amount of enzymes, may, under favorable conditions, act continuously with but the most gradual loss of power.

Digestion begins in the mouth where the food is subjected to a mechanical process or grinding to break it up into smaller particles thus enabling the digestive juices to get at the food more readily. It also aids in mixing the saliva of the mouth with the food. Chewing or mastication is the only conscious work of digestion and all the subconscious processes depend upon how well this has been performed.

Simultaneously with the chewing of the food the digestive juice of the mouth is poured out upon and thoroughly mixed with it. Saliva, as it is called, is a colorless, odorless, tasteless, ropy fluid secreted chiefly by the parotid, submaxillary and sublingual glands. It is contributed to by the secretions from the bucal, palatine, lingual, molar and tonsilar glands. In man it is normally alkaline in reaction, although, during fevers, while fasting, when there are digestive disturbances, and between midnight and morning it may become acid. About 1500 grams, or between one and two quarts are secreted in twenty-four hours.

Its secretion is not a simple filtration due to blood pressure but is accomplished by the action of the cells composing these glands. In common with all the cells of the body these exercise a selective power by which they select from the blood stream the elements needed in the manufacture of saliva and reject the rest. The salivary glands are under nerve control which secures coordination.

The active principle in saliva is an enzyme known as ptyalin which acts upon starches, converting these into a form of sugar known as dextrines. Ptyalin is lacking in the saliva of all carniverous and some other animals. In these the saliva, is not a true digestive juice, but acts, solely to moisten the food thus enabling the animal to swallow it.

Ptyalin is not present in the saliva when food is taken into the mouth that does not contain starch. The tongue contains various sets of taste buds among which are proteid and starch buds. The function of taste not only affords us pleasure, but is an all important element in the subconscious processes of digestion. Particularly it serves to stimulate the flow of the digestive juices, especially those of the stomach, and to suit their character to the food eaten. The nerve impulses set into motion by the taste of food sets the mechanism into action necessary to digestion. The character of food eaten determines through the taste buds the character of the digestive juices released to act upon it. Saliva will be poured into the mouth but no ptyalin will be present if the food eaten contains no starch. Even sugar, if put into the mouth will not occasion the release of ptyalin although, the mouth will quickly fill with saliva.

After food is masticated it is swallowed and enters the stomach where the work of digesting the starch continues until sufficient gastric juice has been poured into the stomach cavity to render its contents acid. The enzyme, ptalin, is destroyed by acid in a minute percentage. The reader is asked to keep this fact in mind as we shall have occasion to refer to it in dealing with food combinations.

In the stomach the food is slowly mixed, by the movements of the stomach, with the gastric juice. This is a clear, colorless fluid, strongly acid in reaction and possessing a characteristic odor. It is secreted by many small glands situated in the walls of the stomach, and contains an enzyme known as pepsin which acts upon proteins and acts only in an acid medium. Besides pepsin it contains two other enzymes—renin, which coagulates the casein of milk and gastric lipase, a fat-splitting enzyme. It also contains mineral matters and hydrochloric acid. The hydrochloric acid (commercially known as muriatic acid and used as a soldering acid) is very powerful and literally eats to pieces the food it permeates. It would soon destroy the stomach except for the fact that its walls are continually protected by an alkaline secretion. This alkaline bath in which the stomach is kept in analagous to the water bath some furnaces have to be kept in to prevent them from melting. It sometimes happens that the alkaline protection becomes weak in some spots and then the acid eats a hole in the inner coat of the stomach producing an ugly sore or ulcer. This acid also counteracts putrefaction and enables the pepsin to work; it aids in regulating the sphincters of the stomach and assists in awakening the pancreas to activity.

Gastric juice is secreted much in response to stimuli from the higher centers. As we noted before, taste buds aid in regulating its secretion. Through the medium of taste the flow of gastric juice is regulated. For instance if starch or other non-protein foods are eaten a gastric juice will be secreted which differs from that secreted when proteins are eaten. The sight and smell of food also aid in regulating the flow of gastric juice.

In the well known experiments upon Saint Martin it was found that a piece of metal could be introduced into the stomach but it would not occasion any flow of gastric juice. If, however, someone entered the room with a platter of steaming steak, the instant the man's eyes fell upon this the gastric juice would begin to flow into the stomach. When no gastric juice was needed none was supplied. Pavlow, introduced into the stomach of a sleeping dog (through a fistula) 100 grams of flesh. After an hour and a half the flesh was withdrawn by means of a string to which the meat had been tied. The loss of the meat was only six grams. This same amount of meat (100 grams) was again introduced into the stomach through the fistula, after the dog had been allowed to see and smell the meat. Under these conditions the weight of the meat was reduced 30 grams in the same time. The reader will readily perceive the importance of such facts in diet. They teach us that food must be seen, smelled, tasted if digestion is to proceed normally. But the food must not be so disguised by condiments, spices, etc., as to deceive the senses as this will prevent the setting into motion, through the nerves, of the mechanism necessary to digestion.

The flow into the stomach of gastric juice is apparently in advance of the actual arrival of food and seems to be proportional to the pleasure afforded by eating. This should teach us that the pleasure we derive from eating is only a means to an end and not the end itself.

Pepsin, is a protien splitting enzyme, which, as noted above, acts only in an acid medium, and converts proteins into peptones. Beyond coagulating the casein of milk rennin appears to have no other function. Gastric lipase has but little effect upon fats.

The secretion of gastric juice is hastened or retarded by a number of factors the chief of which are here given:

Accelerated by:
  (1) hunger
  (2) pleasureable taste
  (3) sight and smell of food
  (4) thoughts of food

Retarded by:
  (1) fear, worry, anxiety, anger and other destructive emotions
  (2) failure to taste food
  (3) absence of hunger

(5) joy, happiness, etc.
(6) effects of food on lining of stamach
(7) ingestion of water
(8) secretagogues arising
as by-products of the
process of digestion.

(4) lack of proper sali-
vary digestion
(5) pain, fever, etc.

When the work of digestion is completed in the stomach the food is poured through the pyloric orifice into the small intestines where it undergoes further changes. There are three digestive juices which are poured into the intestines all of which are alkaline in reaction.

The first of these, the pancreatic juice, is secreted by the pancreas and enters the intestines just below the union of the stomach and duodenum or upper portion of the small intestine. This juice, the secretion of which is excited by the action of the acid contents received from the stomach upon the walls of the intestines, is poured out about the time the contents of the stomach pass through the pyloric valve.

Pancreatic juice contains three enzymes. One of these known as diastase or amylase resembles ptyalin and continues the work of digesting starches and sugars converting these into a form of sugar known as monosaccharides. It is not destroyed by the acid contents of the stomach as is ptyalin. A second, known as trypsin, is a protein splitting enzyme, but unlike pepsin, does not require the cooperation of an acid to accomplish its work. In fact, it is destroyed by a strong acid. By its action the peptones are converted into amino-acids. The third enzyme known as liapase causes fats to undergo cleavage forming fatty acids and **glycerine.**

The second of the juices poured into the intestines is bile. This is secreted by the liver and enters the intestines at about the point where the pancreatic juice enters. Its secretion goes on continuously but is accelerated after meals. It contains no enzyme and is, therefore, **not a true** digestive juice; but acts chiefly by producing a **favorable** environment for the action of the pancreatic enzymes. If it is prevented from entering the intestines the ability to digest and absorb foods, particularly fats, is reduced. Bile increases the solubility of the fatty acids by emulsification, accelerates the action of the pancreatic liapase, stimulates intestinal activity, counteracts putrefaction, and assists in the union of water and oils.

The third or intestinal juice is secreted in abundance by small glands situated in the walls of the small intestines. It contains an enzyme known as erepsin which co-operates with trypsin in the final stages of protein digestion. This juice also completes the preparation of carbohydrates for entrance into the blood.

Finally, when the work of digestion is completed in the intestines the carbohydrates have been reduced to a form of sugar known as monosacchanides, the fats have been converted into fatty acids and glycreol and the proteins have been reduced to amino-acids. Water and salts undergo no change. The waste portions of the food are separated from the usable portions and are sent on into the large intestines or colon to be expelled.

So long as the body is normal the digestive secretions are sufficient protection against the fermentation and putrefaction of food which would otherwise be set up by microbes. However, if the vital powers are lowered so that the secretions are deficient in quality or insufficient in quantity, or if there is disease which impairs the digestive powers bacterial fermentation sets in and we have indigestion. The fermentation produces toxins of various kinds which when absorbed into the blood and lymph serve to poison the body. Some of these poisons are the ptomains, leucomains, indol, phenol, cresol, leucin, tyrson, ammonia, sulphurated hydrogen, fatty acids, oxalic and uric acids, alcohol and the Xanthin bodies. Of these, indol is the most easily absorbed and is most readily recognized in the urine.

The chief causes of gastro-intestinal indigestion are overeating, enervation and bad combinations. Enervating influences are anything that lower nerve force and includes such things as overwork, underwork, extremes of cold and heat, use of stimulants, sexual excesses, etc. Anything that enervates lessens digestive power and becomes an indirect cause of indigestion.

Overeating, overworks the digestive organs as well as introducing more food into the system than is needed. Food eaten in excess is bound to accumulate as waste and decompose as poison. The injurious effects of working after eating will be discussed in a later chapter.

From the differences in the results of fermentation and those of digestion it should be apparent that, although, the enzymes are spoken of as ferments, they do not produce fermentation. Rather the digestive juices and their enzymes act as powerful solvents—for, (and keep this fact in mind) digestion reduces food stuffs to the diffusible state without depriving them of their organic qualities while fermentation renders it diffusible by reducing it to the inorganic and therefore useless state. Digestion is solution; fermentation is disintegration.

Before food can be of any value to the body it must be carried to the cells. In order to do this it is necessary that it be removed from the intestinal canal and taken up by the blood and lymph. The process by which this is accomplished is termed absorption.

Some absorption takes place in the stomach and a small amount, chiefly of water takes place in the colon. The small intestine due to its peculiar structure is specialized for the work of absorption. The greater part of the food is absorbed from this.

Some part of the process of absorption may be explained by the laws of diffusion and osmosis, but only a small part of it may be so explained. We are forced to make due allowance for the fact that the cells lining the small intestines are living. The walls of the intestines do not behave like a dead membrane. Every epitheliel cell lining the digestive tract is in itself a complete organism, a living being, with the most complete function. These exercise a selective capacity by which, in a normal condition, they permit the absorption of good food and prevent the absorption of a whole series of poisons which are readily soluble in the digestive juices. It is a physiological not a physical process. One of active selection and absorption and not mere osmosis.

This is well illustrated by the following well known facts. Certain substances which are rated by ordinary standards, as highly diffusible are not allowed to pass through the intestinal lining. Magnesium sulphate (epsom salts) and grape sugar will serve as an excellent example of this. When a test is made with parchment or any ordinary membrane the sugar is found to be less diffusable than salts. In the intestines this is reversed. The sugar is readily absorbed while the salt is excluded almost entire.

This selection of the good and useful and rejection of the injurious and useless is done by the cells lining the walls of the intestines as *these take up the food from the intestines and secrete it into the blood stream.*

Some of the salts seem to be absorbed in the stomach. However, most of these together with the monosaccharides, amino-acids, fatty acids and glyctrol are absorbed from the small intestine. By this is meant these compounds disappear from the intestine. It by no means follows that they enter the blood as such. It seems probable that they undergo some changes during their passage through the cells. This is known to be true of the fatty acids and soap for these are changed in their passage through the cells and enter the blood as neutral fat.

Proteins belonging to one class of animals will not nourish another class of animals, if injected directly into the circulation without undergoing digestive changes. The protein (albumen) of an egg if injected directly into the circulation acts as a poison and is immediately expelled. The proteins of nuts, wheat, cheese or milk, mutton, beef, eggs, chicken, etc., are all different and distinct but each and all of these may be used to nourish the human body. However, before they can be so used they must first be converted into a particular class of proteins. If they are not so converted they not only do not nourish the body, but if they are forced into the blood stream they act as real poisons.

In spite of the many changes the proteins of the various foods undergo in the stomach and intestine they still remain the protein peculiar to those foods—eggs, beef, mutton, beans, etc. However, during their passage through the intestinal walls these proteins undergo some change (of a nature wholely unknown) which fits them for entrance into the body. For no sooner than these have passed through the intestinal wall into the circulation, than their nature is changed. They are now "human proteids."

Once the food is in the blood stream it is carried to all parts of the body to nourish the cells and to be used for the various purposes which food serves. The food material may be conveyed directly to the liver, or if may be carried through the lymphatic system. It appears, as a general rule, that the proteins and fats are conveyed directly to the liver while the carbohydrates are sent by the other route. When the food reaches the cell it is subjected to still further changes which are apparently due to enzymic action, before they are finally incorporated by the cell.

CHAPTER 3
Uses of Food

If the processes of digestion seem complex and but little understood the processes of nutrition are much more so. While nutrition is claimed to be purely chemical, it is acknowledged, by even the most materialistic, to be different in many ways from the other chemical processes known to us. This is particularly true of the final stages of the process by which the pabulum is transformed into living tissue. By this final act dead matter is raised to the plane of living matter.

Even Prof. Chittenden was forced to acknowledge that this "involves a chemical alteration or change akin to that of bringing the dead to life"; while Dr. Charlton Bastian, F. R. S., London, argued that these facts of nutrition, particularly those of the plant, in which inorganic matter is converted into the organic substances of the plant, prove to us the possibility of the creation of life from the non-living. All of which shows, that, while the digestion of food materials and their conversion into living tissues is considered to be purely chemical, these are far different from any chemical action and reactions known to the laboratory, even though the chemist may be able to discover no difference. It cannot be disputed that if the substances are the same and the processes and changes are identical the products would be, to say the least, very similar. But no chemist can even imitate the work done by plant and animal nutrition. The great mystery of nutrition is still unexplained. We can no more explain today how food material is changed into living human flesh and blood than could the lowest savage of a thousand years ago.

It is certain, however, that much of the changes the food undergoes after being absorbed is due to the action of enzymes. For instance there is antolytir arids, found in the tissues generally, which split the amino-acids into simpler compounds. Then there are guanase found in the thymus, adrenals and pancreas, which changes guanin to Xanthin; adenase, found in the pancreas, liver and spleen, which changes adrenin to hypoxanthin and the okidoses found in the liver, lungs, muscles, etc., which cause oxidation, as of hypozanthin to xanthin, and of xanthin to uric acid. No effort will be made at this place to take these matters up in detail. The reader who may be interested in pursuing these still further is referred to any of the standard works on nutrition. We must devote our attention to the use of foods.

Let us begin with the proteins, since these have been the subject of more discussion than any other part of our food, and are considered, by orthodox scientists, to be the most important of all the elements of our food. All this came about as a result of the mistakes of the early physiological chemists, particularly Liebig and Vogt of Germany. These found that muscle is almost pure protein and water and Liebig thought we should eat muscle to make muscle. Of course, the cow eats grass, not muscle, out of which she makes the muscle Liebig would have us eat, but this simple fact was overlooked.

Voigt followed Liebig with a series of experiments on dogs. This was about 1860. With these he thought he had succeeded in proving the great physiological importance of protein. It was assumed that muscular activity is due to the oxidation of the muscle cells themselves. It was a case of mistaking the machine for the fuel; yet, on the basis of this assumption Voigt, with the aid of his dogs, estimated that the average man requires about 118 grams of protein daily. He seems later to have reduced this standard by nearly one half, but no one took the reduction seriously.

The Voigt standard is now known to be much too high. Protein leaves the body through the kidneys in the form of urea. In fact, the composition of the urine depends more upon the protein (nitrogen) intake than upon anything else. By measuring the excretions and comparing it with the food consumed it is possible to tell whether less protein or more protein is being lost than is being consumed. Examinations of the urine under almost all conceivable conditions of life and activity, have shown that in the healthy adult the nitrogen intake and output is balanced, providing, of course, the intake is not less than the actual needs of the body.

The amino-acids (proteins) have been termed the "building-stones" of the body since these, next to water, form the largest part of all the tissues of the body. However, the body's requirement for these for building purposes is very small. No matter how much nitrogen one consumes above the body's requirements the organism always responds in the same way. That is, it sets aside for excretion all surplus nitrogen. So unless the nitrogen intake is less than the body's requirement the balance is usually struck between income and outgo. Exceptions to this are during growth, following a protracted fast, convalescence, after wasting illness and pregnancy during which periods they excrete less nitrogen than is consumed; and during some diseases in which there is a rapid breaking down of tissue and consequently more nitrogen is excreted than consumed.

Repeated examinations of urine have disclosed the fact that the proportion and quantity of the urinary constituents are modified, by exercise or physical labor, very little. This means that protein decomposition is not materially increased by physical effort and leads to the conclusion that the protein requirements of the average healthy man or women is no greater while engaged in manual labor than while engaged in mental effort.

For years the orthodox scientific world held tenaciously to the high protein standard set by Voigt. Although Hirshfeld had in 1887 by a series of tests placed the protein standard at 47 grams the orthodox chemists never accepted his standard and the low protein diet did not attract much attention until Horace Fletcher startled the scientists out of their lethargy a few years ago. Since then, much evidence has been accumulated by the progressive members of the scientific world showing that protein is not so valuable as formerly supposed. In fact, the evidence is strongly in favor of the statement that protein—and certainly excessive protein—is a physiological burden and destroys health. Among those who have helped in this work and whose name is seldom or never seen mentioned is Dr. Thomas Powell.

The diet of Horace Fletcher was examined and measured by Prof. Chittenden in his laboratory at Yale and found to contain about 44 grams of protein. This led Prof. Chittenden to perform a series of tests. He fed a diet to a squad of athletes, which diet contained only 63 grams of protein. These men gained 35 per cent in endurance on this diet during a few months.

Perhaps the most exhaustive series of dietetic experiments ever performed by any man were performed by Dr. M. Hindhede, director of the Hindhede Nutrition Laboratory which was established by the Danish government in recognition of his brilliant achievements in the field of dietetics.

He has shown that the elaborate nitrogen balance—studies on which the old high protein standard was supposed to be based are meaningless and profitless. "These results," he says, "which are confirmed by many other experiments of mine on low protein diet, suggest, at least, that an active man of between twenty and thirty years of age, seventy kilograms (154 lbs.) in weight, can easily establish equilibrium on twenty-five grams of digestible protein, which is only 24 per cent of the old academic standard of 105 grams."

"It may, therefore, be said that the whole protein problem over which the world has been worrying itself for the past fifty years has been but one huge mistake; for if we are to judge by the results of the equilibrium experiments, it would seem to be practically impossible to avoid getting protein enough."

"If we take the trouble to study the innumerable equilibrium experiments the only comment we can make is what a waste of time and labor." That there was much of such waste of time and labor will be seen when we consider that a bulletin of the U. S. Dept. of Agriculture collected 2,299 of these tests.

The experiments of Hirshfeld have already been referred to. He was a young man of 24 years and performed heavy labor, weight lifting, mountain climbing, etc., on a diet containing less than half the amount of protein that was claimed to be necessary. He lost neither weight nor strength while the "nitrogen balance" showed that he did not lose body protein. Dr. Hindhede says of his work: "It is strange, indeed, that Hirshfeld's investigations have been allowed by science to drift almost into oblivion. He was a young man (twenty-four) who could make little impression against the weight of Voigt's authority."

Hindhede raised four athletic and wide-awake children on a diet so low in protein that it has been said "it would frighten a cooking school teacher into blind staggers." He has proven that a high protein diet is not required by growing children.

But this was not the end. Hindhede found that the excess proteins, after entering the blood, underwent decomposition and recomposition giving as a final result nitric acid, phosphoric acid and sulphuric acid. There was also an excess of uric acid and amonia compounds. He contended that in order to neutralize the acids formed by the decomposition of excess proteins, the body was forced to give up its mineral salts. Thus the teeth, bones, cartileges, nails, hair, etc., were leeched of these elements.

These powerful acids destroy the liver and kidneys to such an extent that one may safely say no man ever died of uremia whose kidneys had not been, for years, gradually destroyed by the powerful acids resulting from excessive protein intake.

Dr. Thomas Powell had previously brought out these same facts. He called protein the "arch destroyer" and referred to it as pathogen (disease producer).

It was long thought that muscular tissues are oxidized or decomposed in the development of muscular power and that they are rebuilt from food, particularly protein. This, if true, would have given rise to even larger protein requirements than the standards called for. Anyway, during these many years we have been feeding upon beefsteaks, eggs and other high protein foods all the while claiming that we did not want to suffer from malnutrition and become lean, pale, individuals like the vegetarians nor did we want to rear dwarfed offspring like the rice eating **Japs and Chinese.**

The life insurance companies have discovered that the lean folks, (the skinny) live about twenty years longer than they should. Every school boy knows how the Japanese Jenriksha men pull the beef-fed Englishman through the hills and mountains of Japan at the rate of forty miles per day.

Several years ago a seventy mile walking race was staged in Germany. There were eight vegetarians and fifteen meat eaters. The first six men in were vegetarians. Most of the meat eaters never finished the race. Of course the pretended worshipers of the high-brow will say this is alright for the physical worker but the mental worker must have meat. This is Mr. Arthur Brisbane's famous argument. He thinks it saves energy in digestion. This energy can then be used in mental work. It would seem that he could see that energy saved in digestion could also be used in physical effort also. Meat eaters should have more endurance, more strength, than the vegetarian.

Again Mr. Brisbane should be able to see that the manual laborer can work off the excess protein more readily than the inactive mental worker.

That the protein requirement of growing animals is not high is shown by the fact that milk, the natural food of young animals, is very low in protein when compared to meat or eggs. Cow's milk, for instance, is about three and one-half per cent protein. The calf is a very active and rapidly growing animal, in fact, more active and of much more rapid growth than the human infant. As the calf grows older it adds grasses to its diet and these are much lower in protein content.

The cow will from grasses alone, secure all the proteins

required for her and her calf, both during pregnancy and during the period of lactation.

Milo Hastings says in Physical Culture for March 1916:

"The human youngster grows so slowly, after the first year or two, that the amount of protein needed for growth is so small in proportion to the other elements of the diet needed for heat and energy that the active child eating a diet of cereals, fruit, and vegetables in sufficient quantities to keep up childish activity, must of necessity consume more protein than is needed or can be utilized in growth.

"A young pig may gain a pound a day, but a young human rarely gains an ounce a day. In fact it takes him fifteen years to gain a hundred pounds. Eggs are about the same composition as the human body, and if for fifteen years a child ate no protein but that contained in one egg a day he would have eaten six times the protein equivalent of his own body. One sixth of an egg a day supplies the growth protein for the human youngster. On the plan of rearing young America on two pounds of meat, milk, eggs, legumes and cheese and bread a day, which plan our orthodox food chemistry prescribes, the growing child must pass through his liver and kidneys and utterly waste enough protein to build about five thousand pounds of human flesh.

"This thing figured out becomes a farce. The stuffing process of raising children is better suited to make pigs that would gain three hundred pounds of flesh in a year. Nature needs eighteen years of experience to bring a human brain to maturity, and so she provided a trap door through which to dump out the pig diet and keep us human still. How much physiological harm the dumping process works upon the child's organism we do not yet know—probably much less than most of you, after reading these lines, will imagine. The adaptibility of our physiological machine is a never ceasing source of wonder."

It is evident that there is no danger of anyone ever consuming too little protein. In fact this is just what

Hindhede found in his studies of the dietetic habits of nations. He found that in the degree to which a nation lived on a low protein diet, in that degree did they suffer less from disease. During the world war his opportunity came to demonstrate on a large scale, the truth of his findings. He was made food administrator over Denmark. His experiment involved a whole nation of millions of people and covered a period of three years. No other investigator had ever had such an opportunity. He reduced the death rate in Denmark forty per cent in one year's time by diet alone. He used a low protein diet. He concludes that the average adult human body may require twenty grams of protein daily but that the requirement may be even less than this.

His assistant, Dr. Madsen used an experimental diet containing but twenty-one grams of protein with only favorable results.

Turning now to carbohydrates let us state in a general way their uses in the body. They are used chiefly in the production of heat and energy. At least this is the orthodox theory. Instead of, as formerly held, the muscle cells being consumed in muscular activity, it is now claimed that sugar (glycogen or muscle sugar) is oxidized in the cells giving rise to energy. Fat is an available second choice. The monosaccharides are converted into glycogen in the liver.

There is a fascinating theory that the energy in food is stored up sun beams. No work on diet or plants is complete without an account of how the plant stores up the sun's rays. Coal which was once plants, is supposed to be the sun's rays stored away. All the light, heat and energy coming from these things are claimed to have come originally from the sun.

The fact is the leaves of the plants are so constructed that they focus the sun's rays upon structures within the leaf, much the same way as the lense of the eye focuses the light upon the retina. The leaves breathe in carbon dioxide from the air where the carbon is wrested from the embrace of oxygen by the power of the solar beams. Hydrogen, also is wrested from oxygen in this way. In other words, it has been shown "that those elements which had been united by the lower court, of chemical affinity, are divorced, or forced assunder, by the higher court of solar chemism." Sunlight is an essential factor in plant nutrition, just as it is in animal nutrition. There is no evidence that plants store up the sun's rays although they do store up the carbon and hydrogen.

The body stores up carbohydrates and does not eliminate all of the excess supply as is the case with proteins. Some of these are stored in the liver as glycogen, some in the muscles as muscle sugar, while some is converted into fat and stored as such. It is only after this is done that any excess is eliminated.

We hear much of starch poisoning these days. Hindhede found that starch poisoning was seldom, if ever, met with among those people whose diet is predominantly carbohydrate, if they lived on natural instead of denatured starches and sugars. Starch poisoning by denatured carbohydrates is due to the fact that these have been robbed of their mineral elements and this causes them to leech the tissues of their salts. It also leads to carbohydrate fermentation.

To illustrate what we mean by denatured carbohydrates leeching the tissues of their mineral constituents let us look for a minute at the process of sugar manufacture. Nature has placed in the natural sweets enough of the organic mineral elements, water and oxygen to satisfy their "desire" for these elements. In the process of manufacture of commercial sugar these other elements are extracted giving "free" and "unsatisfied" sugar. So great is the affinity of sugar for iron that it must be made in copper kettles as it abstracts the iron from iron kettles and literally "eats" holes in them. In the body the denatured starches and sugars do likewise. They leech the tissues of their mineral salts. "Free" sugar also has an almost insatiable "desire" for oxygen.

Carbohydrate fermentation, gives rise to carbon-dioxide and alcohol and results in chronic auto-intoxication which resembles, in every way, the symptoms of chronic alcoholism. The alcohol produces chronic irritation in the system and results in the formation of scar tissue. Previous to the formation of the scar tissue there is the usual disturbances caused by irritation. It also causes capillary congestion which results, in turn, in atrophy of brain and muscles. The irritation of the mucous surfaces results in the overproduction of mucous giving rise to catarrh.

The mineral salts, or ash, are most of them alkaline and are used for a number of purposes. They form an essential part of every tissue in the body, and predominate in the harder structures, such as bones, teeth, hair, nails, etc. They are the chief factors in maintaining the normal alkalinity of the blood as well as its normal specific gravity. They are also abundant in all the body's secretions and a lack of them in the diet produces a lack of secretions. They are also used as detoxifying agents, by being combined with the acid waste from the cells. The wastes are thus neutralized and prepared for elimination. Their presence in the food eaten also aids in preventing it from decomposing. Acidosis produced by the fermentation of proteins and carbohydrates often comes because the mineral salts have been taken from the food thus favoring fermentation.

The body has no method of storing up mineral salts as in the case of carbohydrates. A fixed amount is kept suspended in the blood. After the absorption of a fresh meal there may be an excess in the blood but this excess is promptly eliminated.

The body has power to extract salts from the tissues of the body in the event of a lack of them. Sodium, for instance serves to combine with uric acid and other acids which form as the result of our excessive protein consumption, neutralizing these. If one is eating a diet of meat, eggs, cheese, etc., and not consuming sufficient sodium to offset the acids formed by these the blood is forced to draw upon the other tissues for sodium with which to combat these acids. Nature is often forced to draw upon the tissues in this manner in those living upon the conventional denatured diet.

During pregnancy in women this is especially true. Calcium (lime) is used in large quantities in building bones. If the food is lacking in this the mothers blood will also lack sufficient lime for the formation of the bones of her unborn child. The child can receive its food supply from no other source than the mother's blood. Nature always favors the child above the mother hence the harder structures of the mother's body are forced to give up their lime to the embryo. As Nature always favors the most vital organs, the salts are extracted from those parts that can be most readily dispensed with. The teeth, hair and nails usually have to give up their salts first. Thus while "primitive" peoples and animals that live on natural foods, continue to keep their teeth through life, civilized man with his denatured diet is fast becoming a bald and toothless race. We shall have more to say upon this later.

Let me again emphasize the very important and fundamental fact that these salts must always be taken in the organic form as found in fruits and vegetables since they cannot be assimilated in the inorganic form. Many eat common table salt (sodium chloride), while many doctors advise it on the theory that it is good for one and necessary to maintain health. However, sodium is no exception to the above rule. It can no more be utilized by the body when supplied in the inorganic form than any of the other salts. One may as well eat pig iron or rock lime to supply iron and lime to the body as to eat common table salt to supply the body with sodium. We shall discuss this matter more fully in the chapter devoted to condiments.

The laboratory men and commercial exploiters of the public's ignorance have within recent years been telling us from the housetops of a mysterious something which they call vitamines to which they ascribe wonderful powers. Minute quantities of these things are supposed to work wonders for one, while, if they are lacking in the diet it works havoc with the one eating such a diet.

However, recent experiments by PHYSICAL CUL-

TURE'S ''Food Research Laboratory'' have shown that the addition of small amounts of vitamine containing food is not sufficient to accomplish the work which has been claimed for them. It was found that life, health and growth were sustained in an ideal way only when those foods containing the vitamines predominated in the diet. On the other hand trouble followed the continued use of a diet which contained only small amounts of the vitamine containing foods.

The commercial exploiters have found ways to extract the vitamines from their natural storehouse and have put them up in various forms for our use. We can have them as a yeast cake, in paste form or as chocolate coated wafers. Great things are claimed for them.

They will give you bright sparkling eyes, a peach-like complexion, beautiful figure, broaden your shoulders, develop your muscles, fill you full of pep and vim, give you health and strength, etc. At least, they do this in the advertisement. But you can no more gain these desirable qualities by eating these chocolate wafers or yeast cakes than by any other method that neglects the individual habits of living. The miracle monger will always seek for short cuts to these things, at least, as long as there is money in it.

If there are such things as vitamines, if they are anything more than mineral salts, you can supply your body with all that it requires (if it requires them from an outside source) by eating fresh fruits and fresh green vegetables. Experiments with the supposed vitamines have shown that those same processes of milling, refining, canning, pickling, preserving and cooking food that are known to rob the food of its mineral salts, or to so alter them chemically as to render them useless, also destroys their vitamines.

Whether there are or are not such things as vitamines these experiments have served to bring home to the orthodox food scientist, the value and importance of natural, 'unprocessed foods. Some of them in view of the results of the experiments, have succeeded in overcoming their fear of germs to such an extent that they advise the eating of some fresh uncooked fruits or vegetables daily.

CHAPTER 4
Effects of Denatured Foods

No discussion of dietetics would be complete without some consideration of the effects of denatured foods. Observations and experiments upon both animals and man have shown that a diet deficient in organic mineral salts produces disease. Indeed many articles of food have been shown to be actual poisons due to their lack of these all important elements.

Two kinds of substances are taken into the body; namely, base forming (alkaline) and acid forming foods. A proper balance between these must be maintained if health is to be preserved.

The blood is normally slightly alkaline in reaction. The waste from the cells is acid in reaction. These wastes if not neutralized and eliminated reduce the alkalinity of the blood. This condition is commonly referred to as acidosis, or an acid condition of the blood. The blood cannot become acid during life, for if it should lose its alkalinity even to the point of neutrality death would result in a few minutes. The condition really present is a lessened alkalinity or hypoalkalinity of the blood.

These acids are very irritating and poisoning to the cells and tissues of the body. They must be neutralized and eliminated. The neutralization is accomplished by combining them with organic mineral elements. It is a rule of chemistry that when an acid acts upon a mineral a salt and another acid is formed. In the body the resulting salt and acid are less irritating and more easily eliminated than the original acid.

There is only one source from which to obtain the mineral salts and that is from the food eaten. If there is a deficiency of these the body is forced to draw upon its own tissues for the mineral elements with which to neutralize the acid waste of the cells. This devitalizes and destroys those tissues, giving rise to serious deficiency diseases.

A plant, in order to maintain health and normal growth must find in the soil a certain minimum of each of the elements required in plant nutrition. If, for instance, only one-half the required amount of potassium is present, then no matter how abundant the other elements the plant cannot utilize them in a normal way. The rate of growth is slackened and the ultimate development of the plant is depressed.

In the Museum of Natural History (New York) is an exhibit showing the effects of soil deficiency on plant life. These plants, all of the same kind, were reared in soils lacking some element. The exhibit has to be seen to be fully appreciated. They range in size from about three inches to about eighteen inches in height. Their color ranges from a pale yellow to dark green. The leaves of some are broad, of others narrow. Some of the leaves are kinky. All of the plants except one is defective both in size, color and features and all except that one were raised in soils lacking some food element. For instance one was raised in a soil lacking iron, (the plant has "anemia") another in a soil lacking potassium, another in a soil lacking nitrogen, etc.

This is of interest as showing the extreme importance of the elements in the food of plants. These elements are of equal importance to man.

About eighty years ago Dr. Magendie of Paris starved one full pen of dogs to death by feeding them a diet of white flour and water, while another pen thrived on whole wheat flour and water. He fed another pen of dogs all the beef tea they could consume, and gave the dogs of another pen only water. The beef tea dogs all starved to death. The water fed dogs had lost considerable weight and would have starved also if the experiment had been continued, however, they were alive after those fed on beef tea were all dead. They were fed and all recovered.

Dr. Chas. E. Page of Boston says, "Pigeons, chickens

and mice will all flourish on graham flour, but all will die within three weeks on white flour."

Dr. P. L. Clark of Chicago says, "If two puppies are taken from the same litter both in sound, normal health, and one is fed white flour products and water, and the other whole wheat flour products and water, in the course of twelve to sixteen weeks the puppy which has been fed white flour products and water will be dead and the other, fed the whole grain products, which properly nourish the body, will be normally developed."

What do these things show? Simply this, that foods which have been deprived of their mineral contents not only do not nourish the body but actually poison it. We would not be doing our full duty if we did not point out here that whole wheat products alone will not sustain life, health and growth in a normal manner. Recent experiments have shown that after a shorter or longer period the normal rate of growth slackens unless the animal is fed in addition to whole wheat products, some green foods. These experiments even show that if life and growth are to continue in an ideal manner the amount of green foods required is greater than the amount of whole wheat consumed.

A colony of mice fed on the best grade of white flour will all develop constipation in three days and die within a month. An equal number of mice fed on whole wheat flour will flourish and gain weight.

Why is this so? Because, in the process of milling about 30 per cent of the grain is thrown away and with it practically all of the mineral salts. White flour is of so little value as a food that bugs, weavels, and worms will not get into it except when forced by extreme hunger to do so, and then it kills them in a short time. They will readily eat whole wheat flour and do well on it. It has been truthfully said "we boast of having the whitest flour in the world. We have also the thinnest hair and the poorest bones, teeth and nerves as a result."

A series of experiments were made with plants. Analyses were made of the elements entering into the composition of various plants. These plants were placed in water containing all of the elements necessary to healthy growth of each particular plant. Each of the plants were found to thrive and grow in such a solution. One of the elements was then removed and each plant was left in the water with one missing element. In a short time the plants begun to turn yellow and wither away. Had they been left in this solution they would have died. But it was found that if the element was put back into the water, the plants would immediately gain in strength and vitality and would soon be growing again in a normal way. It was found that it did not matter what element was withheld—if any element was lacking the plants did not thrive. Why do we expect to do better? Do we possess the power to live and grow in a normal way if one or more of these sixteen elements are lacking in our diet? We do not. This we shall amply demonstrate in the course of this chapter.

The principal base-forming elements are potassium, sodium, calcium, magnesium and iron. The principal acid-forming elements are nitrogen, carbon, hydrogen, phosphorus, sulphur and chlorine. Both proteins, carbohydrates and fats contain large amounts of acid-forming elements. Of the mineral salts the base-forming elements are often referred to as positive elements while the acid forming ones are referred to as negative elements. In all or nearly all natural foods Nature has placed more of the positive than of the negative salts as the following representative list will show.

	Positive elements	Negative elements
Human milk	7.04	4.79
Cow's milk	13.08	11.39
Carrots	15.64	6.10
Radishes	10.30	4.25
Spinach	31.35	26.23
Tomatoes	20.70	7.05
Apples	2.21	1.34
Oranges	12.46	2.85
Bannas	10.63	6.25
Dried figs	42.24	14.43

Meats, eggs, most nuts, most grains and dried beans

contain more negative than positive elements. All natural fruits, all green vegetables, milk and the blood of all animals contain more positive than negative elements. Thus it can readily be seen that if foods are eaten as Nature prepares then without any additions or substractions the body would at all times be given enough of the base-forming elements to neutralize the acids formed within. The rest would be simply a matter of power to digest and assimilate.

But the factories, refineries, mills, canneries, bake shops, cooks, etc., have seen to it that we get but little natural foods. Not only have they been very busy subtracting, from them, their valuable mineral elements but they have also learned to add to them many irritating, injurious and poisonous chemicals, dye stuffs, preservatives, etc., until thousands are yearly killed and many more are weakened in body and mind. We are fast becoming a race of glass eyes, bald heads, false teeth and wooden legs as a result. As one well known Nature Curist has so truthfully remarked: "We wake ourselves with caffein, move our bowels with cathartics, coax an appetite with condiments, seek rest in nicotine, go to sleep with an opiate, and die just when we should begin to live."

It is estimated that over half the human family lives on rice. However, it is whole and not denatured rice. Nearly all the rice sold in America is polished with talc after its bran, which contains nearly all its mineral elements has been removed. The remnant which is practically all starch contains more or less talc for our system to battle with.

Experiments on pigeons, chickens, rats, guinea pigs, etc., have shown that these animals when fed on white flour, polished rice, degerminated corn meal, etc., develop diseases in every way resembling rickets, beri beri, pellagra, neuritis, multiple neuritis and acidosis in man. These diseases were soon cured when the whole grains or the polishings from the grains were added to the food. For instance pigeons fed on polished rice for a few weeks develop multiple neuritis. If they are fed whole rice or the bran and waste portions, (the grindings) the disease soon disappears.

The great English physiologist, Prof. Starling testified before the Royal Commission on Vivisection that "the last experiment must be upon man." If the feeding of denatured foods to animals will produce such diseases will they also produce the same or similar diseases in man? The answer is yes and the proof of this is plentiful. We can only hope to give a few of the many notable examples in the space of this chapter. But enough will be given to convince the intelligent reader that there is something wrong with the conventional diet.

In 1914, 4,000 men engaged in the building of the Medina-Mamora Railway in South America were killed by acidosis, beri beri and tuberculosis induced by an acid forming diet of meats, white flour, degerminated corn meal, polished rice, tapioca, corn starch, farina, cakes, jellies, jams, glucose, sugar, syrups, lard and canned goods. The project had to be abandoned.

All around the workers, in the woods, the monkeys subsisted on the fruits and nuts that grew in abundance. These were strong and healthy, and free from the ailments from which the men were dying. However, the men spurned the monkey food. Just as the man in civilization refuses to eat celery, lettuce, etc., and refers to them as grass and fodder. The only members of the above crew of men who remained to tell the story were saved by a diet of acid fruits.

Why does not the average individual suffer in this way? He does, but not to the same extent these men did. This is due to the fact that he consumes enough base forming foods, fruits, fresh vegetables, milk, etc., to protect him to a great extent. However, the American people are still consuming far too many acid forming foods. This is shown by the steady death rate from consumption, the rapid increase in nervous afflictions, degenerative diseases and by our lowered resistance to epidemic influences.

Nor is it enough that we consume large amounts of the protective foods with our acid formers. This is too much like taking an antidote with the poison. We should cease taking the poison. If we consume more acid forming foods than the body requires and these are offset by the base forming foods this still entails a hardship upon the organs of digestion and those of elimination.

In 1915,, twelve convicts in a Mississippi penitentiary volunteered as subjects for a dietetic test. Dr. Goldberger, who made the test wanted to prove that pellegra was caused by carbohydrate foods.

These twelve men were fed on demineralized and de-germinated corn products with the result that they all developed the disease and underwent intense suffering. Some of them even attempted suicide.

They were placed on a normal diet with the result that their usual health was soon re-established.

It should be carefully noted that these men were fed on denatured and not natural carbohydrate foods. It is extremely doubtful if such results would have been obtained if natural carbohydrate foods had been used. Certain it is that it would have required much longer to have brought these results about. Natural, whole corn, is not a perfect food. Anyone fed upon this exclusively for a sufficient time would be expected to develop some ''deficiency'' disease. People do not confine themselves to an exclusive diet of this kind and it may be objected that if one secures a variety of foods such results will not occur. This objection is answered by the case given above of the South American Railway builders and by the fact that many who do secure a variety of foods have pellegra and other ''deficiency'' disease. Mere variety is not sufficient. The food eaten must possess sufficient amounts of all the food elements required by the body, in an assimilable form. If it does this and is a mono-diet such results will not follow. Note, for instance, babies are fed the first year of their life upon milk exclusively. It is a period, too, of rapid growth. Yet if the milk is whole and from a normal mother or even from a normal cow they do not develop deficiency diseases.

A very striking case which proves that even a varied

diet of denatured foods will produce the same effects as those observed to follow a denatured mono-diet occured during the war. We refer to the experiences of the German raider, the "Crown Prince Wilhelm."

This cruiser, after having been upon the high seas for 255 days and sinking 14 French and British merchant men was forced to put into port at Newport News because 110 of her crew were stricken with beri-beri. The crew was dropping at the rate of about two per day. The ships physicians were unable to deal with the situation. So, also, were the American physicians. None of them knew what to do.

The men presented symptoms of weakness, irritability, muscular atrophy, paralysis, dilation of the heart and pain upon pressure. Their diet had been very similar to that eaten in the average American household. It consisted of fresh meat, white flour products, canned vegetables, potatoes, sweet biscuits, cheese, oleomargerine, tea, coffee and champagne. Much fresh fruits, fresh vegetables and whole wheat had been captured by the raider from the French and English merchantmen but these had all been sent down to the fishes while only the more "staple" foods were retained for use.

Had it not been for the excellent work of Alfred W. McCann, a well known Nature Cure dietitian, these men might all have died. At least most of them would have perished. As it was, only one failed to recover. Mr. McCann prescribed a diet very rich in base forming elements with the result that improvement was immediate and rapid. All protein, sugar, fat and white flour was excluded from the diet. In two weeks the most severe cases were up and the men rapidly regained their health. No drugs were given.

The lesson is plain. If we desire health we must stop shoveling denatured carbohydrates, proteins and fats into our digestive tract and give our bodies natural foods. The cases given may be extreme but the conditions of those we see around us assure us that they are not exceptional. In fact, almost everyone we meet is suffering in some way from mal-nutrition due in a large measure to the failure to supply the body with proper foods.

Nature has prepared for young mammals a perfect food for the first period of their lives. This food, milk, if coming from a healthy mother fed upon natural foods is adequate to sustain life, health and growth in an ideal way, even during the period of most rapid growth. But the fear of germs that always accompanies acceptance of the germ theory has caused man to tamper even with milk. In an effort to kill supposed disease germs there is a widespread practice of subjecting milk to a high degree of heat. This impairs the food value of the milk. This fact became so obvious that in the larger cities, where pasteurization is required, provisions have been made whereby certified milk can be had to feed infants upon. It produces constipation and does not sustain growth in a normal way. Rickets and scurvy are common in infants fed upon pasteurized milk. The death rate among babies so fed is also greater than those fed upon whole milk.

Dr. Fraser, a Canadian physician writing on germs, says concerning the effect upon the health of the people the rejection of the germ theory would have:

"It would discourage the use of half-cooked (pasteurized) milk for infants—in Toronto, where no provision is made for getting natural milk, the average infantile death rate is twenty-nine per cent higher than the rest of Ontario."

This is a rather serious increase in the infantile death rate over those cities where babies are fed natural milk. Surely if pasteurized milk is so worthless as a food for infants it cannot be regarded as a wholesome food for adults. What are the facts? These are just what one would suspect them to be. In adults it produces constipation, is hard to digest and does not give the results one gets from natural milk. The experience of all those institutions where the milk diet is used has been that pasteurized milk is practically worthless as a curative diet.

The oldest, most common and most popular method of denaturing food is that of cooking. Note above what is done for milk when heat short of boiling is applied to it. For many years Nature Curists have been warning the public of the waste of food, loss of health and strength and the unnecessary expense, caused by cooking food. It is only here and there that one has heeded the warning.

Orthodox food scientists in their experiments with vitamines have discovered that uncooked foods are far superior to cooked foods as growth promoters. They contend that cooking destroys the vitamines. These men now advocate the use of some uncooked food daily.

Whatever cooking may do to the hypothetical vitamines, there are some things that it does to food that can be seen. Cooking changes food both physically and chemically.

The power of heat to bring about physical and chemical changes is too well known to need any discussion here. When heat is applied to foods it brings about such changes as:

(1) Coagulation (hardening) of the proteins of meat, eggs, milk, etc., making them tough and indigestible.

(2) The destruction of the elementary plant form, tearing down its structure and changing its composition.

(3) Certain destructive changes in the element grouping, in foods, returning part of these elements (especially the organic salts) to their inorganic, and therefore useless state, so that a large part of the value of their mineral content is lost.

(4) Changes in flavor and odor of food.

(5) Drives part of food off into air as gasses.

(6) Where food is boiled through two waters and first water is thrown away most of the soluble mineral elements are sent down the drain pipe.

(7) In cases of seeds, such as nuts, beans, peas, grains, etc., the germinating principle is destroyed so that cooked seed will not germinate.

Such changes cannot take place in food without impairing its food value. In fact, we have already seen that it does this in the case of milk. At the outset of the war in Europe a French Scientist fed some pigeons on roasted whole corn. It was found to produce the same results that followed the use of denatured corn products. Pigeons fed on whole raw corn thrived and grew.

Nature Curists have proven in thousands of cases that the change from a diet of cooked to uncooked foods is always, if properly done, followed by improved health.

At about 145 degrees Fahrenheit certain properties of plant life are destroyed. A leaf of cabbage, for instance, if immersed in water that can be easily borne by the hand, will wilt, showing that part of its cellular life is destroyed at that low temperature. The heat to which such foods are subjected in cooking may be increased or prolonged until all the properties of the plant are destroyed. Many articles of food which are baked in an oven are subjected to a very intense heat ranging from 300 degrees F. to 400 degrees F. Much of their food value is destroyed, thereby. Bread that is browned in an oven is half destroyed, being partly charcoal and ashes. If it had been left in the oven twice as long it would have been entirely destroyed. At every step in the process of cooking from the time the food is put in or upon the stove until it is destroyed entirely, if it be allowed to cook that long, destructive changes take place that impair its food value and unfit it for use by the body.

While cooking does alter and change food in many ways, wasting much of it, it does not add anything to the food. Cooking even breaks down the natural resistance of food to fermentation so that foods after being cooked ferment sooner than they do in the uncooked state.

It is often argued that cooking adds to the palatability of food. This is, at least, not true with most foods and we have noticed that the others are not palatable after being cooked unless they have been flavored, spiced, sweetened, peppered, salted, etc., or have had mustard, catsup, horseradish, or some form of dressing added. The fact is, we are always kidding ourselves into believing that the things we are in the habit of doing are the very things we should do; that the things we have learned to like are the things that are best for us, and we consciously or unconsciously resist any proposed change, even, if there are plenty of evidences that the change would be for the better.

Habits have a powerful grip upon most people. The cooking habit is no exception. When the art of cooking was first discovered is not known. One thing is certain, however, cooking is not natural and man survived the period of time that intervened between his introduction upon the earth and his discovery of the black art of cooking. It is reasonably certain, too, that, at first, only a few articles of food were cooked and the custom of eating cooked foods spread slowly. Since uncooked foods constituted the greater part of the diet and served as "protective" foods man was deceived. He could not see the harmful results of eating cooked foods. Today it is hard to convince his degenerate descendants of its evil consequences.

CHAPTER 5
The Failure of the Calorie Fallacy

In the foregoing chapters on diet nothing has been said of the calories so much talked of by orthodox food scientists and regular physicians. In the colleges, sanitariums, hospitals and publications of old school physicians the caloric value of food is the only standard recognized. Government food bulletins talk very learnedly about callories. Professional nurses and professional dietitians appear to know all about this new god. Even restaurants and hotels have begun to remind us of the caloric value of foods.

Medical men and orthodox food scientists are agreed that an individual requires so many calories per day and if he doesn't get this amount he will suffer. In medical institutions the patients diet is figured up in cn.ories and he is fed according to this standard. Yet we dared ignore the calorie in our previous chapters and even dared to insist upon fasting and low calorie foods.

To understand why we did this let us get a look at this little fetich of the orthodox. A calorie is a unit of measurement, just as the inch and yard are units of measurement. It is the amount of heat required to raise the temperature of one gram (about 20 drops) of water one degree. Barnes has shown that with the production of one calorie of heat in a steam engine enough energy is obtained to lift a weight of three pounds one foot into the air. The caloric value of foods is obtained by burning them in the calorimeter and measuring the heat liberated.

Insisting that man derives all his energy from the food eaten and neglecting all the other important functions performed by food the orthodox food scientist considers those foods that give off most heat per pound to be the best foods for human consumption.

Ridiculous as this may appear to a man of average intelligence this is food science in this twentieth century, according to the worshipers of the great god Mumbo Jumbo. The human body is more than a mere furnace or fire box into which we must continue to shovel fuel. The fuel value of food is the least valuable thing about it. White sugar is a very high grade fuel having a fuel value of 1750 calories per pound as compared to 165 calories for butter milk, 100 calories for tomatoes and 95 calories for spinach. Yet animals fed on white sugar and water soon die. The nutritional value of food can no more be measured in calories than the value of water in the system can be stated in pounds or quarts.

In measuring the caloric value of food only the combustible portions are considered. That portion of the food that does not burn commonly referred to by the orthodox food scientist as "ash" (meaning ashes) and which is made up of the mineral content of the food is not even considered. By such a standard oleomargarine with 3410 calories per pound is one of the greatest of foods while lemons with 155 calories, oranges with 150 calories and strawberries with 150 calories are practically worthless. Salt pork with 3555 calories per pound is a food for the gods by this standard while celery and lettuce with only 65 calories each per pound and skim milk with but 165 calories consume more energy in digestion than they produce when oxydized. Yet neither oleomargarine nor salt pork will sustain life, health or growth. Animals fed on such a diet soon perish.

Osborn and Mendell fed animals on a diet of denatured starches and fats, refined sugar and refined proteins and found that when so fed they rapidly declined in health. The addition of inorganic salts to the food was found to be absolutely valueless.

When the whey of milk was added to the diet their decline in health ceased. The refined sugars, starches, fats and proteins have a very high caloric value while whey possesses very little food value. Whey contains none of the fats or proteins of milk but does contain iron, phosphorus, calcium, potassium and other organic salts. These tests prove that organic mineral salts are of more importance than heat units. Indeed, it can easily be shown that those foods that are the most deficient and worthless of all are the very foods which rank highest in fuel value.

Consider white bread with 1200 calories per pound and refined corn meal with 1635 calories per pound and then think over the fact that high as these foods are in caloric value, they not only will not sustain life but actually produce death in animals fed upon these exclusively quicker than starvation itself. White sugar, oleomargarine, polished rice, salt pork, etc., do the same. Animals fed on these foods or tapioca, corn syrup, corn grits, cream of wheat, macaroni, puffed rice, corn starch, corn flakes, and other such foods possessing a high fuel value sicken and die.

If the fresh juices of vegetables are added to the refined foods the animals survive but do not regain their normal weight and strength nor their resistance to disease. These vegetable juices contain no fuel value. These animals are restored to normal vigor and health only after they are fed unrefined foods such as cabbage, spinach, celery, lettuce, whole grains, whole milk, etc. These foods are so low in caloric value as compared with the refined starches, sugars, proteins, etc., that the orthodox scientist regards them as being practically valueless.

A pound of apples gives but 190 calories while a pound of watermelon only yields 50, but either of these foods is superior to the refined high calorie foods.

McCullum's experiments have shown that some foods will sustain growth while other foods will not. It is assumed that those foods that sustain growth and development contain certain substances to which the term vitamine has been applied. These substances are found abundantly in spinach, lettuce, cauliflower, cabbage, celery and milk. All of these foods are low in fuel value. The high calorie foods already mentioned are absolutely lacking in this respect. They will neither sustain nor promote growth. Grass and grass seeds, oranges, lemons, grapefruit, tomatoes, in fact all fresh fruits and green vegetables, all of which are very low in caloric value, are rich in growth promoting elements.

Prof. Sherman says of the calorie: "In connection with such comparisons of food value, while of primary importance, is not alone a complete measure of its nutritive value, which will depend in part upon the amounts and forms of nitrogen, phosphorus, iron and various other essential elements furnished by food." We may add that the value of any food to the individual is partly determined by its digestibility and by the individual's present nutritive needs and powers of digestion and assimilation. It is obvious that no part of food that is not digested can be of use however high its caloric or other value. Again food eaten, when not required or when the digestive apparatus is not prepared for the work of digestion can only produce harm.

In determining the fuel value of foods, not only are the growth promoting substances wholly ignored but also those elements which, though absolutely worthless from the calorific standpoint are absolutely essential to the regulation of the specific gravity of the blood, the functioning of the blood corpuscles, the contractibility of the muscles, the preservation of tissue from decomposition, the chemical reaction of the internal secretions, for maintaining normal alkalinity of the blood and for use in preparing the cell wastes for elimination.

Iron and manganese which are the oxidizing agents of the blood have no caloric value. Florine which forms such a hard protective shell around the teeth and calcium which forms a large percentage of the normal composition of bone are wholly lacking in heat producing properties. Sodium, magnesium, sulphur, potassium and other elements that are used in the processes of assimilation and elimination cannot be substituted by calories.

Think for a minute over the lesson of the German Raider, The Crown Prince Wilhelm. The crew was fed on a large variety of high caloric foods such as:

Breakfast:—Oatmeal with condensed milk, fried potatoes, white bread, cheese, sausage, corned beef, smoked ham, fried beef, beef stew, oleomargarine, coffee, white sugar and cookies.

Dinner :—Beef soup, pea soup, lentil soup, potato soup, pot roast, fried steak, roast beef, salt fish, canned vegetables, potatoes, white bread, cookies, soda crackers, white sugar, condensed milk, oleomargarine.

Supper :—Fried steak, corned beef hash, cold roast beef, beef stew, white bread, potatoes, white sugar, cookies, oleomargarine, coffee and condensed milk.

Nearly every one of these foods possess a high caloric value but every one of them are lacking in the organic mineral elements and growth promoting factors. After two hundred and fifty-five days on a diet like this, this ship steamed into Norfolk with many of her crew dead, 110 ill on their bunks and many others about ready to break down. Their ailment which was similar to beri-beri or pellagra was cured by a diet that possessed almost no fuel value whatsoever, but was rich in organic salts.

The amount of heat and energy required by various individuals varies so greatly with the conditions of climate, occupation, age, size, temperament, etc., that food values based on the caloric standard are of no practical value. Aside from this most of the heat produced in the body is used in maintaining normal body temperature and not for the production of energy. If health is destroyed, if the nutritive functions are impaired, to stoke up on fuel foods is not only valueless but is positively harmful. This is easily proven when we compare the results of such treatment with those obtained by the fast or by a low calorie diet which is rich in the organic mineral elements.

The burning of food in the body is a vital or physiological process and does not take place in a dead body. On the other hand, if the functions of the body are impaired this process is impaired also and foods that are high in fuel value cannot be properly cared for. This fact is ignored by the calorie worshipers.

To declare that man requires a given number of calories per day and to feed these all the while ignoring the individual's condition is the height of folly. In a state of nature demand reaches forth to supply and satisfies itself. The calorie feeders force the supply even when there is no demand or when there is lack of ability to properly care for the supply. Along with this their standard of measuring food values wholly ignores the most important elements of the food and the further fact that not all the food elements that are combustible are burned in the body. Those proteins that are used in building new tissue are not used for the production of heat and energy, even if we grant that man derives his energy from food.

It should be easily seen that a system of feeding based on the caloric or fuel value of foods must inevitably lead to mischief. And this is exactly what it has done for it invariably causes patients to be stuffed with fuel foods that are deficient in the other and more vital elements. These patients are forced to eat beyond their digestive capacity in the effort to feed them the standard amount of calories. A standardized treatment without a standardized patient is a farce. And a standardized patient is an impossibility.

It is estimated that one slice of bread containing about one hundred calories would enable a man to lift one hundred pounds three feet—once. Or, if he lifted it over his head, he would consume two slices of bread. A meal containing a thousand calories would enable him to lift the weight to a height of six feet only five times. He would then be forced to eat and digest another meal before he could lift the weight again. The days diet of a moderate eater would enable him to lift a hundred pounds to this height only fifteen times and leave him with no energy for further exertion. The writer has lifted over this amount to arms length over head, or over seven feet, more times than this after a three days' fast and then performed much more work during the day.

The whole thing is absurd when viewed in this light. The farmer or mechanic would require the digestive apparatus of a cow to enable him to eat enough calories to perform his daily tasks.

We do well to bear in mind that the above figures represent only the energy expended in lifting the weight and includes no energy consumed in eating and digesting the food, in carrying—on the processes of the body, the work of the heart, lungs, bowels, etc.—and takes no account of the process of thinking. If energy to do these things is derived from food we can never account for the frequent gains in strength made while fasting. The calorie fallacy is a complete failure.

CHAPTER 5

Condiments

The use of condiments is a well nigh universal evil. Condiments of some nature are indulged in by almost all people, "civilized" or "savage" upon our globe. Many condiments now in use have been used from remote antiquity. Man seems to have acquired many of his harmful practices early in his career.

Many condiments now in use are manufactured articles and were not used until very recent times. The others began to be used at some earlier date, but it is not to be supposed that man learned to use each of these at the very beginning of his career. He probably learned their use by accident. As he spread over the face of the earth he continued to add to his variety of condiments until today he has quite a large number. Today the average individual looks upon their place in the diet as quite the natural thing and is ever ready to defend their use.

Upon what grounds are they usually defended? It is claimed that they:

(1)   make the food more palatable;
(2)   increase the appetite;
(3)   stimulate the flow of the digestive juices.

So far as we are aware it is never claimed that they are foods. But almost every one declares that he cannot eat without them. Their food would not taste like anything. They would not enjoy eating. They do not stop to inquire why these things are so.

Does their use really render the food more palatable? Yes to those accustomed to them. But not so to the one untrained in the use of them. What they really do is to cover up the fine delicate flavors that exist in food so that the condiment user tastes the condiment but not the food. He who is accustomed to the use of unseasoned, unspiced food knows that those who use condiments are missing many fine delicate flavors that are far more pleasing to the sense of taste than any condiment can be. Real pleasure in eating comes from tasting the natural flavors of those foods man is adapted to by nature.

Condiment users cannot enjoy an unseasoned, unspiced meal because their tastes have been perverted by this very practice. These things so deaden the sense of taste that it is not able to find the natural flavors of food. Their use is truly habit-forming and the longer they are used the more one requires to satisfy his taste. They pervert and impair the sense of taste.

Those peoples whom we are accustomed to refer to as primitive, and among whom condiment using is not developed to the extent it is among "civilized" nations, far excel us in the power and keenness of taste. This is true because we, by the use of condiments, which are injurious to every fiber in our body, are slowly and surely destroying our sense of taste. Such perversions of taste as clay eating, and filth eating are frequently met with, while tobacco chewing by men and pickle eating by women are very common. Salt eating is an almost universal perversion in both sexes.

It requires no argument to convince any save those guilty of the practices that clay eating and filth eating represent perversions of taste while many readily admit that tobacco chewing is a perversion of this sense but few there are, indeed, who will admit that salt eating, pickle eating, the use of pepper, mustard, vinegar, spices, etc., are also perversions of taste. Nevertheless it is true. Hereafter, when anyone complains that he or she could not relish food without the "seasoning" you may put it down that that person's taste is perverted. They are no longer capable of enjoying the natural taste of food. Why? Because they have cultivated an artificial taste for stronger flavors.

Condiments are often used to cover up the unpleasant taste of foods that have begun to spoil. This is the case in hotels and restaurants. They are used, too, to give taste to foods whose natural flavors have been destroyed by cooking. Many foods taste flat, insipid when they are cooked. Few would eat them without some kind of seasoning. But this is no evidence of the value of condiments. Rather it is only added evidence of the harmfulness of cooking. If a food that can be relished before cooking cannot be relished without the addition of seasonings after cooking this should lead us to see the fallacy of cooking. If a food cannot be relished either before or after cooking without the addition of condiments it would be far better for us not to eat it.

In this connection let us say that many foods may be relished by the natural taste in their natural state that the perverted taste would turn down. The perverted taste is not a reliable guide. Some foods may even be relished after being cooked and without the addition of condiments, by the unperverted taste. Before a food is condemned because of unpalatableness let us be sure that it is unpalatable to the unperverted taste.

Does the use of condiments increase the appetite? Yes, and for this very reason their use should be condemned. The desire for food should arise out of actual physiological needs. When these needs are not present no food should be taken.

Why should hunger be stimulated by the use of condiments. Appetite is counterfeit hunger, a false desire for food. It may be created and increased by the use of condiments. But this leads to over eating and over eating leads to disease. So great is the power of condiments to increase one's appetite that many say that it is almost impossible to overeat if one does not use them.

If no natural desire for food is present, then there is no necessity to take food. If there is a natural desire for food, condiments are not needed in order that we may enjoy our food. If there is a real need for food in the system, no condiments are needed to give us a desire for food. We will be hungry. An artificial hunger (appetite) serves no useful purpose.

Do condiments stimulate the flow of the digestive juices? Yes, or at least some of them. They are irritating to the lining membranes of the mouth, stomach, etc., and much juice is poured out upon them to counteract their influence. It is doubtful, however, if they increase the secretion of enzymes.

It is claimed by the advocates of condiments that by adding to our gustatory enjoyment, increasing the appetite, and stimulating the flow of digestive juices their use improves digestion.

Although we have shown that they do not add to the joys of eating in any true sense and that the increased appetite is an evil rather than a good, we may admit that by their use there may be a temporary improvement in digestion. We have seen, however, that if we are to continue receiving the false pleasure and increased appetite from their use we are forced to use them in increasing quantities. So also with the stimulation of the flow of the digestive juices. If they are to continue to have this effect we must use more and more of them, for they are truly weakening to the secreting glands.

If the practice is continued the glands may become so weakened that they are no longer able to discharge their duties. It is the tendency of all stimulation, to exhaust. Exhausted digestive glands cannot be calculated to improve digestion. Indigestion is the inevitable end.

In the living world there is a law known as the LAW OF DUAL EFFECT, which has been formulated thus:

"The secondardy effect upon the living organism, of any act, habit, indulgence or agent, is the exact opposite and equal of the primary effect."

Advocates of the use of condiments have been in the habit of looking at the primary effects of their use and wholly ignoring their secondary effects. They may temporarily make the food eaten more palatable but in the end they make it impossible to enjoy unseasoned food. Their use may temporarily increase the appetite which leads to overeating but in the end this must bring disease with loss of appetite. They may temporarily increase the secretion of the digestive juices but ultimately they exhaust those glands by overworking, over stimulating them. They are like alcohol that appears to give us strength. This is the first and temporary effect. The second and lasting effect is one of weakness, exhaustion.

Nature has arranged so that the use of natural un-seasoned foods, eaten when required by the body and under proper conditions will stimulate the secretion of the digestive fluids in a perfectly normal, natural way and such stimulation is never sufficient to impair the functional vigor of those glands. Artificial means of stimulating them to activity are not necessary. They are always harmful.

If such glands are unable to furnish enough secretions to meet the system's needs they require rest, not stimulation. Just as stimulation, which appears to give us strength, weakens us; so rest and sleep, which appear to weaken us, really strengthens us in the end.

We learned in a previous chapter of the part played by taste in adapting the digestive juices to the food eaten. If this is to be done properly it is necessary that we taste the food thoroughly. If it is disguised with condiments the sense of taste becomes confused. There cannot be the mutual adaptation of juices to food that follows the taste of the food alone. This factor is more important than it may seem to those unaccustomed to think in physiological terms.

Besides the effects of condiments already mentioned these do other things to us that are by no means desirable. They are one and all irritants and as a consequence produce inflammation in the digestive tract. As their use is continued there follows a hardening (toughening) of the mucous membrane lining the alimentary canal. This enables us to use more and more of the condiments.

As an illustration: The Mexican is a great user of cayenne pepper. He is schooled in its use from childhood. A Mexican can eat on one "hot tamale" enough cayenne pepper to "set the whole insides afire" if eaten by the non-user. Yet the Mexican enjoys his firery meal. If you, dear readers, are already addicted to the use of cayenne pepper and have forgotten its influence upon the normal lining of the mouth and throat you may test it or any other condiment upon the lining membrane of your nose. Whatever burns and inflames the lining of the nose will do the same for the stomach. Whatever will thicken and harden the mucuous lining of the mouth and throat will also thicken and harden the lining membrane of the stomach. Non-irritating condiments, such as catsup and certain salad dressings are to be condemned because these disguise the taste of food thus interfering with the adaptation of the digestive juices to the food eaten.

Should the non-user attempt to duplicate the feat of the Mexican, not only would his mouth and throat seem to be on fire but he would feel distress in his stomach. There would be an intense and insatiable thirst. But this is not all. Next day with the movement of his bowels he would experience the same irritation and burning in the rectum, showing that cayenne pepper is indigestible and loses none of its irritating properties during its passage through the digestive organs. It has been twenty to thirty hours in the stomach, intestines and colon, irritating and inflaming these. It has hindered rather than improved digestion. It soon ruins digestion. Its continued use produces a thickening, toughening and reddening of the walls of the stomach and intestines and of the lining membrances of the nose and throat. Black and white pepper have the same effects, only being less irritating than red pepper are milder in their effects. Spices, nutmeg and other "firey" substances produce like effects. The differences in their effects are in degree, not in kind.

These effects are by no means desirable ones and the use of substances that produce them are to be condemned. If by the use of condiments you have so perverted and palsied your sense of taste that you can no longer appreciate the finer flavors of natural food, if everything tastes flat, insipid and unsatisfactory unless highly seasoned, you may be sure that the integrity of your digestive system has been impaired and its powers of digestion greatly weakened.

Mustard, pepper, ginger and all heating spices and condiments, are not only not necessary but are decidedly mischievous in their effects on the digestive apparatus. Dr.

Beumont's renowned experiments upon Alexis St. Martin, which he begun in 1825 and continued without interruption, till 1833, an account of which was published in 1833 under the title "Experiments and Observations on the Gastric Juice and the Physiology of Digestion" are known to all students of physiological science. He found by repeated and careful experiments, that when precisely the same kinds of foods were taken at the same hour on successive days, and in almost exactly similar conditions of the stomach, food which had been dressed with liberal quantities of strong mustard and vinegar was three-quarters of an hour longer in digesting than that which was taken without any condiments. All this difference, was noted in the same stomach, which was accustomed to the use of such condiments and which was, therefore unable, due to loss of tone and vigor as a result of their use, to properly perform its function on pure unstimulating food, as a healthy stomach would have done. The doctor also found that when mustard and pepper were taken with the food these remained in the stomach till all the food was digested and continued to emit a strong aromatic odor to the last; and that the mucous surface of the stomach presented a slightly morbid and turgid appearance towards the close of the digestive process. These important facts have too long been overlooked. Consider them, reader.

The stimulation produced by these various substances, being due to their powers to irritate, is always and necessarily exhausting to the tissues upon which they act, just in proportion as they are unfitted for the real wants of the system and unfriendly to its interests. Whatever may be the real character of the stimulus, every stimulation to which the system is subjected, increases, in proportion to its power and influence, the tone and action of the parts upon which its influence is exerted, and so long as the stimulation lasts, there is always an increased feeling of strength and vigor in the system or part, whether any nutriment has been imparted to it or not.

But the apparent increase in strength and vigor is neither real nor lasting. As soon as the stimulation ceases there is a feeling of weakness and lassitude. By so much as the stimulation exceeds in degree that which is necessary for the full and healthy performance of the function of the organs stimulated, by just so much does the expenditure of vital power and waste of organized substance exceed, for the time, the recuperating and repairing powers of the system, and as a consequence the exhaustion and debility which follow the stimulation are always and necessarily equal to the excess.

In the normal undepraved condition of the mouth and stomach their sensibilities enable them, with the nicest discriminating accuracy to perceive and appreciate both the quality of the stimulus and the degree of stimulation. But the habitual use of unnatural stimulants so deprave the sense of taste and the sensibilities of the stomach that these often wholly lose their powers of discrimination to such an extent that they are unable longer to perceive the quality of the stimulus and retain only the ability to appreciate the degree of stimulation. By such means their delicate susceptibility to the action of their natural and appropriate stimuli (food) is impaired so that natural foods fail to excite sufficient action in these organs to maintain their normal tone and satisfy the demands of the system.

There is a pernicious fallacy abroad that our daily trespasses against the laws of life are as the dropping of water upon a rock—wearing, indeed, but so slow and gradual, so imperceptible that they make scarcely any difference in the duration and comfort of our lives. The truth is the reverse. Nothing is more certain than that these daily transgressions are wearing indeed, but when we consider that the average duration of human life is only about one-third to one-fourth what it should be and this short life is filled with pains, discomforts and disease just in proportion to the extent of our transgressions we may see how fast they wear.

The effects of our habitual transgressions are cumulative. They are comparable to the falling snow. One snow flake will not stop a train but after a few hours of heavy snowing the snow plows have to be called into operation before the trains can run. This fact is not only true of the use of condiments but equally so of any of our transgressions of the laws of life. For instance; it is not probable that one drink of whiskey would have any appreciable effect upon our health or length of life but its continued habitual use even in moderate quantities results in disease and premature death.

Condiments do more than merely impair the digestive organs and deprave the sense of taste. That part of them that enters the circulation exerts the same irritating, stimulating influence upon the other organs of the body. In this way they help to destroy the nerves and harden the arteries. They excite the system, producing a feeling of well being which, in accordance with the law of dual effect, is always followed by a feeling of lassitude.

If you have cultivated the condiment habit and can no longer relish the natural flavors of foods you should begin, at once, to cultivate an appreciation for the more delicate flavors of foods and learn to relish your foods for their own sakes rather than for the seasonings that have been added. You will soon learn to relish wholesome foods and as the years pass you will relish these more and more. In fact, after the passage of sufficient time you will come to appreciate the fine, delicate flavors of foods much more than you now relish the taste of condiments. You will also find your digestion to be better.

Of all the substances added to our food common salt (chloride of sodium) is the only one that is claimed to be indispensible. We do not intend here to notice the flimsy, unfounded, arguments that are advanced in favor of salt eating. We wish rather to call the reader's attention to a few facts concerning its use that utterly condemn the practice.

It should be borne in mind that the body is not capable of utilizing any inorganic substances except water and the oxygen of the air. Common salt is an inorganic substance, and a powerful irritant. Some say it is an irritant poison. Get a small bit in the eye or the raw exposed surface of a cut or wound and be convinced of its irritating powers. It causes sharp pain in the cut or wound. If salt is taken into the system it has the same effect upon the tissues and nerves of the internal economy. Its effects upon the nerves must be great.

It is a stimulant and like all other unnatural stimulants wastes the vital powers. Its stimulating influence upon the flow of saliva is well known. It is used in some institutions in a form of bath known as the salt rub, because of its stimulating properties. The writer remembers one patient to whom a salt rub was so stimulating that it left him exhausted and depressed for the rest of the day. A teaspoonful of salt given to the non-user or to a child, increases the heart beat ten or more times per minute. Such stimulation is never justifiable and is only a waste of vitality.

Dissolve a tablespoonful of salt in a glass of water and drink it. What happens? If the sensibilities of the stomach have not been greatly impaired by the previous use of salt the irritation occasioned by this dose produces vomiting. To protect the delicate lining of the stomach much mucous is poured out.

Or it is discharged into the intestines where more mucous is secreted to envelop the salt and protect the lining of these from its acrid irritating qualities and it is hurried on to the colon and expelled. It occasions a diarrhea. In either case it is hurriedly expelled from the system because the organic instincts recognize that it is wholly innutritious and indigestible and an irritant.

If salt is taken in small quantities it is not met by such a violent reaction. Part of it finds its way into the blood to be eliminated by the skin and kidneys. It is excreted as salt, having undergone no change in its passage through the system. The sweat of the salt eater is salty, it tastes of salt. The writer has many times seen the shirts of salt users who were laboring hard in the heat of summer and sweating profusely, become stiff with salt. Salt could be seen upon the shirt which smelled of brine. Such sweat is irritating to the skin and its glands. The sweat of the non-user is not salty, and does not taste salty.

The tears of the salt user are salty and are irritating to the eyes. The tears of the non-user are not salty and are not irritating. It cannot be possible that nature intended that the tears which are intended to lubricate and cleanse the eyes should be irritating to these.

Salt is wholly innutritious and affords no nourishment to the system. It is both indigestible and unassimilable. It enters the body as a crude inorganic mineral substance, is absorbed unchanged as a mineral substance, goes the rounds of the general circulation as an unassimilated mineral and is finally eliminated as such.

It is an irritant to all the tissues and organs of the body and is met by these everywhere with vital resistance. This reaction against it constitutes the stimulation produced by salt and is therefore always followed by a commensurate degree of debility and atony of the parts affected—stomach, intestines, absorbents, arteries, veins, heart, skin, kidneys, etc.

The use of salt, the same as the use of spices, etc., depraves the sense of taste and weakens or utterly destroys our powers of discriminating between the various food substances eaten. The one who habitually uses salt does not relish his food if no salt has been added. It is true also that the longer the use of salt is continued the more salt is required to produce the desired effects. Salt disguises the natural taste of food thereby hindering the precise adaptation of the digestive juices to the nature of the food eaten. It cannot, in any true sense, improve or aid digestion as is often claimed. Rather it interferes with the normal action of the digestive organs and impairs their powers and sensibilities. It always, in proportion to the freedom with which it is used, diminishes gustatory enjoyment.

The sense of taste is not only a very important and necessary factor in adapting the digestive juices to the food eaten but it is also a guide to the amount of food to eat. A perfectly normal taste is a perfect and reliable guide as to when to cease eating providing one is eating

natural unseasoned food. A perfectly normal taste is rare.
However, if the taste is stimulated and confused by rich
spices and condiments, dressings and flavorings it cannot
serve this true function. Salt is an equal offender in this
respect with these other articles.

In view of these facts does it seem possible that common table salt is necessary to life and health? What then,
becomes of the common arguments that it is universally
used among mankind and certain animals and therefore
necessary? They are seen to be false. Even if we grant
that the salt eating habit is universal among men it does
not prove to be more than a universal deception. However, it is not true that salt is universally used among
mankind. Dr. R. T. Trall remarked in his "Hydropathic
Encyclopedia," Vol. 1. Page 336: "Millions of the human
race have lived healthfully, and died of a good ripe old age,
without employing it at all; * * * furthermore, hundreds
of thousands of human beings now live in the enjoyment
of good health, who have never used salt either as a food
or a condiment."

Richard T. Colburn, in "The Salt Eating Habit,"
says: "I think it would not be difficult to show that there
are whole nations and tribes of people who do not eat salt.
I am told by an Italian, who has lived among them, that
the Algerines do not. I was myself informed while in the
region that the Indian tribes inhabiting the banks of the
Columbia and Puget Sound do not. It is noteworth also that
those tribes are among the most graceful, intelligent and
industrious tribes in North America, and are fine in personal appearance. I think there is little doubt that the
inhabitants of the island of the Pacific ocean lived from a
period of vast antiquity, until the discovery by Europeans,
without putting salt crystals on their food. It has continually happened that hunters, tourists, soldiers and ex-
plorers have been left for weeks, months and years without
a supply of salt, by accident or otherwise, and have survived without apparent injury. Finally, there are many
persons in the United States who have voluntarily abandoned the use of salt for periods ranging from one to

twenty years (and for aught I know longer), not only without injury but with increased health, strength and activity. So far from being natural to man, the instincts of children, especially when born free from an inherited bias in its favor, go to show by their rejection of it that it is unnatural. Like the taste for coffee, tea and various seasonings, it is an acquired one; few if any children but will prefer unsalted food.

"It should not be overlooked that the manufacture and distribution of salt as an article of commerce is a thing of history, and has attained its enormous dimensions within the past century and a half. It is inconceivable that in past times the population of the world, made up as it was largely of pastoral and nomadic people inhabiting the interior of the great continents, should have supplied themselves with salt as an ingredient of food as we do. The ommission of any mention of it in the older chronicles and even among the more perfect records of the classics, except at the luxurious tables of the rich, goes to confirm this supposition."

Sylvester Graham, who possessed one of the keenest and most analytic minds among the early Nature Curists said: "It is a little remarkable that some have contended for the necessity of salt as an article in the diet of man, to counteract the putrescent tendency of animal food or fresh meat, when there is not a carnivorous animal in Nature that even uses a particle of it, and few if any of the purely flesh-eating portions of the human family ever use it in any measure or manner and most portions of the human family who subsist mostly on vegetable food wholly abstain from it."

The author once addicted to the salt eating habit and unable to enjoy his meals without an unusually liberal helping of the mineral, has not used salt now for years and is better in every way without it. Foods that were once flat, insipid, tasteless and unsatisfactory without salt now yield up their many fine delicate flavors which taste a thousand times better than salt. Not only is this true, but foods containing but small amounts of salt are no longer relished.

As to the lower animals there is no real warrant for the assumption that certain of these, including deer, buffalo, cattle, horse, sheep, etc., require and seek salt.

Mr. Colburn says: "I have diligently inquired of old hunters and pioneers for confirmation of the story that deer and buffalo are in the habit of visiting regularly the salt springs or 'licks,' in order to eat the salt. I have not been able to find one who has ever seen the licking process himself. There is reason to believe that hunters do take their positions at certain brine springs to find their game, and that the deer at certain seasons of the year resort to them—precisely why is not determined. Nothing of the kind is now claimed of the buffalo; that is a tradition."

The present writer has been over considerable stretches of this fair land and has never seen a "salt lick." What is more we have inquired of a few old hunters ourselves and have been surprised to find that most of these did not even know what we were talking about. One of those of whom we inquired had hunted deer over Texas, New Mexico, Colorado and Arizona and said he had never heard of a "salt lick."

If it is true, as Mr. Colburn seems to think it is, that deer do frequent brine springs at certain seasons of the year it is not possible that all deer do so for there are vast stretches of land in this country that are or were at one time inhabited by deer where no such springs exist. This is especially true of the plains country of our great southwest where a spring of any kind is a novelty.

Sylvtster Graham wrote: "As to the instinct of the lower animals, it is not true that there is any animal in Nature, whose natural history is known to man, which instinctively makes a dietetic use of salt." It is not even claimed to be true of all animals; in fact, Salt is commonly considered to be fatal to chickens, pigeons, hogs, etc.

Speaking of domestic animals Mr. Colburn wrote: "It is a common notion that salt is necessary to the well-being, if not the preservation, of horses and horned cattle. It is,

I am persuaded, a great mistake. In the first place, although it is undoubtedly true that some domestic cattle will eat salt, and follow impatiently to get it, it is not true of wild cattle. I am assured by many of the great herders in Texas, Colorado, and California, that the native cattle are not fed salt, never see it, and will not eat it if offered. Of course it is a transparent absurdity that salt could be hauled hundreds of miles to feed these great inland herds; and it is not done as is supposed."

In the early days of the cattle industry which had its beginning in Texas and spread from there throughout the west, it is true that salt was not hauled to the cattle and horses. With the coming of the railroads many ranchmen do supply salt for their cattle and stock, not from any need for it on the part of the cattle but simply because popular superstition holds that they require it. No evil effects have been observed to result in cattle deprived of its use.

On the other hand cattle have to be taught to eat salt. It is put in their food, sprinkled on hay after being dissolved in water, etc., until they acquire the salt eating habit. Often when a man possesses but one or a few cows he sprinkles the salt on their backs where it works down through the hair and causes the cows to lick it off. In this way they acquire the habit. Cattle with the salt eating habit are like humans with the same habit—they like salt and will eat it if offered. However, the writer knows from extended experience and observation that cattle do not instinctively turn to salt under any condition but must be taught its use.

It is claimed that salt-fed cattle will fatten faster than those not so fed. This may be true. At least the experiments of Boussingault point to the fact that this is true for a time. His trial showed that ten cattle salted and fed alike in other respects gained in weight some forty pounds in about one-hundred days over ten un-salted cattle, and that, otherwise, both classes were equally good in health at the end of this period. This same might prove true in the case of healthy human beings although, so far as we know, no such experiment has ever been conducted. But one thing is certain, everyone who indulges in salt does not gain weight. Many of them loose weight. Again, it should be borne in mind, that, if it were an actual gain in healthy flesh due to temporary stimulation of the digestive organs of the cattle one hundred days would hardly be a sufficient length of time in which to show the real and lasting effects of salt eating.

But it was no gain in healthy tissue—in muscle, in health, in power. Rather it was a gain in fat. And it is a well-known fact that fat is a disease and not a desirable acquisition.

At this point we can hear the salt addicts saying: "But there are many old men and women who have lived in average health to a good old age and have eaten salt regularly all their lives. If salt is injurious, why have not these suffered?"

It is the old story all over again. The average person is unable to see beyond the point of his nose, at least, he is unable to see anything beyond that point which he does not want to see. In the first place he points to an old man or woman whose age ranges from sixty-five to eighty. This is far short of the age to which man should attain. Again, what passes for average health is not health. It is a diseased state. The average man isn't fit for life's duties after he passes forty or fifty. Most of those who reach eighty or more haven't seen a well day in thirty to forty years. Still less of them are anything but a burden to themselves. They belong to the unburied dead. Lastly these individuals are exceptions. Comparatively few individuals reach eighty years. If only one in a thousand reached that age, however, the addict would see only that one and could not be made to see the nine-hundred-ninety-nine who perished long before. Just why mankind insists on forming his rules on exceptions is not clear, unless, it is that he delights in being a slave to his habits.

This same argument could be brought forward in support of almost any bad habit to which men are addicted. We can point to many old men that have been users of tobacco all their lives. But this does not prove the value of tobacco. We can point to many such old men who have indulged in alcoholic drinks all their lives. But this does not prove the value of alcohol. The same is true of coffee, tea, opium, arsenic and other poisons. But this not only does not prove them to be useful, it does not even prove them to be harmless. As has been remarked: "Our attention is called to the few old survivors of the habit. They resemble the few old survivors of many battles. They survive, not because war is harmless, but in spite of its fatality."

We have not space here to dwell upon other inorganic substances that are used in food in the form of baking powders, cooking soda, etc. While most of these do not seem to be as harmful as salt they are harmful to an extent and absolutely useless to the vital economy. The manufacturers of the various brands of baking powders usually advertise the harmfulness of other brands. What they say of the other powders is usually true but what they neglect to say is that their own powder is as harmful as the ones they are kicking about.

CHAPTER 7
Fruitarianism - Vegetarianism

"And the Lord God planted a garden eastward in Eden and there he put the man whom he had formed.

"And out of the ground made the Lord to grow every tree that is pleasant to the sight and good for food; And the Lord God took the man and put him into the Garden of Eden to dress it and to keep it.

"And the Lord God commanded the man, saying, of every tree of the garden thou mayest freely eat."

In these few words the writer of Genesis explains to us that man was originally a gardener or rather a horticulturist and lived upon the fruits of the trees. In this many of the ancient myths, legends and traditions agree perfectly with Moses. These also picture man as living in a state of perpetual bliss with health, strength and a very long life so long as he remained on his fruit and nut diet and as becoming depraved, weak, short lived and diseased when he forsook this and took to a diet of meat. This early age of man was called the "Golden Age."

Moses tells us that man's first transgression was the eating of a forbidden meal. He has kept this up even down to the present day. Indeed today the forbidden meals seem to be the ones most desired. It is a significant statement of Moses when he said: "And the Lord God said, Behold, the man is become as one of us, to know good and evil: and now lest he put forth his hand, and take also of the tree of life, and eat, and live forever, therefore, the Lord God sent him forth from the garden of Eden, to till the ground from whence he was taken." Moses evidently thought that there was one fruit in the orchard that was such a perfect food that it was capable of sustaining the body in such a degree of perfection that life would continue forever.

After man's transgression Moses represents God as

saying to Adam that because he had disobeyed His command: "Thou shalt eat the herb of the field."

Whatever one's attitude towards the Bible and the Mosaic record may be we cannot escape the fact that here was an early recognition of the truth that man's natural diet was the fruit of the trees of the garden and that in the absence of these the herb and especially the "green herb" of the field is a next best choice. The unperverted instincts of early man may have led to the recognition of this fact.

This same fact is observed in those lower animals belonging to the frugrivorous group. In seasons or localities where there is a scarcity of fruits these animals take easily and naturally to the tender shoots of the herb of the field.

All the facts of comparative anatomy and physiology prove that man is naturally a frugriverous animal that his natural food is the fruit of the trees of the garden. We are aware of the fact that the orthodox scientist attempts to place him in a class with the domestic hog, that is an omnivorous animal. However, this arises not out of any frank consideration of the true facts of anatomical and physiological science but rather it arises out of the old fallacy that whatever the majority of mankind are in the habit of doing is the right thing for all to do. There is an inclination in all of us to consider those conditions under which we grow up to be the natural condition. We become strongly prejudiced in favor of such conditions and allow our prejudices to form the basis of our opinions. We may think we arrived at our positions by due processes of reason and logic but the fact remains that in most instances we were simply born to them.

Most of our so-called thinking processes are devoted to finding excuses for going on believing as we already do. Meat and eggs after they have been "touched up" by the art of the cook have a powerful appeal to the gustatory sense of many and it must be admitted that meat eaters are strongly prejudiced in favor of its use. They like it and do not want to give up its use. For this reason every excuse is sought to serve as a reason for making a burial ground of our stomachs. But the fact remains that man was never intended as a corpse eater and should not now be swallowing the carcasses of dead animals.

Man is not fitted by nature to rend and tear as are the beasts of prey. He does not relish the sight, taste or smell of fresh blood and the warm quivering flesh of his freshly killed victim. Killing is really repulsive to the higher nature of man.

There are many anatomical and physiological differences between man and the carnivero such as the relative size of the liver and length of the digestive tract, the differences in the structure of their teeth, their differencs in natural equipment for securing food, the differences in the character of their digestive juices, of the chemical reaction of their urine, differences in thyroid activity and many others which unfit man for a diet of meat. We cannot dwell upon these differences but must pause to say that while it is true that man possesses a wonderful power and range of adaptability which has enabled him to use considerable meat, it is not possible for him to so alter his anatomy and physiology to such an extent that he will be able to take care of a meat diet with the same degree of efficiency that he does the diet he is adapted to by Nature. Although man has included meat in his diet for thousands of years his anatomy and physiology, and the chemistry of his digestive juices are still unmistakably that of a frugivorous animal.

Not only is this true but there is ample evidence that the use of meat, particularly its use in the usual quantities is detrimental to man's health and strength of mind and body. This is due chiefly to four factors:

First: Meat is very rich in protein and its use in the usual quantities means the intake of considerable more protein than is required with the consequences we have previously noted. This same objection applies to the liberal use of eggs.

Second: Meat contains considerable quantities of the end products of metabolism which are held up in the tissues at the time of death. These wastes are poisonous and irritating and lend to meat a stimulating property that is usually mistaken for added strength.

Third: No matter how carefully handled, meat very readily undergoes putrefaction and it is impossible to get it so fresh that more or less putrefaction has not already taken place. It also putrefies as readily in the digestive tract and the putrefactive poisons it forms in the stomach and intestines are the same as those it forms when allowed to putrefy in the ice box.

Fourth: The conditions under which animals are kept that are intended for use as food and the manner in which they are fed to fatten them are not conductive to health. It is very seldom, if ever, that a fattened animal is killed that is free of disease and the eating of diseased meat is not conductive to health.

Any animal to live upon a meat diet must be equipped to overcome the difficulties these things present. Some of the lower animals will make a feast off the rotting carcass of an animal that has been dead for days while others will eat only freshly killed prey which they have killed themselves. Those that feast off the rotting carcass—buzzard, opossum, hyæna, etc.,—do not die of ptomaine poisoning but such a feast would be dangerous to man. Of course many do eat rotten meats (''ripened'' poultry, for instance) without so suffering but there is no doubt but that their health would be much better if they did not eat such food. Man, if in good health, can take considerable putrescent matter into his stomach without any appreciable injury but this is no reason why he should make a habit of doing so.

There can no longer be any doubt in the minds of those who are willing to look at this matter with an unbiased mind that an intelligently planned diet free of meat, fish, fowl, eggs, milk, cheese, etc., is conductive to greater health and strength of body and clearness of mind. Hindhede, in his study of the dietetic habits of the nations of earth found that the people of most nations are practically or wholly vegetarians and that the nearer they approached this ideal the less disease and weakness existed among them. Other students of this subject have shown this same to be true.

The experiments of Profs. Chittenden and Fisher of Yale and those of Horace Fletcher demonstrated that a higher degree of strength and endurance may be maintained on a fleshless diet while the facts of history testify in very eloquent tones to the superiority of a fleshless diet.

The Greeks and Romans conquered the world on a vegetable diet. Their soldiers marched for miles each day, carried heavy armor and fought with such heavy armor in violent hand to hand combats that required strength, endurance, speed, agility, quick wits and precision.

The early German tribes that overran and conquered Rome were practically vegetarians. The Hindoos, Chinese, etc., have been vegetarians from time immemorial. The peasantry of Europe are yet practically vegetarians seldom tasting animal food.

We take the following miscellaneous excerpts from "Fruits and Farnacea" by Smith and Trall:

"The peasantry of Norway, Sweden, Russia, Denmark, Poland, Germany, Turkey, Greece, Switzerland, Spain, Portugal, and almost every country in Europe subsist principally and most of them entirely on vegetable food. The Persians, Hindoos, Burmese, Chinese, Japanese, the inhabitants of the East Indian Archipelago, and of the mountains of the Himalays and in fact most of the Asiatics, live upon vegetable productions."

"The people of Russia, generally, subsist on coarse black bread and garlics. I have often hired men to labor for me. They would come on board in the morning with a piece of black bread weighing about a pound and a bunch of garlics as big as one's fist. This was all their nourishment for the day of sixteen or eighteen hours labor. They were astonishingly powerful and active, and endured severe and protracted labor far beyond any of my men. Some of these Russians were eighty and even ninety years old and yet these old men would do more work than any of the middle aged men belonging to my ship."

"The Chinese feed almost entirely on rice, confections and fruit; those who are enabled to live well and spend a temperate life, are possessed of great strength and agility."

"The Egyptian Cultivators of the soil, who live on coarse wheaten bread, Indian corn, lentils and other productions of the vegetable kingdom, are among the finest people I have ever seen."

"The Greek boatmen are exceedingly abstemious. Their food consists of a small quantity of black bread, made of unbolted rye or wheat meal and a bunch of grapes or raisins or some figs. They are astonishingly athletic and powerful; and the most nimble, active, graceful, cheerful and even merry people in the world."

"From the day of his irruption into Europe the Turk has always proved himself to be endowed with singularly strong vitality and energy. As a member of a warlike race, he is without an equal in Europe in health and hardiness. His excellent physique, his simple habits, his abstinence from intoxicating liquors, and his normal vegetarian diet enables him to support the greatest hardships and to exist on the scantiest and simplest food."

"The Spaniards of Rio Salada in South America, who come down from the interior and are employed in transporting goods overland, live wholly on vegetable food. They are largely, very robust and strong; and bear prodigious burdens on their backs, traveling over mountains too steep for loaded mules to ascend and with a speed which few of the generality of men can equal without encumberance."

"In the most heroic days of the Greecian army their food was plain and simple produce of the soil. The immortal Spartans of Thermopylae were, from infancy, nourished by the plainest and coarsest vegetable aliment; and the Roman army in the period of its greatest valour and most gigantic achievements, subsisted on plain and coarse vegetable food. When the public games of Ancient Greece —for the exercise of muscular power and activity in wrestling, boxing, running, etc.,—were first instituted, the atheletae in accordance with the common dietetic habits of the people, were trained entirely on vegetable food."

The superior value of a diet of fruits and vegetables were recognized by such early sages as Pythagoras, Plutarch, Plato, Socrates and others. The laws of the Spartans forbid the eating of flesh. Of the training of the early Greek athletes the historian Rollin says:

"Those who were destined to this profession frequented from their most tender age the Gymnasia or Palaestrae which were a kind of academies maintained for that purpose at the public's expense. In these places, such were under the direction of different masters, who employed the most effectual methods to inure their bodies for the fatigues of the public games, and to form them for the combats. The regimen they were under was very hard and severe. At first they had no other nourishment but dried figs, nuts, the recent curd of milk, a new cheese and boiled grains, or a coarse kind of bread called maza. They were absolutely forbidden to use wine, and required to observe the strictest continence." In later times when animal food came into general use a portion of flesh meat was introduced into the diet of the atheletae but according to the testimony of early Greek writers it was soon found that the free use of meat made them "the most sluggish and stupid of men," and, therefore, those who had the training of the atheletae withheld meat from them entirely, till a short time before their public performance, and then it was introduced in very small quantities at first, and gradually increased. In spite of all this care, the stupefying effect of the flesh meat was so apparent, and especially on the mental powers, that the stupidity of the athletae became proverbial

In 1907 thirteen British physicians issued a remarkable manifesto in which they said:— "We, the undersigned medical men, having carefully considered the subject of vegetarianism in its scientific aspects and having put its principles to the test of actual experience hereby record an emphatic opinion that not only is the practice based on a truly scientific foundation but it is conductive to the best physical conditions of human life."

A few years ago a walking-match was held in Germany in which fourteen meat-eaters and eight vegetarians started off for a seventy mile hike. All the vegetarians reached the goal, "in splendid condition," the first requiring but fourteen and a quarter hours. The first and also the last meat eater to arrive came in "completely exhausted" and demanded brandy to "revive" him, just one hour after the last vegetarian arrived. All the rest of the meat eaters had dropped out of the race after the first thirty-five miles had been covered.

In 1902 the famous Karl Mann of Berlin, a vegetarian, won the Berlin-Dresden walking contest covering the distance of 125 miles in 26 hours and 52 minutes. He was examined by a committee of physicians at the close of his walk and again 24 hours later and declared to be in a most excellent condition.

In the next four days following his walk he was kept so busy writing, lecturing and being interviewed that he says he slept but 21 hours during the four days. Thus he proved that the highest degree of physical and mental energy can both be obtained at one and the same time from a diet which strictly excludes flesh, fowl, alcohol, coffee, tea, cocoa, chocolate and every other stimulant. Mr. Mann takes but two meals daily and excludes besides the above mentioned articles, milk, eggs, cheese, butter and pulse from his diet.

In 1906 Mr. Mann again won the Berlin-Dresden walking contest over 31 competitors. The thirty-two contestants left Dresden at 7:30 A. M. on May 18th, in bad weather. Of these, part were fruitarians and vegetarians and part were meat eaters. The first six to arrive in Berlin were fruitarians and vegetarians. Mr. Mann who came in first, covered the distance in 26 hours and 58 minutes, just six minutes more time than he required to cover the same distance four years before. He was fresh at the finish while of the meat eaters who were well known and tried athletes it is said they "arrived utterly exhausted."

In describing the remarkable feats of strength performed by the "hercules of Hindustan" Prof. Bastana Koomar of Calcutta, India and Extension Lecturer of the

University of Wisconsin says: "The average American is apt to jump to the conclusion that this Hindu Hercules eats nothing but the very best cuts of porterhouse steak, the rarest game birds and the most high priced eggs to make him so strong as that.

"Nothing of the kind. Ram Murti is a strict vegetarian. He never eats meat in any form, nay, not even eggs."

When Geo. W. Patterson, the well known Chicago athlete climbed Pike's Peak a few years ago he said in the Denver Times :

"Raw food is the best strength builder and enabled me while carrying 30 pounds of luggage on a very inferior running wheel, to readily draw away from the apparently strong meat eating wheelman going up to Palmer Lake.

"But the climbing of Pike's Peak was the real test. My companion, though a vegetarian and of about equal physical ability, ate partly cooked food. Three meat eaters were with us from the half-way house nearly to the timber line; one of these was an experienced mountain climber of fine physique against whom I thought I stood no show, as I had never been above Hog's Back, near Morrison, before; and to get into such altitude was a decidedly new experience. But at the timber line even the best man slowed down, and his mouth breathing became very labored, while a dozen raisins and dates had so strengthened me that I felt I must go faster to reach the summit before daylight, so I went on alone the last three miles in a little over an hour, making the last half mile faster than any before, over frozen ties and finishing on a brisk run. The down trip showed as much superiority of the food as the ascent had.

"As to the cold or disease resisting qualities of the food, I can say that I took a bath in the cold stream at night above the halfway house, rubbing off with the hands only, in a drizzling rain, then lying down for over three hours in a damp, deserted mine to sleep, with only one extra suit of summer underwear on in addition to the ordinary summer clothing. Neither this nor three hours standing in the cold at the summit left the slightest trace of a cold, in fact, I do not believe one can catch a cold or take any other disease unless the system is filthy inside from accumulated unneeded food, which will not digest without exceptional effort. The best cure for this condition is a short fast, followed by a very light fruit and then raw food diet. Of course using unlimited fresh air, distilled water, contact with the earth and sunshine, good healthful, all-around exercise, preferably in the mountains, air, sun, and cold water baths.''

Otto Carque quotes a northern explorer as saying: ''Many labor under the impression, that they cannot keep warm during the winter months, especially in Alaska, unless they eat an abundance of meat and animal fat. This is an erroneous idea, as has been amply and practically demonstrated. Our houses are not plastered and are not made extra warm, yet I wear thin clothing most of the winter and keep comfortable. I have no difficulty in finding good nourishing food. At present I am following a strict vegetarian diet. My health is none the less robust, and perhaps it is to that regimen I owe my keen sensibility to impressions and a hopeful, contented disposition.''

The Dallas Morning News (Dallas, Texas) for May 20, 1923 carried the following news item from Cristobal, Canal Zone.—''Athletes from the Panama Canal Zone may be America's hope in the marathon race to be held at the Paris Olympiad in 1924.

''During the recent maneuvers of the Forty-second Infantry in the jungles, several of the regiment's long distance men were detailed as runners to deliver messages from the camp to divisional headquarters at Balboa. The runners carried messages over the jungle trails in the heat of the blazing tropical sun in a manner that would be utterly impossible for an American.

''The Forty-second Infantry is composed of natives of Porto Rico, all naturalized Americans. Sergt. Cabalero is the Isthmian long-distance champion and Antonio Cruz and Carlos Moreno have finished a close second and third in recent races. These men are descendants of Indian and

Spanish settlers. They live simply and train on a diet of rice, bread, beans and tropical fruit.''

From every source comes unmistakable evidence of the superiority of the no-animal-food diet in building health, strength, endurance and body symmetry. In this country it used to be thought that the manual laborer could not get along without meat or eggs for each meal, and this idea still prevails to some extent. However, a new idea is fast supplanting this. It is now held in many quarters that while vegetarianism or fruitarianism will do for the physical worker, the mental worker should have meat. It is contended that the eating of meat saves digestive energy which may then be utilized in mental effort. The idea is absurd on the face of it. First mental efficiency like physical efficiency depends upon health and pure blood and a proper training of the mind and it has been demonstrated over and over again in millions of cases that pure blood and health are better maintained on a fruit or vegetable diet than upon a meat diet. Second, if any appreciable quantity of energy is saved in the digestion of meat it should make itself apparent in greater physical as well as mental endurance.

The prodigious mental labors of Geo. B. Shaw who is a strict vegetarian points to the fact that a meatless diet is good also for the mental worker. Thomas A. Edison and Nicolas Tesla do not find meat a necessary article of diet. Isaac Newton lived on coarse bread and water while demonstrating the principles of calculus, the new mathematical method he perfected in application to the revolutions of the moon. Nearly all of the ancient sages were vegetarians or fruitarians and all of these agree that such is man's natural diet. The truth is there is as much evidence that this diet is as conductive to strength and clearness of mind as to physical strength and endurance. Over two thousand years ago the Grecian schools of philosophy taught it as a well established fact of experience, and it became a generally received doctrine, that ''eating much and feeding upon flesh, makes the mind more dull, and drives it to the very extremes of madness.'' Theophrastus, who studied under Plato and Aristotle and succeeded the latter in the Lyceum is authority for that statement. We are informed that his auditors became two thousand and that he died at the age of one-hundred and seven.

Diogenes asserted that the proverbial stupidity of the athlete, to which we have already referred, was wholly due to their excessive use of the flesh of swine and oxen. The Calmucks, Tere Del Fuegians, and indeed all portions of the human family that feed principally upon flesh foods are remarkable for their mental stupidity, sluggishness and indocility.

The cause of vegetarianism and fruitarianism is making rapid strides in the world today because it is founded on correct principles, appeals to the reason of the average man and works in actual practice.

It is not to be denied that man was created with a constitutional adaptation to ''every green herb bearing seed, and every tree, in which is the fruit of a tree yielding seed'' so that a pure and proper vegetable diet is essential to the highest and best condition of human nature. But God has also given man a constitutional capability of adapting himself, within certain limits, to things that are not compatible with the highest and best condition of human nature, but which, as it constitutes more or less of an infraction of the laws of his being, will sustain his physiological and psychological interest only with more or less disadvantage and deterioration.

Many noting this constitutional capability of adaptation have contended that man by reason of his superior powers of intellect and reason is capable of rising above the laws of his nature and by the exercise of his rational and voluntary powers may adapt himself to those things that are not naturally adapted to his needs so as to make them equally as congenial to his nature as those things to which he is by nature adapted. This view represents a rather superficial and entirely erroneous conception of the whole problem. This principle, if correct, furnishes a legitimate excuse for indulgence in any and all unnatural practices to which man may be able to adapt himself, including even, drug habits, condiment eating, etc. But it is false to think that the reason of man lifts him above the laws of his own being and enables him to transgress these with impunity.

If man is not organized to eat flesh in its natural state and if animal flesh is not congenial to the highest physiological and psychological interest of his nature, then no power of reason can enable him to render it suitable food for him or make him naturally an omniverous animal. It can make him artificially an omniverous animal only with detriment to all his physiological powers.

This physiological power of adaptibility is by no means confined to man but is common to the horse, cow, sheep, dog, cat, lion, tiger, etc., and perhaps to the whole animal kingdom. In the higher classes, at least, both the carniverous and herbiverous as well as the frugivorous animals possess a wide scope of adaptibility to various kinds of food substance. Not only has the dog and cat been taught to live upon vegetable foods but so have the eagle, the lion, etc. Sheep, horses, cows, etc., have been trained to live upon a flesh diet. If then the power of adaptibility which man possess makes of him an omniverous animal like the domesticated hog, then the same power possessed by these other animals prove them to be likewise. The truth is the reverse and no lion, eagle or tiger, in a state of nature ever feeds upon vegetable food, nor does the horse, sheep, rabbit, deer, or buffalo in a state of nature feed upon flesh food. These animals are led instinctively to eat only those foods to which they are constitutionally adapted and reject all others. Man should know that in him reason has not been substituted for instinct but superadded to it, not for contrary but for the same and higher accordant purposes.

The old idea that the human body is not subject to law still warps and twists the reasoning of many. Men who believe that the movements of the stars of heaven are ruled by fixed and unalterable law give voice to ideas that are founded on no other than the idea of physiological lawlessness. An excellent example of this is contained in a short item by a well known authority on diet, and published January 24, 1925. He says: "Many people do not seem to be thoroughly nourished without meat as an occasional part of their diet, though milk and eggs are often a satisfactory substitute. * * * Meat eaters usually have a greater tendency to physical ailments of various kinds. A meatless diet, if you can be thoroughly nourished on it, will usually develop a greater endurance, and I believe the time will come when it will be proved that non-meat eaters live to a greater age than those who eat meat."

Does it not seem a bit strange that some are so constituted that they are forced to lower their endurance, subject themselves to various physical ailments and shorten their lives in order to be well nourished? Does it not strike the reader as being absurd that the physiological laws and requirements of many demand meat, even though its use is an evil, while these same laws and requirements of many more do not require this evil, in order to be "thoroughly nourished." This is physiological lawlessness with a vengeance. But this is not all. In the Jan. 24, 1925 issue of The Graphic is an item by Milo Hastings explaining the world-old fallacy that what is one man's food is another man's poison. He says:

"Did you ever stop to think when you saw a very fat man and a very thin underweight man sit down and eat the same meal? If so, common sense would tell you that both cannot be eating right, and that if the meal is correct for one of them, it must be 'poison' for the other."

Any ranchman would know better than this. If he wants to fatten a herd of cattle, hogs or horses he feeds them, all alike, upon the same food. And they all grow fat upon it. That is, they all grow fat upon it, if they are all healthy animals. If one or more of the animals fail to fatten the ranchman knows immediately that there is something wrong with the animal, not with the diet. He knows, too, that as soon as the animal is restored to health this same diet will fatten him. The writer was born and reared in Texas and has had considerable experience in feeding animals and much opportunity to observe the feeding by others.

The reader who has read and understands the chapter entitled *"Man Shall not Diet with Food Alone"* will readily grasp the thought I here intend to convey. All these ideas that chaos reigns in the realm of physiology should be ignored by the intelligent reader.

If a man does not seem to be "thoroughly nourished" on a vegetarian or a fruitarian regimen it is not the fault of the regimen but of the man. There is nothing in meat, except the wastes of the animal, that is not in the fruits and vegetables. The man who does not seem thoroughly nourished without meat is in the same class as the man who does not seem thoroughly fed unless he has had his smoke after eating. I do not appeal to that old fiction called "common sense" but to facts and logic.

A theory has recently arisen in certain Nature Cure quarters, where there is a decided trend toward spiritism and occultism, that while vegetarianism or fruitarianism and the uncooked food plan are good for people in general there are many cases that must have flesh foods, eggs, etc., to maintain health. Health is referred to as a positive and disease as a negative state of body or mind. The negative or acid-forming foods, meat, eggs, cheese, refined foods, etc., are correctly credited with being the cause of the negative condition. To remedy such conditions the eating of negative foods is stopped and fruits and vegetables chiefly uncooked, that are rich in the positive organic mineral elements are fed to counteract and overcome the negative or acid condition.

Thus far, all is well, but it is contended that many, after being restored to health by this diet, have to return to the old disease building diet, because, it is claimed, the continued use of positive foods, after these have corrected the negative condition, builds a negative condition and produces symptoms of abnormal psychicism in some. In order, then, to overcome or prevent such a negative condition negative foods are fed while the positive ones are reduced.

The whole thing is a subversion of the laws of diet and is built, not upon sound principles of physiological science, but upon the incoherent and childish mutterings of spiritism and occultism. In part, it is an attempt to supply an excuse for the indulgence in flesh food, alcohol, etc., by those making these claims, its other purpose is securely hidden away in the inner chambers of occult philosophies.

The very fact that such results are observed only by and among those who dabble in crystal gazing, table rapping, and frequent the darkened chambers of the seance room and have never been observed elsewhere should lead us to view the theory with suspicion. For it is a well known fact that symptoms of abnormal psychism develop very frequently in those who dabble in the occult no matter what their diet. In fact it has been the writer's observation that a majority of these people sooner or later develop abnormal nervous and mental symptoms.

Mediumship is admitted by all spiritists to place a tremendous strain upon the nervous system of the medium and these ladies are often exhausted for days following a "trance." Other practices of these people such as "healing," "entering the silence," "crystal gazing," "table rapping," "fortune telling," etc., also place more or less strain upon the nervous organization of the operators. It is far more reasonable to ascribe the abnormal symptoms to these and other practices of which they in common with the rest of mankind are guilty rather than to place the blame upon a natural and healthful diet which has already proven its value in their case by restoring or greatly improving their health.

To say the least it is absurd to claim that a positive diet after building positivity will in some cases build negatively while a negative diet that once built a negative condition will restore a positive condition after it has been lost. We should study diet in the light of Nature and physiological facts and not allow mysticism and occultism to lead us astray.

As an instance of the misleading tendency of these pseudo-philosophies we present the following. In the summer of 1921 we listened to a nationally known lecturer upon New Thought, Occult science (?) etc. During the course of her lecture she told of a child that had died as a result of excessive candy eating. She said: "Had the child been in perfect harmony with the higher thought, the overeating of candy would not have injured the child. But the 'world-thought' is; too much candy injures children, and the child succumbed to this world-thought." Such talk is utter foolishness and arises from a very superficial view of the laws of nature. It is also the world-thought that water will drown a man if he fills his lungs with it and is not rescued in time but no amount of harmony with the "higher thought" will set aside the laws of nature and prevent the water from drowning the man. The "world-thought" that water will drown one like the "world-thought" that excessive candy eating injures children (grown ups also) came only after the effects had been witnessed. Man did not first get the idea that water will drown us, and then, begin to be drowned later but men were drowned first and then we knew what the water would do.

If "world-thought" was that opium or alcohol were congenial to man's psychological and physiological interest neither "higher thought" nor "world-thought" nor the two combined would prevent the use of these substances from producing their ruinous effects. We have no intentions of denying the real and legitimate powers of mind but we do desire to make it plain that no mental or occult system can be made to take the place of obedience to the laws of our own constitution, physiological and psychological. Such ideas as the one this lady presented enter our heads at a time when there is nobody on duty upstairs.

In conclusion let us reiterate the statement made many times before in former chapters that correct eating or abstinence from eating cannot be made to atone for our transgressions of natural laws in other departments of life. Proper food will not compensate for a lack of exercise nor take the place of sexual temperance. Life is a many-sided affair and if we expect to enjoy it in the highest it is necessary that we keep all sides in order.

Do not get the idea that by merely dropping meat and eggs from your diet all your troubles will vanish. It is as easy to make oneself sick by the improper use of vegetables and fruits as by the use of flesh foods. Follow the rules for eating and combining given in a later chapter and then observe all the other rules and principles that govern life.

CHAPTER 8
How to Eat

Man is a creature of habit. During the many ages that have elapsed since his introduction upon the earth he has accumulated many harmful habits and practices and left behind or perverted his natural instincts. Man's instincts, originally perfect and a safe guide in life are today like a pair of assayer's scales that have been thrown upon an ash heap for some time. These scales are so delicately balanced that they will weigh the amount of lead or carbon used in writing one's name. After lying out on an ash heap for a few months and becoming corroded with rust they will weigh nothing accurately. So man's instincts after six thousand years on the ash heap of sin and sensuality are today very unreliable guides. Probably, in none other is this more true than those instincts that relate man to his food. For this cause, reason and science have to be called to the aid of instinct that we may learn again, how to eat.

All eating should be done to serve the actual needs of the body for nutritive material and should never be indulged in for mere pleasure, as a social function, merely from meal time habit or for some other reason. If we do this we cannot possibly over eat. Over eating is our greatest and most common dietetic error. This overworks the stomach and intestines, the liver, kidneys, heart, lungs, glands, in fact, the whole physiological economy and occasions a tremendous expenditure of nervous energy.

The prevailing idea that the body is a machine that needs only to be supplied with fuel as an engine requires to be supplied with coal is a very mischievous fallacy. While it is claimed that food is burned in the body to produce energy there are many reasons to doubt this. From the minute we arise in the morning until we retire at night we suffer a gradual decline in power, notwithstanding our constant ingestion of food. In fact, it can readily be shown that the more food one eats the more power he will lose. We are thoroughly tired after a long day of grinding toil but we can no more recuperate our strength at the table than at the grog shop. Rest and sleep, even if no food is eaten, will replenish our strength. There is usually, if ones does not eat a very heavy meal, a feeling of exhiliration and renewed strength following the ingestion of a meal but this is stimulation not added power.

Eating for strength, then, really means eating in moderation. For over eating not only puts a heavy tax upon the system in the effort to digest the food; it clogs up the system with an excess of nutritive matter and toxins. The undigested portions of the food undergo fermentation and putrefaction generating poisons of various kinds.

Disease is inevitable. Stronger constitutions, or those with very strong digestive powers may endure this abuse longer than their less fortunate friends but even these must sooner or later give down under the strain. Sylvester Graham has well said: ''A drunkard may reach old age, but a glutton never.''

We should not only eat to supply the real needs of the body but we should eat only such foods as really supply those needs and that are, at the same time, devoid of any injurious properties. The food should be fresh and wholesome and as near the natural state as can be obtained. All denatured foods—foods that have been milled, refined, canned, preserved, embalmed, treated chemically or otherwise tampered with, should be excluded. All dried foods that have been bleached by chemical process or treated by chemicals for any purpose during the drying process, white sugar, white flour, degerminated corn meal, polished rice, canned goods, most so-called breakfast foods, embalmed meats, etc., should be excluded from one's diet.

Observe those two rules—eat only to supply the actual needs of the body, and eat only fresh, clean, wholesome, natural foods—and all other rules of diet become of secondary importance. However, if we observe these other rules they will aid us in observing these two primary rules —of moderation and naturalness.

The first rule in any truly natural system of feeding should be: EAT ONLY WHEN HUNGRY. If we do this we eat only to supply the demands of the body. We cannot repeat too often the admonition, do not eat if not hungry.

Hunger is the voice of nature saying to us that food is required. There is no other true guide when to eat. The time of day, the habitual meal time, etc., these are not true guides.

But there is a vast difference between hunger and what is called appetite. Appetite is a counterfeit hunger, a creature of habit and cultivation, and may be due to any one of a number of things; such as, the arrival of the habitual meal time, the sight, taste or smell of food, condiments and seasonings, or even the thought of food. In some diseased states there is an almost constant and insatiable appetite. None of these things can arouse true hunger for this comes only when there is an actual need of food.

One may have an appetite for tobacco, coffee, tea, opium, alcohol, etc., but he can never be hungry for these since they serve no real physiological need.

Appetite is often accompanied by a gnawing or "all gone" sensation in the stomach, or a general sense of weakness, there may even be mental depression. Such symptoms usually belong to the diseased stomach of a glutton and will pass away if their owner will refrain from eating for a few days. They are temporarily relieved by eating and this leads to the idea that it was food that was needed. But such sensations and feelings do not accompany true hunger. In true hunger one is not aware that he has a stomach for this, like thirst, is a mouth and throat sensation. Real hunger arises spontaneously, that is without the agency of some external factor and is accompanied by a "watering of the mouth" and usually by a conscious desire for some particular food.

The hungry person is able to eat a crust of dry bread and relish it. One who only has an appetite must needs have his food seasoned and spiced before he can enjoy it.

Even a gormand is able to enjoy a hearty meal if there is sufficient seasoning to whip up his jaded appetite and arouse his palsied taste. But he would be many times the better for it if he would only await the arrival of true hunger before eating.

If this plan were followed, what would become of our present three meals a day plan? It would be relegated to oblivion where it truly belongs. It should be known that the three-meals-a-day custom is really a modern one. So far as history records none of the nations of antiquity practiced it. At the period of their greatest power the Greeks and Romans ate only one meal per day. Among the many things that have been offered as an explanation for their physical, mental and moral decline has been their sensuous indulgence in food which came with power and riches. Whatever other factors may have contrived to bring about their decline (and certain it is there were many factors) there can be no doubt that their excessive indulgence in the pleasures of the palate contributed its fair share.

Herodotus records that the invading hosts (over five millions) of the Persian general, Xerxes, had to be fed by the conquered cities along their line of march. He states as a fortunate circumstance the fact that the Persians, including even the Monarch and his courtiers, ate but one meal per hay.

The Jews from Moses until Christ ate but one meal per day. They sometimes added a lunch of fruit. We recall reading once in the Hebrew scriptures these words (quoting from memory) ''Woe unto the nation whose princes eat in the morning.'' If this has any reference to dietetic practices it would indicate that the Jews were not addicted to what Dr. Dewey called the ''vulgar habit'' of eating breakfast.

In the oriental world today extreme moderation as compared to the American Standard, is practiced.

One should always seek to eat at such times and under conditions that will insure the best results in digestion. Some things enhance digestion while others impede it. If the following two rules are adhered to this condition will be met.

Rule 2. NEVER EAT WHEN IN PAIN, MENTAL DISCOMFORT OR WHEN FEVERISH.

Any or all of these hinder the secretion of the digestive juices, divert the nervous energies away from the digestive organs and impair digestion. If pain is severe or fever is high all desire for food is lacking. If these are not so marked a slight desire may be present, especially in those whose instincts are perverted. Animals in pain instinctively avoid food.

Any food eaten, while there is fever will only add to the fever. The feverish person needs a fast not a feast.

In the chapter on digestion it was learned that certain mental states enhance digestion while others retard and impair the process. The illustration is an old one of the person who sits down to enjoy a hearty meal, after a hard day's work. He has a ravenous desire for food. Just as he is about to begin eating some one brings him the news of the loss of a loved one through death, or of the loss of a fortune. Instanly all desire for food is gone.

Why is this? Because the body needs all its energies to meet this new circumstance, and it requires much energy to digest food. Food eaten under such conditions is not digested. It will ferment and poison the body.

A very interesting experiment once performed upon a cat will be of aid to us here in making this rule clear. The cat was fed a bismuth meal after which his stomach was viewed by means of the X-ray. The stomach was observed to be working nicely.

At this point a dog was brought into the room. Instantly, fear siezed hold upon the cat. His muscles became tense and motionless, his hair "stood on end." The stomach was viewed a second time and seen to be as tense and motionless as the voluntary muscles. Digestion was at a standstill. The dog was taken from the room whereupon the cat became calm and settled, with the result that the stomach resumed its work.

These facts, more of which could be given, illustrate

nicely the effects of the mental state upon digestion and teach us, very forcefully, the folly of eating when in mental distress. Worry has a similar effect. It practically stops the flow of gastric juice and inhibits the normal peristalic movements of the stomach.

Allow me to repeat: Never eat when in pain, mental or physical discomfort or when feverish. If the eating of a meal is followed by bodily discomfort or by distress in stomach and bowels do not eat until this is past. This is the natural way and is instinctively followed by the lower animals.

Rule 3. NEVER EAT DURING OR IMMEDIATE-LY BEFORE OR AFTER WORK OR HEAVY MENTAL AND PHYSICAL EFFORT.

Many who read this rule will throw up their hands in holy horror and exclaim: "But I cannot work without food! I must eat to keep up my strength!" All of which reveals how little real knowledge of food and feeding they possess. The ancient Romans displayed more knowledge when they said: "A full stomach does not like to think."

The fact is, if digestion is to proceed normally almost the entire attention of the system must be given to the work. Blood is rushed to the digestive organs in large quantities. There is a dilation of the blood vessels in the organs to accommodate the extra supply of blood. There must be a consequent constriction of the blood vessels in other parts of the body in order to force the blood into the digestive organs and to compensate for their own loss of blood.

But if the brain and muscles are to work they, too, require an increased blood supply. In order to supply them there is a dilation of the blood vessels in the brain or muscles and a contraction of the blood vessels in the viscera.

Every part of the body cannot be supplied with extra blood at the same time. If one part gets an extra supply some other part must get less.

The same is true of the nervous energies. Those organs that are working must be supplied with nerve force. If one is engaged in mental or physical effort his nervous energies are diverted from the digestive organs and digestion suffers.

The animal in a natural state lays down and takes a rest, perhaps some sleep, after eating a meal. Some years ago an experiment was made by feeding a dog his usual meal of meat and then taking him out for a fox hunt for a few hours. The dog was then killed and the stomach opened. The meat was found to be in the same condition as when eaten. Another dog fed at the same time and left at home to rest had completely digested his meal.

The dog in the chase was using all his blood and nervous energies in running. Digestion simply had to wait. In spite of the fact that this principle is well known there are still many who pose as diet experts who advise that the heartiest meal of the day be taken in the morning. The reasons given are (1) The body after a night of sleep is better able to digest the meal than in the evening after the day's work is done, and, (2) The food eaten at this time will supply energy for the day's work.

It is true that we have more energy after the night's rest than after the day's work. It is not true, however, that the digestive organs have rested during the night. It is also true that real hunger is not produced by a night of restful repose and to eat a heavy meal in the absence of hunger would be contrary to the first law of natural dietetics. All of this aside, the digestion of a meal eaten in the morning would have to wait upon the other work. We can force our mind and muscles to act and thereby withdraw the blood from the stomach but the stomach cannot force these other organs to cease their activities and permit the blood and nerve force to be sent to it.

If food supplies energy, it can do so only after it is digested and absorbed. Under normal conditions the digestion of a meal in both the stomach and intestines requires from ten to sixteen hours. If one is working, either mentally or physically much longer time is required. Food taken in the morning could not, therefore, supply any energy for the day's work. On the contrary, if the food is to be digested, that part of the energy required to do the work of digesting it is taken from the day's work. Any-one who will test this out may soon satisfy himself of the correctness of this principle. Let him give up the morning meal for a few weeks and note the results.

The morning meal is best omitted altogether. At most it should consist of an orange or unsweetened grape fruit. The noon meal should be very light. The evening meal should be the heaviest meal and should be taken only after one has rested a little from his day's toil.

During sleep the blood is withdrawn from the brain and muscles. So, also, the nerve force is withdrawn from the muscles. The viscera receive the blood and much of the nerve force. Digestion may proceed without hindrance. If one is sleeping there is no fear, worries, anxieties, etc., to interfere with the work of digestion.

Of course, if one has had a full meal for breakfast and a full meal for noon he has already had too much food and will be very uncomfortable if another full meal is had in the evening. Three dinners in one day are two too many. But this is the popular practice, especially among the la-boring classes. As a result, they become, old and stiff and wornout early in life.

If one goes into a restaurant in the early morning in any one of the larger cities and observes the clerical and professional world breakfasting he at once discovers one of the reasons why there is so much inefficiency, weakness and disease among this class. They may be seen in large numbers eating a breakfast of eggs and toast or rolls, with coffee. No time is taken to properly masticate the food. It is washed down with coffee, while the ''eater'' nervously fingers the pages of the morning paper.

After a breakfast of this kind they rush off to work and get through the morning some way. It is from this class we get most of our patients.

Eating between meals is a common practice. Often we hear people say they do not eat much. Indeed, they don't compared to what is usually consumed by others, if we compare only what they eat at meal time. But these people often eat more food between meals than at any other time.

A cow with seven stomachs and eating grass requires the larger part of a day to consume enough food. But a man or woman with only one stomach and consuming concentrated foods may eat in this way in one day enough food to satisfy the actual needs of the body for a whole week. The digestive organs are given no time to rest.

Rule 4. DO NOT DRINK WITH THE MEALS.

This is a very important rule and should be adhered to strictly. It has reference to the use of water, tea, coffee, cocoa or other watered drinks while eating. Milk is a food, not a drink.

Laboratory tests have determined that water leaves the stomach in about ten minutes after its ingestion. It carries the diluted and consequently weakened, digestive juices along with it, thereby interfering seriously with digestion. It is often argued that water drinking at meals stimulates the flow of gastric juice and thereby enhances digestion. The answer to this is (1) It is not the natural way to stimulate the secretion of digestive juices and results sooner or later in an impairment of the secretory power of the glands; and, (2) It is of no value to digestion to increase the secretion of the digestive fluids only to have them carried out of the stomach into the intestines before they have had time to act upon the food.

Water taken two hours after a meal enters the stomach at a time when the gastric juice is there in abundance and the reactions are proceeding nicely. The water sweeps these on into the intestines and retards digestion. Take your water ten to fifteen minutes before a meal and at least four hours after meals.

Drinking at meals also leads to the bolting habit. Instead of thoroughly masticating and insalivating one's food the one who drinks with his meals soon learns to wash it down half chewed. This practice should be avoided at all costs. Milk is a food and should be slowly sipped and held in the mouth until thoroughly insalivated before swallowing. No other food should be taken in the mouth with the milk. Thoroughly chew, insalivate and taste all food before swallowing. Food that is treated in this way can be swallowed without the aid of a liquid.

Cold drinks, water, lemonade, punch, iced tea, etc., that are often consumed with meals impair and retard digestion. Cold stops the action of the enzymes which must wait until the temperature in the stomach has been raised to normal before they can resume their action. When the cold drink is first introduced into the stomach it is shocked or chilled. After it is sent out of the stomach and the reaction sets in there is a feverish state resulting in great thirst. Ice cream acts in these same ways. Eating ice cream is like putting an ice pack to the stomach.

Hot drinks weaken and enervate the stomach. These destroy the tone of the tissues of the stomach and weaken its power to act mechanically upon the food. The weakening of its tissues in this way often helps in producing prolapsus of the stomach.

Water in coffee, tea, cocoa, lemonade, etc., is water still. These drinks also stimulate the appetite and lead to overeating. Aside from this the first three named each contain powerful poisons that act as stimulants. Their habitual use impairs digestion, wrecks the nervous system and injures the kidneys. The coffee and tea user, as a rule, perspires excessively in summer.

Drinking with meals is not natural and is not practiced by any of the lower animals. Anyone who would have the most perfect results in digestion will find the pursuance of this rule of not drinking with meals, will do much to give these desired results.

Rule 5. THOROUGHLY MASTICATE AND INSALIVATE ALL FOOD.

This is our last, but no means least important rule for eating.

Digestion really begins in the mouth and if we neglect this important step in the process we cannot hope to secure ideal results in the remaining steps. In our study of digestion we learned that the flow of the gastric juice of the stomach depends largely upon the taste of the food. Experiments have shown that if food is put into the stomach and this has not been tasted no gastric juice is secreted. If, however, the food is tasted and not allowed to reach the stomach there is an abundant secretion of this juice. This should emphasize the importance of thoroughly tasting the food before it is swallowed. It should be known that food must be chewed and thoroughly insalivated before it can be properly tasted. In fact, the longer one holds the food in the mouth the more tastes he discovers.

We also learned that certain substances arising as by-products of salivary digestion aid in accelerating gastric digestion. These by-products cannot arise if there is no salivary digestion. It is therefore very necessary that we thoroughly masticate and insalivate our food before swallowing it.

Food that has been completely broken up by chewing is readily accessible to the digestive juices but foods that are swallowed in chunks require much longer time for digestion. Much energy may be saved in the digestive process if we but take a little time and chew the food. Besides this, swallowing food without chewing it leads to overeating, hurried eating and all the train of digestive evils that arise from these. Allow me to repeat: Thoroughly masticate and insalivate all food before swallowing.

Let us now turn our attention to food combinations. Much that is written upon food combinations is untrue and misleading. Too much effort has been spent in trying to make it appear mysterious and hard to understand. While, almost everyone who writes upon food combinations have varying rules, the truth is that the rules for combining food are few and simple. These are based upon the facts which we have already learned about foods, their digestion and use. In the following pages we shall try to make the rules so plain that a child may understand them.

The best rule for combining food that has ever been set down is "don't do it." That is the rule advocated by many of eating only one article of food at a meal or as it is termed the mono-diet. There can be no doubt about this practice assuring best results in digestion and if due care is exercised in selecting the food for each meal a sufficient variety can be had to supply all the needs of the body. At the same time this method of eating would tend to prevent overeating.

To follow this rule is not absolutely essential to health and strength; besides by giving a little attention to how we combine our foods and by eating according to the rules laid down we may get practically the same results.

The greater the variety of food eaten at any one meal the more it complicates the digestive process. The number of articles taken at one meal should be limited. Simple dishes and few of them—not more than four. This is not the general practice. But the general practice leads to disease. The average person has learned that we require a variety of foods and attempts to obtain his variety all at once.

The enzyme ptyalin acts only in an alkaline medium. It is destroyed by a mild acid. Therefore: NEVER EAT CARBOHYDRATE FOODS AND ACID FOODS AT THE SAME MEAL. By this we mean, do not eat bread or cereals or potatoes, etc., with oranges, grapefruit or pineapple or peaches, etc. The acid not only prevents carbohydrate digestion by destroying the ptyalin but it favors carbohydrate fermentation. The fermentation destroys the food and gives rise to carbon dioxide and alcohol.

The flow of gastric juice depends chiefly upon the taste of proteid food. If no protein is tasted no gastric juice is secreted. If much gastric juice (which is acid) is poured into the stomach it prevents carbohydrated digestion. For this reason: NEVER EAT A CONCENTRATED PROTEIN AND A CONCENTRATED CARBOHYDRATE AT THE SAME MEAL. That is; do not eat meat or eggs or cheese, etc., with bread or cereals or potatoes or cakes, etc. To do so will not only cause the suspension of carbohydrate digestion in the stomach but the carbohydrate is forced to remain in the stomach until protein digestion is complete. It is then poured into the intestine in a half prepared state, not having undergone salivary digestion. It will likely have already begun to ferment.

An acid process (gastric digestion) and an alkaline

process (salivary digestion) cannot be carried on at the same time in an ideal way in the stomach. In fact, they cannot proceed together at all for long as the rising acidity of the stomach contents soon stops carbohydrate digestion completely. Carbohydrate fermentation then ensues.

The eating of two concentrated proteid foods or of two concentrated carbohydrate foods at the same meal complicates the digestive process and leads to overeating of proteins or carbohydrates. There are grounds for believing that when two proteins or two carbohydrates are eaten together the enzyme responsible for their digestion will not attack one protein until the other protein is digested or will not attack one carbohydrate until the other carbohydrate is digested.

Certain it is that if two such foods are taken at the same meal we are sure to consume an over supply of that kind of food. For this reason: NEVER EAT TWO CONCENTRATED PROTEIN FOODS NOR TWO CONCENTRATED CARBOHYDRATE FOODS AT THE SAME MEAL. This is to say; do not eat meat and eggs and cheese or eggs and cheese at the same meal and do not eat bread and potatoes, or bread and cake or bread and cereals, or potatoes and cake or potatoes and cereals, etc., together. The eating of meat and milk or eggs and milk is condemned by many and in this they are correct. Moses also condemned this practice.

The practice of eating starches that have been disguised by sweets is also a bad way to eat carbohydrates. If sugar is taken into the mouth it quickly fills with saliva but no ptyalin is present. Ptyalin is essential to starch digestion. If the starch is disguised with sugar, jellies, jams, syrups, etc., the taste buds are deceived and carbohydrate digestion is impaired.

Soups, which are usually swallowed without mastication and insalivation should not contain starch. Mr. Fletcher advocated masticating soups.

Finally, THE BULK OF EACH MEAL SHOULD CONSIST OF FRESH FRUITS OR FRESH GREEN VEGETABLES. This for the following reasons:

First: It prevents overeating of the concentrated foods.

Second: It assures an abundant supply of the positive organic mineral elements without which the other elements cannot be utilized.

Third: If such things as vitamines exist, it will supply an abundance of these.

Fourth: These foods supply the bulk to the food so necessary to normal peristalsis.

Fifth: Neither last nor least, these foods resist putrefactive changes in the stomach and intestines thus helping to keep them clean and aseptic.

All fresh fruits and green vegetables should be taken uncooked if the above results are desired as the cooking impairs the food. They may be eaten separately or as salads. No dressings or other means of disguising these salads and deceiving the sense of taste should be used on them.

Some uncooked food should be consumed at each meal. A good rule is to eat a large fruit or vegetable salad at the beginning of each meal as this will prevent overeating of the more concentrated foods.

Any vegetables or fruits that are cooked should be cooked in their own juices, and these juices should be retained and eaten. We once read of a lady who ate spinach to supply her system with certain mineral salts which were lacking in her diet. She boiled the spinach and poured the water it had been boiled in down the sink. Most of the soluble salts in the spinach went down the drain pipe with the water. The lady got very little of them. The reader should now know better than the lady referred to and should not make this mistake.

It is the present custom of writers on diet to sprinkle their pages with sample menus. Apparently they give little attention to the rules of combinations which they lay down. For no one can find any evidence in the sample menus that those rules have been applied.

As a general rule the chief meal of the day should consist of a fruit or vegetable salad (all salads should be

uncooked and devoid of all dressings, condiments, seasonings, etc.) one or two cooked non-starchy vegetables and
then the proteid or starch food that is to accompany the
meal.   Either fruit or vegetable salad will combine well
with all non-starchy foods, including all protein foods.
Fruit salads should be combined with the protein meal
but never with the starch meal.   Acid fruits may be taken
with milk contrary opinions notwithstanding.   Hunger
makes the best sauce to spread over a meal.   Use it, but
no other.

Sample menus are not necessary.   Any intelligent
reader can easily follow the rules given above and plan
his or her own menus.   These rules are not complicated
or hard to apply.   We advise that both the rules for eating and the rules for combining foods be followed as closely as circumstances and conditions will permit and then
the meal should be forgotten about.

Don't become a "diet bug."   Once your meal is swallowed let it digest.   To be continually worrying because
you did not get a correct combination, or couldn't get the
food you wanted and had to take what you didn't want, or
for some other cause, does not help matters one bit, but
it does interfere with digestion.

Keep cheerful and forget it.

CHAPTER 9
Feeding of Infants and Children

We have heard many reputable physicians say that infant feeding is the hardest problem with which they have to deal. This despite the fact that about all the time spent in Medical Colleges in the study of diet is devoted to infant feeding.

Every old grandmother knows all there is to be known about the care and feeding of infants. She may have given birth to ten children and half of these may have succeeded in reaching maturity but this terrible death rate does not convince her that her pet superstitions about infant care are not "law and gospel." The fact is these people usually know about as little about caring for a baby properly as the physician does.

When we see or even think of the many senseless abuses to which many thousands of babies are forced to submit we do not wonder that the death rate among infants is so terribly high. A great part of these are actually killed—murdered. Many mothers feed their children so much and so often that the baby is in a constant state of discomfort or actual suffering. Every time it cries from this cause it is fed again. One soon comes to believe that babies are incapable of crying except when hungry. As the crying continues some soothing syrup which invariably contains opium in some form is given. Very often an alcoholic is administered and in many other ways baby is drugged.

Then there is a widespread superstition that if a mother allows the baby to "taste" some of each food she eats, her milk will not give baby the colic. We have seen many mothers begin feeding their babies in this way by the time they were a few weeks old and long before they were really capable of properly caring for such foods they were eating, corn, oatmeal, beans, meat, eggs, etc. Such crimes against infants would be tolerated by no stock raiser towards his young animals. He knows only too well that the consequences to the animals would be disastrous.

The crimes daily committed in the care (?) of infants are so many that we cannot begin to enumerate them here. Let us look for a minute at the results of our present methods.

Over four hundred thousand children under ten years of age die in American homes each year. Those that do not die are forced to suffer from many diseases ranging from a diarrhea, cold or slight skin eruption to a severe fever such as pneumonia or typhoid. Although it is an exploded idea that every child must have its share of the so-called children's diseases few escape these under present day methods. Measles, scarlet fever, chickenpox, whooping cough and other such complaints are all too frequent.

Many children fail to develop normally, both mentally and physically. Not only do they develop defective teeth, but many are afflicted with enlarged tonsils and adenoids, sore throat, defective vision, defective hearing and many other troubles too numerous to mention. Infantile paralysis is becoming more and more frequent.

In the year 1909 there died in New York City alone 20,716 children under two years of age. Of these deaths 5,126 are ascribed to diarrheal causes. In 1910 in this same city 5,456 deaths of children under two years of age are recorded for the sixty-day period from July 2nd to September 3rd. Of these deaths, 2,886 are ascribed to diarrheal causes. More than one-sixth of all the babies born in France do not reach the age of 12 months. A frightful mortality.

Now if we assume that the mothers and physicians of New York City are as intelligent and as capable of caring for infants as the mothers and physicians of other cities and that the death rate in other large cities is equally as high as in New York we come face to face with the terrible fact that every year nearly 10,000 infants under two years of age die in the ten leading American cities during these two months. We cannot for a moment believe that such a state of affairs is natural. It is due solely to our barbaric methods of caring for children.

We pride ourselves on having reduced the infant mortality so much during the last twenty-five to fifty years, and there can be no doubt that the death rate has been materially lessened but it is altogether too high yet. It is about time we begin to look for a method to bring the death rate down as low as possible.

Infants and children are not addicted to the many weakening and enervating practices so common among adults. For instance we cannot accuse any infant of bringing on enervation and toxemia by the tobacco habit or by sexual excesses or over work or jealousy, etc. Babies are subjected to many adverse influences but probably the worse of these is over-feeding or improper food.

Think of 2886 children under two years of age dying every sixty days during summer in New York City of stomach and intestinal disorders which are in almost every case due to over-feeding or improper food. Add to this the fact that nearly all of the ailments to which children are subject arise from gastro-intestinal putrefaction brought on by improper feeding and you begin to realize how important it is to know how to feed the baby to avoid disease. It has been definitely proven that Infantile Paralysis arises in almost if not every instance from some ailmentary disorder—from the fermentation and putrefaction of food in the stomach and intestines. The problems of fresh air, sunshine, proper clothing, exercise, sleep, cleanliness, etc., for the baby are each of great importance and no one need expect to have a healthy child where these are neglected, but the feeding problem is perhaps of greatest importance.

All children, except sick ones, should be fed upon a diet of growth. It is during this period of life when growth and development are proceeding rapidly and nutrition is at its highest (except during pregancy) that the greatest amount of building material is needed. At only three other periods are such food requirements the same or nearly the same. These are after a fast, after an acute disease and during pregancy.

And yet Nature teaches by her own prescription for a diet of growth that orthodox standards are much in error. Nature produces milk for the young mammal that is perfectly adapted to its needs for growth and development and has placed in this fluid all the factors and elements supplied by food that are necessary to maintain normal health, growth and activity. She has not, of course, arranged that the young animal be fed upon this food during its entire period of growth. In fact, no animal in a state of Nature partakes of milk after it is weaned. So after the young animal is weaned it is forced to supply its food requirements from other sources and this food, except in the case of the carnivero and nut eating animals is a low protein food, with the green non-starchy foods preponderating. This should furnish us with a clue to how to feed our own young but probably this does not appear scientific enough to the laboratory gentlemen, who can learn nothing from animals in a state of nature but must have been under artificial conditions.

If Nature has prepared milk for the young animal it is quite obvious that milk is its natural diet during the period in which it is provided. The fact that shows clearly and convincingly the splendid food value of milk is that during the period of most rapid growth in the lives of mammals, milk is the sole food. So efficient is it as a food that a baby ordinarily will double its weight in 180 days with no other article of food. A calf or colt will double its weight in sixty days and a pig in ten to fifteen days on milk alone. It is equally apparent that the milk of the species to which any young animal belongs is the one best adapted to it. That this is very true in the case of human infants is amply demonstrated by the following facts:

Statistics compiled by the Child Hygiene Association of Philadelphia covering 3,243,958 infants who died during their first year of life showed fifty out of every one hundred bottle-fed babies died during their first year of life as compared to but seven deaths during their first year out of every one hundred breast-fed babies.

This fact caused one eminent woman specialist to write the following: "The first and most important duty of motherhood is the breast-feeding of her baby. Next to the right of every child to be well born comes the right to his best food, his own mother's breast milk. Mother's milk is the only perfect infant food; it cannot be imitated; and anyone who advises a mother differently is guilty of a serious crime against a helpless baby. When a baby is denied his mother's milk and put upon a bottle he loses half his chance to be kept alive, and nine-tenths of his chances to grow up into a normal healthy man or woman."

Statistics show that only two breast-fed babies contract the so-called contagious diseases where five bottle-fed babies do so, and that where such diseases are contracted the chances for recovery are greatly increased in the breast-fed baby as compared to the chances of the bottle-fed ones. Adenoids and enlarged tonsils are also more common among bottle-fed than among breast-fed babies.

From war torn Europe came unmistakable evidence of the superiority of breast feeding over bottle feeding, which was equal to that which came from Paris in 1871. During the siege of Paris at that date no cow's milk was available and infants had to be breast fed with the result that the infant death rate took a big drop.

Just before the entrance of the United States into the war in 1917, Lucas reported that the infant death rate in Belgium was unusually low. This he ascribed partly to the fact that the scarcity of cow's milk had forced an increase in breast feeding.

Shortly after the evacuation of Lille, Calumet of the university factulty wrote about infant welfare in that city under German occupation. The Germans had confiscated all the cow's milk so that breast feeding became almost universal. Those mothers who were unable to supply sufficient milk for their infants got other mothers to aid them. So marvelous were the results and so deeply did Calumet feel about the subject that he pleaded against the establishment anywhere in France of any infant welfare depot that would give away or sell or in any way promote the use of cow's milk.

Following the war Dr. Gini of Germany issued a report on infant welfare in that nation during the war. In normal times only 15 to 20 per cent of the babies in Berlin and Breslau are breast-fed. In August and September of 1914 there was a heavy death rate. After October of that year the percentage of breast-fed babies in these two cities almost doubled. With this increase in breast feeding came a corresponding fall in the infantile death rate. The reports from Dusseldorf, Bremen and Wiesbaden were to the same effect.

No such improvement was noted in the rural districts of Germany due to the fact that the farmers had cows and continued to supply milk to their families and to the further fact that the campaign for breast feeding did not extend to the rural districts.

Dr. Gini thinks that in every warring nation in western Europe except Italy the infant death rate was low during the war.

As superior as the mother's own milk is to any other food for the baby it can be so impaired as to be actually harmful. As an instance of this; experiments by the Pediatricians Society of Chicago showed that many cases of colic in babies stopped when the mother ceased eating eggs, meat and other protein foods.

Sugar eating by the mother, if carried to excess, disturbs the balance between proteids and carbohydrates, delays starch digestion resulting in indigestion followed by fermentation and acidosis. This reduced alkalinity of the mother's blood causes her milk to build a fat baby with a lowered resistance to disease.

In severe and instrumental deliveries resulting in injuries, infection and the breaking down of much tissue the blood and tissues, including milk, are so deranged and impaired that the baby is often made sick. These babies may suffer with convulsions and in such cases if no other cause is discoverable, every effort should be made to find if the mother's blood is deranged by septic poisoning. If there is septic infection or pyemia (pus in the blood) the child should be taken from the breast at once. If the mother is dysemic (a deficiency of mineral or other elements) her milk will not be of advantage to the child.

Nearly all diseases affect the quality and quantity of the mother's milk. Mothers should for this reason, if for no other, keep themselves well and strong. Her own diet should be of a character that insures a normal wholesome milk supply. Drugs affect the milk.

Before the coming of the white man to America there were no milk animals here. (The deer and Buffalo were here but were not domesticated.)) Indian mothers were forced to nurse their children and because they had no milk from other sources to aid in weaning their children nursed them for two to three years. Among the Sioux Indians it is said mothers were sometimes known to suckle two children at the same time. This same thing has been observed among the Guiana Indians of South America who as a rule nurse their children three or four years.

However, American and English mothers are fast losing the capacity to nurse their babies. Investigations have shown that only 12 per cent of American babies are entirely breast-fed, while 28 per cent are absolutely bottle fed and the residue from both breast and bottle but many of these insufficiently from the breast. These young citizens get a bad start in life and the results show up very plainly when the call for men comes as in the recent war. Less than fifty per cent of the young men of this nation were found physically fit. In New Zealand where breast feeding is the rule the infant death rate is only half of that in America. This is significant and should lead mothers to a more wholesome mode of living to enable them to suckle their own children.

It is as natural for a mother to supply milk for her baby as for a cow to supply milk for her calf. If the mother is unable to do so it is because she is not normal in some way. Perhaps the most common cause for this deficiency is the denatured, demineralized diet upon which so many mothers live. The mineral salts are absolutely essential to normal secretions. Aside from this they must be supplied to the child and if the mother's diet does not contain them her own tissues will be robbed of their minerals. This deranges the mothers health and impairs her milk. Milk deficient in these salts gives rise to rickets. No calf ever has rickets but human infants often do.

There is good reason for believing that the widespread practice of vaccination is partly responsible for the inability of mothers to supply sufficient milk for their babies.

Mrs. Malcolm says: "we may say, aside from their frequent failure to suckle their young, that the civilized mothers do better after the baby comes, while the savage mothers do better up to the time of birth. After that the ignorance and lack of sanitation work for a high mortality."

If civilized mothers will learn to do as well or better before baby comes as the savage mother does and learn to suckle her child as well as the savage mother this coupled with her tremendous sanitary and hygienic advantages and greater knowledge will enable her to reduce the infant death rate to but a small per cent of what it now is. It goes without saying that they should learn to care for baby in every way.

I have little faith, however, in the likelihood of the modern woman ever returning to her primitive vigor and strength. She is not possessed of the desire to do so, nor of the necessary self control to avoid the evils and abuses that have brought about her present condition. Give to a woman a popular cook book and a rational work on diet and she will almost invariably employ the cook book and let the work on diet rust. Teach her the value of exercise and she will ride the cars with her dog. Paint, powder and the dressmaker's art will pass for the appearance of health. Even our athletic girls of whom we read and see so much today are semi-invalids. They have not learned how to live and they will not learn how. Of course, their male acquaintances are not one bit better in these respects. Women can have normal childbirths and supply their children with milk when they learn to live normally. Until then, they will have to depend on artificial foods and that abomination of infant life—calf food.

Cow's milk forms a large, very hard tough curd which is very hard of digestion and constipates the baby. It is excellently adapted to the digestion of the calf. It often forms, when fed to infants, such large hard curds that they have great difficulty in passing them. Painful bowel movements are the result. It is a terrible thing for a mother to fall down on the job of feeding her baby.

Scurvy, rickets, anemia and malnutrition are often caused by the use of artificial foods. Many children seem to thrive on such foods for a while and then disaster overtakes them. Be not deceived by the advertisements of those who have infant foods for sale. These concerns exist for profit and not for baby's welfare.

Pasteurization alters the salts and sugars of milk and impairs its food value. It is hard to digest and results in constipation followed by diarrhea. If baby is to be fed on animal milk feed it fresh, unsweetened, unmodified milk from a cow or goat that is properly fed and watered and housed in clean well ventilated stalls. Lime is an irritant and clogs the system. It is absolutely unusable by the system. Lime water should never be added to baby's milk. The same is true of all other crude inorganic substances that are used. Sugar favors fermentation and indigestion. It is also irritating and creates a false appetite and abnormal thirst. Feed the child natural foods.

If the mother is normally healthy and is properly fed her own milk will be all sufficient for the baby. It will be a complete food and there will be no necessity of feeding orange juice or other fruit or vegetable juices to the baby. However, if there is reason to doubt that the quality of the milk is good, orange juice may be given between milk feedings. It should be diluted with water and warmed but not heated.

The chief cause of digestive disorders in infants and of all those other complaints that grow out of these is overfeeding. The habit of feeding babies every two hours during the day and every time it wakes up and cries at night is a ruinous one. Such feeding over works the baby's digestive organs and introduces an excess of food into the alimentary tract to ferment and poison the child. It weakens and sickens the child producing diarrhea, colic, skin eruptions, and more serious disorders.

Feeding the baby at night prevents both mother and child from sleeping and teaches the child irregularity in sleep. When the mother's sleep is disturbed in this way she is weakened and normal secretions are interfered with resulting in an impairment of her milk. The impairment of the milk reacts unfavorably upon the child. Feeding at night is not only unnecessary, it overfeeds and sickens the child.

This method of feeding which is also the popular one is what really makes the problem of infant feeding a difficult one. There is no way to adapt even the most wholesome and easily digested food to an infant when it is fed in such quantities. With proper feeding it is but little trouble to find a food that will "agree" with the baby.

Three to four feedings (never over five) in twenty-four hours is enough for almost any baby. Exceptional cases that actually require more are rare indeed. No feeding should be done at night. Regularity in feeding as in other things teaches the child regularity in habits. Babies fed in this way develop faster than those stuffed in the old way. Over nutrition actually inhibits function and retards growth and development.

No feeding should ever be done between meals. Water may be given, however. Children often cry when thirsty and instead of water are given the milk bottle or the breast. Every time a child cries it is not hungry.

If the child is sick, if there is fever, diarrhea, etc., it should fast until these are gone. An enema of luke warm water may be given as often as needed during this time. Don't be afraid to let the baby fast. It will not starve to death.

No other food except milk or milk and fruit juices should be given the child for the first year of its life. At about one year of age fruits and vegetables may be added to the diet. These should form one or part of one meal per day. If four feedings have been indulged in up to this time one of these should now be stopped.

No starchy foods or cereals should be given under two years. The sweet fruits may be added at about one year. These should be run through a fine sieve and fed to the child once per day. About an ounce at each feeding. Artificial sweets—candies, cakes, pies, sugar, etc., should never be fed to children.

Nuts and salads may be gradually added to the diet. Meat and eggs if used should not be given to children under five.

Children should be taught early to thoroughly masticate all food and to avoid overeating. If the child does not relish or desire food it is folly to force or persuade it to eat anyway. If the child is uncomfortable wait till comfort returns before feeding. Children fed in this way will grow up strong and healthy and miss the so-called children's diseases. Overfeeding, irregular feeding and wrong food combinations are responsible for most of the diseases peculiar to children. A little intelligent attention to proper feeding will avoid all of these.

It goes without saying that all food fed to infants and children should be fresh and pure. But we do well to remember that the most wholesome food soon becomes poisonous if taken in excess.

Baby should have fresh air both day and night from the moment of birth. A daily sun and air bath will be of immense benefit, also. Daily exercise should be started at an early age, say at one month, and continued with religious regularity. Baby should be bathed in cool water and if soap is used it should be mild and thoroughly rinsed off after using. If a warm bath is required it should be followed by a cool one.

Powders, salves, etc., should be kept off its body. The cool bath and the daily sun bath will so strengthen and invigorate the skin that it will not chaff. Powders will not be necessary.

Clothing should be light and airy and loosely fitting. There is no sense in smothering a child in a lot of heavy clothes or blankets or dressing it up for show when the neighbors call. It makes baby uncomfortable—sometimes actually tormenting it—and irritable, upsetting its digestion and weakening its whole body. Don't be afraid of draughts. A draught is but air in motion and is never harmful.

Baby should be laid on its stomach, not on its back, from the day of birth. In this position their back becomes stronger and baby develops better. It is the natural position.

CHAPTER 10
Feeding in Adult Life

It has often been said that a man will go to much trouble and expense in an effort to learn how to feed and care for his cattle and stock or how to raise prize winning poultry or dogs but he will give but little attention to how he feeds and cares for himself and children. While we believe this fact has been greatly exaggerated we recognize that there is much truth in it. Men are usually too much absorbed in affairs of business to give much attention to these things. They learn how to feed their cattle and dogs properly because it helps to make money.

Few women are capable of really appreciating the principles of diet as set down in these chapters. This does not arise out of any intellectual deficiency but comes simply from the fact that the average woman would much rather prepare some of the artistic taste pleasers that are to be found in the popular cook books. Give a woman a cook book and she will never learn true dietetics. Perhaps this will not always be so. Let us hope for the best.

At present however, it is the general rule for summer tables to be loaded down with a lot of heavy, greasy, heating foods, just as in winter. Meat, eggs, beans, cereals, pies, cakes, etc., weigh down the dishes no matter how hot the day.

Nature furnishes an abundance of cooling foods in the nature of non-starchy vegetables and juicy fruits but these form a very insignificant portion of the meal of the average person. Many are the times we have seen men come in from work at noon when the sun's rays were beating down upon them with intense heat, and eat a large meal of heavy, heating foods and return to work. Many times have we seen these men grow suddenly "sick at their stomachs" shortly after resuming work and have to stop. They are usually relieved by vomiting but seem never able to learn the lesson Nature is trying to teach. For they repeat the same eating performance next day. Many a man has been "knocked out" by the heat and forced to stop work whose whole trouble was caused by eating a big dinner of such foods. Farmers, mechanic, laborers, all do this.

This eating a winter meal in the summer time is a thing that should be avoided at all periods of life. Much "summer complaints" diarrhea, nausea, etc., will be avoided in this way. Man requires more heating foods in winter than in summer whatever his age. Every one who handles milk knows that any cow's milk will yield more butter in winter than in summer. This is usually attributed by farmers and dairymen to various things but is most probably a provision for supplying more heat producing material to the calf at this time. Whether or not the sugar content of milk is greater during winter than in summer we are not in a position to say. It seems likely that it would be.

In summer one should make it a rule to practically exclude all the concentrated heat producing foods. Meals should be light and consist principally of juicy fruits and succulent vegetables.

After complete physical maturity is reached and growth has ceased one's food requirements are very different to what they were in youth. It requires much material to construct and complete a building but after it is completed it may be kept in repair with but small amounts of material. Just so, it is with the human body. It requires less building material after maturity is reached in order to maintain it in repair than it required to build it up from a tiny infant to a mature man or woman.

The adult body requires only a sufficient amount of building material (protein) to maintain repairs and this amount is extremely small if the body is rightly cared for. We have already shown that the amount of protein required by the growing boy or girl is not great. The adult requires much less. But we do not often find them consuming much less, and this is one of the chief reasons why we so seldom find one enjoying normal (not average) health and why the average person is usually broken down at 45 to 50.

What Dr. Havard has called the diet of maturity should then contain but little protein. We can safely say that if the adult person never touched any of the more concentrated protein foods he would never fail to secure all the protein required by his body to maintain repairs.

The diet of maturity should contain enough of the heat and energy foods to enable one to perform his daily labors efficiently. No hard and fast rule can be set down as to the amount required. This is largely an individual matter and the amount required varies from time to time and with the seasons even with the same individual.

Above all, the diet should contain an abundance of those food elements so essential to elimination and normal secretions—the organic mineral salts. This is imperative if one is to maintain health, strength and youth. These keep the body sweet and clean and ward off those disagreeable and annoying symptoms and disorders that usually accompany "old age."

The mature person should heed the rules for eating and for combining which have been given in an earlier chapter. As age advances it is usually best to decrease the amount of food consumed daily. The reduction will have to depend on the amount of activity indulged in. It should be remembered, however, that if one eats properly and cares for the body intelligently there will not be the necessity for being placed on the shelf at forty and Oslerized at sixty. The weakness and decrepitude that accompanies old age results, not from the turning of the earth on its axis but from the habitual and daily abuses to which we subject ourselves. It is not so much the length of time that a man lives as the kind of life that he lives that ages him. As the old saw has it, it is the pace, not the distance that tells on us. A fast life is usually a short one and is interspersed with much sickness and suffering.

Eating should always be for health and strength, to supply the needs of the body and should not be indulged in merely for social pleasure, or for the gratification of taste.

The adult who has just undergone a long fast or who is convalescing from an acute disease should be placed upon a diet of growth until normal weight and strength is acquired. It should not be forgotten that the diet of growth requires, also plenty of the cleansing foods. The digestion of the convalescing patient is usually very poor and care has to be exercised that the digestive organs are not overtaxed. Following a fast the digestive powers are usually at their highest point of efficiency and it is generally possible after the fast is properly broken to put on weight very rapidly. Sometimes, however, when the faster has had some advanced digestive disorder, care must be exercised not to overtax these organs. Such patients have to be content to gain weight slowly and learn to be satisfied with the fact that they are returning to health even if the increase in weight cannot be as rapid as they would like.

Diet plays a most important role in the life of every one from before birth until death and is worthy the intelligent consideration of all who value health. However, we wish to make it clear that diet alone is not sufficient to cure many, if any cases of disease. No intelligent Nature Cure physician would ever attempt to cure a single case without giving careful attention to the many other factors of life and health.

If the reader will remember that often digestive troubles are due to other causes and not to dietetic errors he will readily understand why this is so. Digestive disorders are often overcome by correcting the patient's sex habits or by changing the state of mind. Living is no one-sided affair and if we are to live in health we may do so only by healthful living in all departments of life. The reader who is interested in these other departments should secure my books on Nature Cure.

Eating during pregnancy often forms a difficult problem for many women. This is largely because they adopt the widespread notion that a pregnant woman must eat for two. Indeed, she must eat for two but the amount of food required by the developing child is so small as not to consume the surplus food she is regularly in the habit of eating. Eating for two often means eating enough for six.

Most of the discomforts and distresses of pregnancy are due to this stupid practice of eating for two. Large, fat babies that are too large for safe and easy delivery are the result of eating for two.

The pregnant woman should eat for health. She should eat as she has learned in these pages. There is no special diet for this period. Let your diet be chiefly fruits and vegetables and partake moderately of proteid and carbohydrate foods.

The loss of teeth that so frequently accompanies motherhood is due to a lack of bone-forming elements in the mother's diet. Nature must have material out of which to form the infant's bones. If the mother's diet does not supply this, her own body must. The teeth are usually first to suffer for the baby's sake. A diet of fruits and vegetables will prevent this and assure baby good bones.

Many mothers are unable to nurse their children. This is often due to disease, often to defective diet and often to other causes. Perhaps vaccination is the greatest single cause of inability to nurse the child. However, if she is capable of normal milk secretion the diet that is best for her health and strength will produce the best milk, and an abundance of it, for the child. Here, again, the practice should be, EAT FOR HEALTH.

If the mother will eat as directed in these pages she will have a comfortable pregnancy, safe and easy childbirth and, if she is capable of normal milk secretion, an abundant flow of rich milk.

CHAPTER 11
Feeding in Disease

Few people give any thought to their manner of eating until they have become sick. Many do not even then consider diet to be of any practical importance, but there are many others who run immediately to their almanacs to find out which particular article of food they have been eating is responsible for their symptoms or to find just which article of food will cure them.

This idea that certain foods have special medicinal effects such as are usually ascribed to drugs is widespread. Rhubarb is said to be a blood purifier, celery is as nerve tonic, buttermilk prevents old age, etc. The truth is these ideas amount to nothing more than superstitions. In this chapter we shall attempt to present to the reader a plan for feeding the sick based on experience and knowledge of correct feeding principles.

At the outset let it be distinctly understood that no feeding should be done in acute diseases. So long as pain, fever and other acute symptoms last nothing but water should pass the patient's lips. The reason for this will be discussed in the chapter on fasting. In this chapter our concern shall be chiefly with feeding in chronic disease.

There are two sides to the story of nutrition. One side deals with the building up of the body and the manufacture of secretions. The other side deals with the elimination of waste matter from the blood and tissues. This latter part is accomplished by the use of food substances that never really become part of the body but are held in solution in the blood. The protein wastes of the cells are carried to the liver where they are combined with the above mentioned elements (positive organic mineral elements) which converts them into soluble salts. These salts are then easily eliminated by the kidneys and skin.

My good friend, Dr. Wm. F. Havard, has suggested the following very practical classification of diet:

"1. THE BUILDING DIET or the diet of physical

growth which is also the diet of convalescense, reconstruction and recuperation.

"2. THE MATURE DIET or the DIET OF MAINTENANCE—diet of adolesence.

"3. THE CURATIVE DIET or DIET OF ELIMINATION."

Let us say at this point that actually diet does not cure. The organism does the curing. Diet is one of the materials or agencies used in curing.

A diseased body is one heavily encumbered with toxins and wastes which must be eliminated before the return to health is possible. The cure must begin with the elimination of these morbid accumulations. Often they are retained, due to no fault of the liver, skin, lungs, etc., but to incomplete metabolism. The organs of elimination are confined in their work to such products as have previously been prepared by the liver and other glands for elimination. If these glands fail in their work of preparation the depurating organs must also fail in their work of elimination. If perfect metabolism is to be secured it is essential that the blood maintain a certain alkaline reserve which can be done only if we consume daily a sufficient amount of those foods that are rich in the positive organic mineral elements.

In disease the processes of growth, development and repair are slackened or stopped altogether, indicating that the body is in no condition to properly care for the normal amounts of protein, starches, etc. And we find by actual experience that when these are eliminated from the diet of the sick they immediately begin to improve in health. On the other hand those patients that consume the proteid and carbohydrate foods always improve very slowly, if at all. A true eliminating diet is one that is rich in mineral salts and lacking in the acid-forming proteins and carbohydrates.

It should be understood that the sick person should give careful attention to the rules and regulations for eating and combining. In fact, it is more necessary for him to do so than for the healthy individual. The healthy person with good digestion may disregard all the rules of diet perhaps for years, without any apparent harm but the sick man with weakened digestion suffers perceptibly following every transgression.

We often hear the young and healthy say "I eat what I please, I do as I like. Nothing hurts me." Our years of experience in handling the sick and treating all forms of disease have revealed to us the fact that there was a time in the life of nearly every chronic sufferer when he too did and said the same thing. In fact, it often seems that the only trouble they find with their diseased state is that they can no longer eat and do as they once did without suffering. Apparently, the only reason they desire to get well is that they hope to return to the old "flesh pots." It does not seem ever to have entered their minds that their past conduct is responsible for their present woes.

You dear reader, if you now hold to the idea that you may abuse your rugged health and powerful constitution with impunity, should disabuse your mind of this at once. You may be able to digest pig-iron, as you say, but you'll be better off in every way if you do not force yourself to do so. "Don't be a fool just because you happen to know how."

Extreme moderation is required in feeding the sick. If elimination is to proceed with the greatest speed it is necessary that the amount of food eaten be considerably less than that required by the body in health.

All stimulating and irritating foods should be excluded from the diet. All foods that undergo fermentation very readily should be withheld. No denatured foods,—white flour, polished rice, white sugar, degerminated, demineralized corn flour, canned, pickled, embalmed foods, jams, jellies, preserves, pastries, so-called breakfast foods, etc.,—should be consumed. All foods eaten should be wholesome, natural foods. Condiments of every nature should be tabooed.

Such dried fruits as apples, peaches, pears, apricots, fancy dates, figs and raisins are bleached with sulphurous acid. Crystalized fruit peels, citron, walnuts and almonds are also subjected to this same whitening process. These should never be used, well or sick. The sulphurous acid disturbs metabolism, destroys the blood corpuscles and other cells and overworks the kidneys.

Commercial apple jam and other jams are made up of sulphurated skins and cores. "Chops" as these are called are composed of about 10 per cent fruit, 10 per cent juice. The rest of the jam is composed of about 10 per cent sugar and 70 per cent glucose. The whole is held together and given a jelly-like consistency by phosphoric acid. Amrath, a coal tar dye, gives it a bright strawberry color while it is prevented from decomposing by benzoate of soda. The government allows one-tenth of one per cent of benzoate of soda to be used and requires that it be stated on the label. It is usually indicated in very fine print. Sulphuric acid is present in almost all commercial syrups and molasses. These syrups have little food value and are harmful in many ways.

The so-called breakfast foods have been refined too much and subjected to such intense heat that their food value is practically all lost.

It can easily be seen that the use of such foods by either the well or sick cannot result in anything else but harm. We have not yet discovered a way to prepare foods, to add to them and subtract from them, that will make them better than they are as Nature gives them to us. Our preparations usually only impair their nutritional value. Until such a method is found it is the part of wisdom for us to stick to the natural foods.

Having decided upon the kind of foods that must be fed the sick—wholesome natural foods, rich in the organic salts and lacking in proteins and carbohydrates—let us now begin our feeding.

It is usually beneficial to begin the treatment of a case of chronic disease with a fast. As fasting will be considered in a separate chapter, we will limit our remarks at this place. The duration of the fast must be determined by the condition and progress of the patient. Usually, such fasts are not necessarily long.

The purposes of the fast are manifold. Almost every case of chronic disease is accompanied by a foul gastro-intestinal tract. No health is possible so long as this condition remains. Fasting enables us to get rid of such a condition in the shortest possible time.

It is sometimes found beneficial to precede such a fast with a few days of fresh fruits or raw vegetables. These increase peristalsis and aid in cleansing the intestines and bowels. After the alimentary canal is once thoroughly cleansed and is given a complete rest it will be in a condition to care for the food eaten in a thoroughly normal manner, whereas before such was not possible. As an illustration let us consider for a minute the case of the fat and the emaciated.

We often see an individual who is little more than "skin and bones" consuming large quantities of food in an effort to gain weight. Across the table from him may sit a large fat man fifty to a hundred pounds overweight who consumes much less food. The fat man grows fatter, the skinny man gets skinnier. Why? Because the fat man digests and assimilates what he eats while the skinny man does not. In fact by over-crowding his digestive organs he is making it impossible for his already weakened organs to digest the food eaten.

Digestion cannot be crowded without injury and this is doubly true if one's digestive powers are already low. The normal person may be able to stand a lot of abuse without being killed thereby but even these had better cut out the foolishness.

We take the emaciated man put him on a short fast, clean out his alimentary tract and correct his enervating habits and he gains weight rapidly on much less food than he was formerly consuming. We recall one patient who had suffered for seven years with gastro-intestinal catarrh and was unable to take food of any kind without suffering much distress. After a nine-day fast and about an equal period on oranges he was placed upon a diet of fresh fruits, green vegetables and one glass of milk per day. This man not only lost his troubles and woes but gained thirty-one pounds of solid healthy flesh in four weeks upon this diet. The change in the color of his skin, in the appearance of his eyes and in his mental state was even more remarkable. Constipation which had troubled him for many years was completely cured and remained so.

What had accomplished all this? Just these four things: (1) Physiological rest secured by the fast; (2) Cleanliness of the alimentary canal secured by the fasting; (3) Purification of the blood and lymph secured by the fasting; (4) The correction of enervating habits—physical, mental and emotional.

This patient could now digest and assimilate his food whereas before this was well nigh impossible. He could not gain weight on but little food whereas before any attempt to increase his weight by the stuffing process would have been disastrous. There is no other one thing that whets up the powers of digestion and assimilation like a fast.

The length of time that one should fast depends upon the individual's condition. No two cases are alike. A long fast should never be undertaken by anyone unacquainted with fasting and ignorant of how to properly conduct it unless under the care of a competent physician experienced in handling fasts. Few medical men are capable, because of lack of knowledge and experience with fasting, of conducting a fast. Fasts are always best taken in an institution away from the petty annoyances of friends and relatives.

Feeding after the fast must depend on the individual case. Breaking the fast is a very important matter for if this is not done rightly all the benefits of the fast may be lost. For instructions about how to break the fast see the chapter on fasting.

After the fast is properly broken the best method of feeding the patient consists in placing him or her on a very frugal cleansing diet of fresh fruits and fresh green leafy vegetables. The patient's weight is purposely kept down by the diet to insure perfect elimination and to insure the absorption of any exudates, deposits, tumorous growths, etc., which were not fully absorbed during the fast.

An acid fruit diet may be employed following a fast of only a few days. This diet may be continued for several days depending on the condition of the patient. Obviously a diet of this kind could not be employed for more than a few days following an extended fast.

For this diet, oranges, lemons, grapefruit and acid grapes are the fruits most commonly used. The fruit chosen is taken at regular intervals during the day in varying quantities depending on the individual case.

These fruits are rich in organic salts which are liberated during digestion and supply the body with the elements necessary to the neutralization and chemicalization of the toxins preparatory to their elimination. They are at the same time, extremely limited in the amount of proteins and carbohydrates which they possess and are well adapted to a curative purpose. There is absolutely no foundation to the old medical delusion that acid fruits should not be given in "acid diseases." We often find that to give acid fruits where hyper-acidity of the stomach is present increases the distress in the stomach and for this reason are forced to use a diet of a different kind. However, hyper-acidity of the stomach is not "acid blood," and fruit acids (organic acids) do not enter the blood as acids.

The fruit diet proper consists of the exclusive use of any juicy or acid fruit. The orange, because of its palatableness, is the most popular, at least, in this country. Grapefruit is very popular with some. From three to sixteen oranges (or their equivalent in some other juicy fruit) per day is the usual amounts given. These should be taken at regular intervals, such as; one orange every hour or two oranges every two hours. In cases where but few oranges can be given one every two to six hours are given. The general effects of such a diet are:

(1)   The digestive system is permitted to rest.

(2)   The blood is alkalinized and normalized.

(3)   They promote elimination resulting in a purified blood and lymph stream.

Vegetable broths are sometimes used instead of fruit and with practically the same results. These are used to distinct advantage in those cases where the digestive tract is so sensitive that the acid fruits cause a burning sensation.

Vegetable broths are of two kinds—cooked and uncooked. The cooked broths are made by chopping one or a combination of the succulent vegetables up fine and boiling it. Is it usually strained after cooking to remove the cellulose.

The uncooked broths are made by finely chopping one or a combination of the succulent vegetables and pressing their juices out.

The grape diet has won great renown in Europe in the Nature Cure institutions there. It consists in living for several weeks on nothing but grapes swallowing the seeds and skins. Five to eight pounds of grapes are taken daily, beginning with a pound and increasing the amount used each day until the capacity of the patient is reached. Such a diet purifies the system very rapidly. It thoroughly improves digestion, increases the action of the kidneys and reduces blood acidity. General Booth used this diet to cure inebriates. He was not only successful in breaking the drink habit in this way but found that his patients gained in weight.

Grapes are rich in iron and have been found very beneficial in anemia and chlorosis. Such diseases as dyspepsia, constipation, catarrh, rheumatism, gout, stones and gravels, malaria, liver and lung troubles, including consumption, yield very quickly to the grape diet.

Obviously a diet composed exclusively of oranges or grapefruit or lemons could not be continued as long as the exclusive grape diet. However, they can usually be continued long enough to bring about the desired results. Or else they may be employed for a period and followed by a less frugal diet after which they may be resumed again.

In feeding these diets the rules for eating should be strictly observed. No attention can be given to combinations since no combining is done. The diet is strictly a mono diet.

There should be no great hurry about breaking away from a diet of this nature. The one who is actually desirous of regaining health will stick to the diet long enough to secure the desired results. After the body has been thoroughly cleansed and the forces of the organism recuperated; when all symptoms of the disease are gone, then a gradual return to a normal diet should begin.

Perhaps the diet most often used is as follows:

After the fast is properly broken the patient is placed upon two or three meals per day of fresh fruits and green leafy vegetables. Meals are small in order to secure the maximum of elimination. Much uncooked food is included. No protein and carbohydrate food is allowed unless figs or raisins are included for their laxative effects. A diet of this kind would be fruit for breakfast, a large uncooked vegetable salad and one cooked non-starchy vegetable at noon and fruit for supper. This diet may be used in hyperacidity of the stomach.

A diet of this kind may be continued indefinitely. The meals may be varied from day to day to avoid monotony. The number of articles of food taken at each meal should be limited to two or three. It should be constantly borne in mind that a diseased person cannot be fed like a harvest hand if he or she is to recover health rapidly.

There are many articles of food that the well man and even the sick man may eat without killing him instantly, and many patients think they should be allowed to indulge in these. They hold to the popular idea that they should eat anything that agrees with them, meaning by this, anything that produces no immediate discomfort. However, the problem of the dietitian is to feed what is best for the patient and not merely the things that the patient may eat without immediate evidence of injury. This same rule should be adhered to by the patient after the cure is completed. He should realize that the same course of conduct in eating, and otherwise, that made him sick the first time will do so a second time, if he returns to it. We can maintain health only by healthful living. Therefore, after the cure is completed, observe the rules for eating and combining laid down in the preceeding chapter and no disease as a result of dietetic indiscretions will arise.

Almost everyone thinks diet is the treatment par excellence for all digestive troubles, but few are able to see any connection between diet and lumbago or gout or pneumonia, etc. But diet alone will seldom cure so simple a digestive disorder as indigestion. This is due to the fact that indigestion is not always due to dietetic errors and seldom, if ever, due to these alone. Indigestion may be due to enervation brought on by any cause. It may be due to worry, to lack of sleep, overwork, or other causes as well as to dietetic errors. Or it may be due to any combination of these. Consequently, before the indigestion can be cured the enervating influences must be corrected. Temporary relief may be secured by carefully adjusting the diet to the digestive capacity but such relief is never cure. Coincident with the dietary adjustment must go the correction of all enervating influences.

What is true of indigestion is equally true of constipation. Probably more remedies for constipation have been offered than for any other disorder from which man suffers and not one of them has been satisfactory. Purgatives, cathartics, laxatives, are all very disappointing. These actually make the constipation worse so that drug taking fastens itself upon the victim and he reaches the point where his bowels will not move without a drug. It is the law of dual effect all over again. The first and temporary effect of the drugs is diarrhea, the second and lasting effect is chronic constipation.

The same is true of the enema only perhaps to a less degree. It does not cure constipation but it does fasten itself upon the user as a habit. It offers only temporary relief, not cure.

The wheat bran cure for constipation has proven equally disappointing. It works like a charm with most people when first tried, but as its use is continued it loses its power to excite the bowels to action and the victim finds himself increasing the consumption of the whole wheat bread or bran bread in an effort to produce the desired results. In a short time he is consuming two and three times as much bread as at the beginning. The bread ferments very rapidly and forms much gas. The enema habit, would, in the end, prove more desirable, if nothing better could be offered.

We might proceed through the whole list of so-called cures for constipation but it would only consume space. The truth is constipation is seldom, if ever, due to a deficiency of roughage in the diet. That large quantities of this is required is disproven by the fact that the normal bowel operates nicely on a liquid diet of milk or fruit juices or vegetable broths.

Constipation may be due to over eating, to over work, to mental strain, sexual excesses, loss of sleep or any other enervating influence or any combination of such influences. It may be due to some drug habit or it may be a mere matter of habit. That is one may neglest the calls of nature repeatedly until the bowels acquire the habit of "puting off" the movement. Toleration of the feces is established. Constipation may be due to lack of exercise. It can be cured only by correcting the cause.

Many cases of this trouble have been cured by simply putting the patient to bed and forcing him to rest for a few days. The influence of a lack of rest and sleep upon bowel action may be seen by all who will observe their own bowel action after losing sleep for a few nights. Any other enervating influence affects the bowels the same way.

Only recently we treated an aged druggist who had not had a normal bowel action for over forty years. He had been a slave to the cathartic and enema habits during all this time. He had tried drinking large quantities of water, the rectal dilator, whole wheat bread, and many other cures but all to no avail. His bowels would not move except when forced to by artificial means.

This patient was forced to rest. All enervating habits were corrected, he underwent a fast of nine days followed by a few days on oranges and then a diet of fresh fruits and green leafy vegetables. He was soon having three normal movements daily in spite of the fact that the amount of food he was consuming was small.

What is true of indigestion and constipation is equally true of other diseases. Few, if any cases can be cured by diet alone. While diet is a most important factor it is by no means the only factor.

Feeding in convelesence is usually a very simple affair. The first rule is moderation. The patient who has just recovered from a severe acute disease is in no condition to take care of a full diet and will be harmed by the attempt. Cleansing foods should comprise the bulk of the diet with the addition of small amounts of proteins and carbohydrates. Care should be exercised not to feed any combinations that would put a tax upon the digestive organs. In fact the nearer one approaches a mono-diet meal the better.

The fruit or vegetable salad at the first of the meal is excellent for the chronic sufferer or the convalescent and will tend to prevent over eating of the more concentrated foods.

As soon as normal secretion is established in the convalescent, a "diet of growth" may be employed.

Here is a rule that should always be followed in feeding a patient or in treating him in any other way: Make the functional abilities of the weakest organ or part the physiological standard. Suppose we have a bridge that in its strongest parts is capable of sustaining a weight of fifty tons, but in its weakest parts will sustain only ten tons. Now suppose we use the strongest parts of the bridge as our standard and start across with a load weighing forty tons. When we come to the weak part, that is only capable of sustaining ten tons, there is a collapse, and we go down with our truck and its cargo into the river.

This would be similar to feeding a patient with strong digestive powers as though all parts of the body were equally as strong. If we make the functional abilities of the strongest organ our physiological standard and feed accordingly we will have a break down of our physiological bridge in its weaker parts. If the skin is inactive a heavier burden is thrown upon the kidneys and these suffer. If the lungs are weak, these are not able to perform the work required to furnish oxygen enough to properly metabolize the meal. If the pancreas or the liver is weak, carbohydrate metabolism suffers. If the heart is weak, it suffers under the burdens, etc.

Never stuff a patient merely because his stomach can stand it. Never stuff a patient because no apparent ill effects follow. The breakdown may not come for a week or a month or more. If distress follows a meal—distress in any part of the body—take the hint and do better next time.

CHAPTER 12
Feeding

By fasting is meant voluntary abstinence from all food except water. Restricted or limited diets are not fasts. The so-called fruit fast is a fruit diet, not a fast.

Fasting above all measures can lay claim to being a strictly natural method. There can be no doubt that it is the oldest of all methods of treating disease. It is much older than the human race itself since it is resorted to instinctively by sick and wounded animals.

It is said that the elephant if wounded and still able to travel will go along with the rest of the herd and can be found supporting himself beside a trees while the remainder of the herd enjoys a hearty meal. The wounded elephant is totally oblivious to the excellent food all around him. He obeys an instinct as unerring as the one that brings the bee to his hive; an instinct which is common to the whole animal world, man included.

A dog or cat if sick or wounded will crawl under the wood shed or retire to some other secluded spot and rest and fast until well. Occasionally he will come out for water. These animals, will, when wounded or sick persistently refuse the most tempting food when offered to them. Physical and physiological rest and water are their remedies.

A sick cow or horse will also refuse food. The author has seen this in many hundreds of cases. In fact, all nature obeys this instinct. Thus does Nature herself teach us that the way to feed in acute diseases is not to do it.

Domestic cattle may often be found suffering from some chronic disease. Such animals invariably consume less food than the normal animal. Every stockman knows that when a cow or horse, a hog or sheep, etc., persistently refuses food, or, day after day consumes much less than normally, there is something wrong with that animal.

In the human realm the same rule prevails to the extent that we permit. One of the first things Nature does to the person with acute disease is to stop all desire for food. The well meaning friends of the sick man may encourage him to eat, these may bring in tasty and tempting dishes designed to please his taste and excite an appetite, but the most they ever succeed in doing is to get the patient to nibble a few bites. The *wise* physician may insist that he must "eat to keep up strength" but Mother Nature, who is wiser than any drug peddling biped that ever lived, continues to say do not eat.

The man who is sick but who is able to be about his work complains of having lost his appetite. He no longer enjoys his food. This is because his organic instincts know that to eat in the usual way is to increase the disease. The man thinks the loss of appetite is a great calamity and seeks ways to restore it. In this he is encouraged by physician and friends who alike erroneously think that the sick man must eat to keep up his strength. The doctor prescribes a tonic and stuffing and, of course, the patient is made worse.

Nature indicates both in animals and man that in acute disease no food but water should be consumed, while, in chronic disease, the amount of food eaten should be much less than that consumed in normal health. If this rule were adhered to by all an untold amount of suffering would be avoided and many would be saved from an untimely death. But, thanks to the medical delusion that "the sick man must eat to keep up strength," this rule is not likely to be adopted by the great majority of the people for years to come.

Let us see what happens if we feed in acute disease. The first thing the patient and physician notes is an increase in symptoms. The fever goes up, the pulse beat increases, pain and other symptoms become more intense. The patient is caused much unnecessary suffering and the patient's relatives are caused much needless anxiety.

Food taken under such conditions is not digested. Nature has temporarily suspended the digestive functions. This is necessary in order that her undivided attention may be given to the task of cure. Energy that is ordinarily consumed in the work of digesting, absorbing and assimilating food is now being used to carry on the curative processes. The muscles of the stomach and intestines are in about the same condition as the muscle of the arm.

There is an almost total absence of the digestive juices. What little of these that are present are of such poor quality that they could not properly digest even small amounts of food. Along with the absence of the power to digest and the absence of the digestive juices, there is lacking that keen relish for food which we have noted, previously, is so essential to normal digestion.

If the food eaten is not digested of what value can it be to the sick man or woman? A two hundred pound man may become sick with typhoid fever. He will lose weight no matter how much he is fed until when he is well he is but a shadow of his former self. In fact, the more he is fed the sicker he becomes, the more prolonged is his illness and the more he will lose in weight. What more conclusive evidence is needed to prove that the food eaten does harm and not good? What is true of typhoid is also true of other diseases.

Food that is not digested undergoes decomposition forming a mass of toxins more or less of which are absorbed to further poison and sicken the patient. A veritible cesspool is formed under one's diaphram that is much more dangerous to that individual than any cesspool that may be in the neighborhood.

To get rid of this rotting fermenting mass of food and the toxins it has formed requires a needless expenditure of energy. Nature is trying to conserve energy. This is precisely the reason she has temporarily suspended the digestive functions. It is little less than criminal to force the organism to divide its energies and attention between the work of curing and the added task of eliminating a rotting septic mass from the digestive tract.

The only sensible thing to do is to keep the digestive tract free of all such matter. Nature herself indicates this in the strongest possible manner for not only is all desire for food cut off but the most tempting dishes are not relished by the sick person. There is a positive disinclination to take food.

The amount of work done by the heart, liver, lungs, kidneys, glands, etc., is largely determined by the amount of food eaten. Why should these organs and the stomach and intestines be given more work to do by eating? Haven't they enough work to perform under the circumstances? Nature demands physiological rest not physiological over work. Her call for rest comes in unmistakable terms. Why, then shall the organs be forced to do extra work by the use of stimulants or by feeding? To stop the use of food for a time affords the most complete rest to the whole vital economy.

In disease the body is encumbered by a mass of toxins that must be eliminated before a return to health is possible. One of our rules for treating the patient is to stop the absorption of all toxins from the outside. Feeding during disease does just the opposite. It keeps the digestive tract full of decaying animal and vegetable matter which is constantly being added to the poisons that are producing the disease. Fasting eliminates all this.

Elimination of toxins is absolutely essential to recovery. There is no known method by which elimination can be so effectively hastened as by physiological rest, or fasting. During a fast the processes of elimination reach their maximum point of efficiency. The bowels, skin, kidneys and lungs are each and all enabled to work with more efficiency. Even the digestive tract which before was busy with the work of digestion and absorption becomes actively engaged in the work of elimination. The process has been likened to a spronge. During health the sponge (intestines) are busy absorbing, during a fast the sponge is being squeezed.

Is there danger of starving during a fast? No. And this is doubly true in acute disease. The fast only shortens the length of the disease and lessens the suffering of the patient.

Many fasts are on record lasting from forty to seventy and even ninety days with only benefit therefrom. Many thousands have fasted for the cure of disease in Nature

Cure institutions and in their own homes, the fast ranging from a few days to a few weeks, and always with decided benefit. Of course, there is a limit to the time any one can go without food and live but most curable diseases are cured before this point is reached.

There is a difference between fasting and starving, a difference indicated by Nature. During a fast there is no desire for food, indeed there may be an actual loathing of food. The very sight, taste, smell or thought of food may produce nausea. This lack of all desire for food persists until the point is reached when to go longer without food is to endanger life and then normal hunger returns. This marks the end of fasting and the beginning of starvation. While hunger is absent the individual abstaining from food is fasting—when normal hunger returns the individual abstaining from food is starving. When normal hunger returns the fast should be broken whether the patient is well or not. If necessary a second fast may be taken later.

In death by starvation the following losses have been observed:

	Per cent.		Per cent.
Fat	91	Spleen	63
Muscle	30	Blood	17
Liver	56	Nerves	00

This loss of fat or muscle might occur at any time without any impairment to health. The loss to the liver and spleen were found to be chiefly of water. The loss to the blood is not serious. The stomach is uninjured. These losses appeared during starvation. No such loss would be registered by a properly conducted fast.

Nature always favors the most vital organs. Thus while fat disappears first and then the other tissues in the inverse order of their usefulness and importance to the organism, the brain and nervous system is apparently able, if given rest and sleep, to maintain their substances unimpaired and without injury during the most prolonged fast. During a fast the diseased tissues are broken down and absorbed rapidly. Fasting promotes the absorption of exudates, effusions and deposits in a manner that nothing else will.

Dr. Robt. Walter says in "The Exact Science of Health:"

"No process of treatment ever invented fulfills so many indications for the restoration of health as does fasting. It is Nature's own primal process, her first requirement in nearly all cases. As a means of promoting circulation, improving nutrition, facilitating excretion, recuperating vital power and restoring vital vigor it has no competitor."

Fasting is good in all diseases, however it will not ressurect the dead. All diseases are curable if the proper measures are employed before there has been too much destruction of tissues or organs, or before vital exhaustion is reached and they are all incurable after this point is reached. There are incurable cases but there are no incurable diseases. Fasting cannot be expected to accomplish the impossible; that is, to cure a case after organic changes and vital depletion have reached a point where regeneration is impossible. The proper thing to do is to employ the fast first and such a state will never be reached. Do not neglect your trouble too long. Long fasts are not always necessary. In fact cases requiring long fasts are comparatively few. For every patient we receive who requires a fast of thirty or forty days we receive dozens of others who require to fast but a few days. It is only fair to add, however, that the longer one puts off attending to his health and the worse his condition becomes the longer he will need to fast.

We do not claim that fasting cures disease but simply that it enables the organism to cure itself. What then does fasting do?

(1) It gives the vital organs a complete rest.

(2) It stops the intake of foods to decompose in the intestines and further poison the body.

(3) It gives the organs of elimination an opportunity to catch up with their work, and promotes elimination.

(4) It promotes the breaking down and absorption

of exudates, effusions, deposits, diseased tissues and abnormal growths.

(5) It permits the conservation of energy.

(6) It increases the powers of digestion and assimilation.

(7) Clears and strengthens the mind.

Fasting is good in chronic disease and imperative in all acute forms. Most chronic cases can be restored to health without the fast but all of these will be restored in much less time by the aid of the fast. In all healing crises that arise during the cure of a chronic disease fasting should be employed. Fasting is the speediest and most effective means known of breaking a drug habit, breaking, alike, the tobacco habit, alcohol habit and opium habit.

Contra-indications for fasting are:

(1) Fear of the fast on the part of the patient. Fear may kill where the fast would be of distinct benefit.

(2) Extreme emaciation. In such cases a long fast is impossible. A short fast of one to three days may often be found beneficial, or a series of such short fasts with longer periods of proper feeding intervening may be found advisable.

(3) In cases of extreme weakness or degenerative cases. Even in many such cases a series of short fasts as mentioned above may often be beneficial. In the latter stages of consumption and cancer the fast can be of no value except to relieve the patient's suffering. It may prolong life a few days. However, fasting is of distinct benefit in the earlier stages of both these diseases.

(4) In cases of inactive kidneys accompanied by obesity. In such cases the tissues may be broken down faster than the kidneys are able to eliminate them.

Outside of these, fasting is of decided benefit in all acute and chronic diseases. Of course, we do not advise chronic sufferers to undertake a fast of more than a few days unless they are thoroughly acquainted with the proper methods of conducting a fast, or unless under the care of a competent physician.

The average Allopath is strongly opposed to fasting

because he thinks it impairs the vitality of the patient. These men do not descriminate between the nutritive requirements of the well and the sick, unless it be that they think the food requirements of the invalid are greater than that of the normal man or woman. This is the idea one gets when observing the stuffing methods they usually employ. Any loss of strength or vitality is looked upon by them as an evidence of lack of food or of improper digestion. It is for this reason that the regular profession boasts of no real dietitians. We advise all sufferers who wish to try a fast to seek a physician who thoroughly understands handling fasting cases.

The reader may ask: "How long must I fast?" We answer, no hard, fast rules can be set down to determine the length of time anyone should fast. The length of the fast must depend on the condition and progress of the patient, by the results desired and by any complications that may arise. Let us say right here that complications during a fast are very few if it is properly conducted. Healing crises often occur during a fast but these are in no sense complications.

Complications may take the form of uncontrolable vomiting, extreme weakness, persistent hiccoughs, a very eratic pulse that remains eratic, fear of starvation or an unreasonable and persistent determination to break the fast. Any of these should cause us to terminate the fast However, one should be certain before breaking the fast, that such symptoms are really lasting and are not mere temporary annoyances. An eratic pulse may arise and last but a few minutes, or hiccoughs may develop and continue for a few minutes and then cease. These should not cause any alarm or apprehension. Be sure the symptom is to be lasting, then break the fast.

The first thing in undergoing a fast is the right mental attitude. Nine of the men who went on the hunger strike with MacSwinney broke their fast on the ninety-fourth day and lived. Fear of the fast may kill in ten days or even less. Fear is a powerfully destructive emotion. Banish all fear of the fast from your mind. We have handled many hundreds of cases and have never yet seen injury come from a properly conducted fast.

No special preparation for a fast is required although it is often found advantageous to precede it by a few days on a raw food diet or a fruit diet. The purpose of this being to thoroughly cleanse the digestive tract.

An enema may be taken daily during the first week of the fast. If it is to be a long fast the enema may be used every other day after the first week to ten days. The purpose of the enema is to secure bowel action as these are very sluggish during a fast. The lining membranes of the stomach and intestines pour out large quantities of mucous which if allowed to remain in the bowels decompose, forming toxins which are reabsorbed giving rise to systemic poisoning. Headache is a very prominent symptom when this occurs.

In acute diseases in which there is severe inflammation of the bowels the enema should not be given. To force bowel action under such conditions increases the pain and may even cause a premature rupture of the inflamed portions. The use of cathartics for this purpose in appendicitis often causes the appendix to burst into the abdominal cavity resulting fatally. No appendix will ever break into anything else except the bowels where it will be expelled by the first bowel movement, if not forced to do so by meddlesome treatment. The giving of cathartics in this disease increases peristalsis and this increases the suffering. The pain caused in this way is sharp and excruciating. With each peristaltic wave of the intestines the food stuff in these is thrown with great force against the inflamed wall of the cecum. This increases the pain. To relieve the pain thus produced morphine is administered. This relaxes Nature's defenses and permits the appendix or cecum to reputure into the peritoneal cavity.

In such cases, if fasting and absolute rest in bed were employed such complications would never occur. The disease is made formidable by the feeding, drugging and officious gouging.

Except in a few instances such as dropsical diseases

all the water may be taken that the patient desires. It should neither be hot nor cold.

In acute disease no exercise should be indulged in. In chronic cases some mild exercise should be taken daily. This should be governed by the strength of the patient and the nature of his trouble. Outdoor walking or deep breathing exercises are best for the faster. If he is confined to bed exercises that can be taken lying down may be used.

Bathing during the fast should be regular but not prolonged. Very hot or very cold baths should be avoided. The bath should be followed by a vigorous rub with a coarse towel or friction mitten.

Fresh air is as essential during a fast as at other times. The faster should avoid being chilled.

Breaking the fast is a very important part of the program. By an injudicious breaking all the results of a long fast may be lost.

After a lengthy fast food can be tolerated in small quantities only. After a fast of only two or three days there is no danger from taking considerable food but it is foolish to do so. If one is going to return to gormandizing he may as well not fast to begin with.

The fast is best broken on fruit juices such as orange or grape fruit or on vegetable broths. From a glassful to a spoonful of the fruit juice or vegetable broth should be taken every two hours for the first day. The amount taken will depend on the length of the fast and the condition of the patient. The longer the fast or weaker the patient the less should be taken. After the first day the pulp of the fruit may be eaten. The amount and variety of foods used should be gradually increased day by day until the normal diet is reached.

Fasting is not a substitute for clean living and self-control. A return to the old disease producing habits will build disease all over again. Learn to live sensibly and you may retain your health and strength.

CHAPTER 13
Gaining and Losing Weight

For the purposes of this chapter the people of this world may be divided into two general classes—those who are trying to gain weight and those who are trying to lose weight. The classes are about equally divided and, if one is to judge by the many things that are advertised to increase or decrease one's weight, they are willing to "try anything once." There are a few people who are about normal in weight, but these are so few and so scattered as to be almost negligible. A still smaller and more scattered number exist who are either underweight or over weight and who are wholly indifferent about their weight and make no effort to correct it.

Insurance statistics reveal that fifty pounds of excess weight after the age of fifty cut short one's life expectancy by fifty per cent. But excess weight is also a danger before fifty. Aside from the danger it is very uncomfortable and cripples one's efficiency. Women have more interest in this matter as it effects their good looks than they do in its effects upon their efficiency. Woman does not desire to be fat because it mars her beauty, and for this same reason she does not want to be skinny. The only true physical beauty is that of the well developed, well proportioned body.

Underweight, when not due to an actual lack of sufficient food is due to defects and disease. This also cripples efficiency, mars beauty and detracts from the joys and pleasures of life.

Practically, we should put less emphasis upon weight and more upon health. For, after all, if one is truly healthy and is leading a normal life his or her weight will automatically adjust itself. The healthy man or woman cannot live in such a manner as to produce overweight or underweight without, ultimately, impairing his or her health.

In general terms it may be said that one's health depends upon the body as it was inherited and upon what one has done or is doing with his or her inheritance. Many are born with inherited structural weaknesses which cannot be entirely overcome. However, it is very seldom that such weaknesses are of such a character as to very materially impair one's health if he lives normally. Usually, such weaknesses only determine what disease one will have if he lives in such a manner as to produce disease, but they do not cause disease. To make this more clear—a man who has inherited weak lungs and a normal digestive tract will be much more likely to develop respiratory than digestive diseases. But the weak lungs are not the cause of respiratory diseases.

There is such a close harmony and interdependence existing between all parts of the body—one part with every other part and every other part with the one—that if one part is disordered or impaired the whole body suffers more or less. So great is the dependence of the whole body upon some of its parts, such, for instance, as the brain, lungs, heart, etc., that if they are destroyed death results instantly. Sound health and vigorous function of the body depends upon the harmonious operation of all its parts and not upon the vigorous action of one or two organs. The body is an unit not an aggregate and functions best as a whole rather than by parts.

Life is a state or condition in which animals and plants exist with the capacity of exercising their natural functions. Perfect life is that condition in which these functions are exercised perfectly and depends upon the perfect development of all the positive characters belonging to the respective species. Perfect life means perfect health. Death is the cessation of life. Between these two extremes of perfect life and death are found all those various degrees of health and disease which exist today. Health and disease are simply two conditions of life, and their existence depends upon the conditions under which life exists.

Briefly, if the seed, egg or ovum of a plant or animal is to develop into the being that exists potential in it, certain conditions are essential. These are moist heat, food, air, water, and protection from violence. When the young bird emerges from the shell, it still must have warmth, air, food, and protection from violence plus light. The young plant just coming up through the soil requires the same. Given these and they develop into full grown birds and plants, well developed, healthy specimens of their kind.

This same is true of human beings. They require light, air, water, food and freedom from violence. They, like the bird, also require exercise, rest, sleep and cleanliness. Given these, in a normal manner, and the baby develops into a wholesome, well formed man or woman; provided— other elements are not introduced to retard, sub- vert, and prevent development.

Health is potential in life and under natural condi- tions is, barring accidents, as inevitable as the rise and fall of the tides. Living matter cannot be otherwise than healthy if the conditions of health are present. But it lies within man's power to place himself under conditions other than those of health and this impairs his health. This state we call disease. Health is impaired in a number of ways and impaired health from any cause affects body weight.

Let us suppose we have a patient who is considerably underweight. We want to add twenty pounds of healthy flesh—not fat—to his frame. How shall we do it? It is the customary practice to feed him lots of fat-forming foods. We stuff him just as a farmer does his hogs to fat- ten them. But we fail to fatten our patient just about as often as the farmer succeeds in fattening his hogs. Why?

For the reason that our patient is not underweight be- cause he has not been eating enough. It is more than like- ly that he has been consuming much more food than his body actually requires. This is usually the case. His un- derweight is due to a lack of power to properly digest and assimilate what he eats. If one is eating as much or more than as much food as his body requires and is eating a correct diet otherwise and is underweight and remains so, this is evidence that his digestion and assimilation are im- paired.

If he cannot digest and assimilate what he is eating regularly, how can he digest double or treble that amount? Food that is not digested and assimilated can add nothing to one's weight. All food eaten in excess of one's capacity to digest will not be digested. All food digested in excess of one's abilities to assimilate will not be assimilated. Undigested food undergoes decomposition and poisons the body.

The obvious thing to do in such a case is to find out what is impairing his digestion and assimilation and correct this. Enervation is the chief cause for their impairment. But enervation is, itself, only an effect. Enervation is simply a functional weakness of the body due to lowered nerve force and may be brought on in many ways. However brought on, it always impairs organic function. If one is enervated the weaker organs of his body suffer most. If the digestive organs are weaker his digestion suffers and he loses weight.

Now it is often possible in such cases to employ stimulating methods in conjunction with the increased food intake and force a gain in weight. Such a gain is, however, only temporary and one will often begin to lose what he has gained even while he continues to stimulate his digestive organs and force them to work harder. The lesson is obvious. Instead of forcing the organs of digestion to work in such a manner we should direct our effort at correcting the enervation that is back of the impairment of the digestive function. This accomplished and digestion will again become normal, whereupon a permanent gain in weight is registered without any change in diet, or perhaps with a considerable decrease in the amount of food eaten. I have seen this repeatedly. Many gain weight merely by reducing their meals from three to two daily.

The man with a powerful digestive system may experience no digestive difficulties when enervated but some other organ or organs not so powerful may suffer. The liver, the lungs, the ductless glands, the kidneys, or some other organ may have its function impaired to a noticeable extent. In this event, while digestion perhaps does not noticeably suffer, nutrition will. He will digest his food but be unable to assimilate it. Stimulation of the impaired function may here also result in a temporary gain in weight, but with no more satisfactory ending than mentioned above. The enervation must be corrected before the impaired organ can resume normal function. This done and the stimulation is useless.

There is an added danger in a case of this nature. There is an inclination to make the digestive capacity the standard of the body's ability to properly care for the food eaten. In those cases where the digestion is powerful and some other organ impaired the habit of making the digestive capacity the systemic standard entails a hardship upon the impaired organ. Think of the absurdity of feeding a diabetic patient all the starches and sugars he can digest—of making the functional abilities of his stomach and intestines rather than of his liver and pancreas the standard by which to feed him. The result would simply be disastrous. Think of feeding a consumptive all or more than he can digest instead of using the functional abilities of his lungs as the standard! Or feed a person with defective kidneys all a strong digestion can care for and consider the amount of work this places upon the kidneys. Or suppose the kidneys are sound and the skin inactive. The extra work this throws upon the kidneys must inevitably impair them.

It is not hard to regain one's health and with a return of health comes a gain in weight. But it is very easy to injure oneself in the effort to regain weight in advance of the regain of health. However, so inadequate is the conception of health held by most men and women that if they are not actually in pain or discomfort they think themselves well. So long as they can, by condiments and seasonings, force themselves to eat three square meals per day and so long as they are able to get up in the morning and by the use of tea, coffee, tobacco, alcohol and soda fountain slops, cold baths, etc., force themselves through the days work they are unwilling to believe that they are in other than perfect health. Or, if they are in pain and discomfort and these can be relieved by drugs or baths, massage, electricity, vibration, etc., they cannot believe that they are not justified in eating as though they were in perfect health. Their very efforts at relief and cure prevents them from coming to a knowledge of the simplest and most obvious truths about health and disease.

If a patient is in the throes of fever everyone knows that he cannot be made to gain weight no matter how much he is fed nor how perfect otherwise his diet. It is a matter of common knowledge that in such diseases—typhoid, pneumonia and appendicitis, for instance—digestion and assimilation are impaired and regardless of what and how much a patient is fed he will lose weight. What seems hard for most people to grasp is that there are various degrees of digestive and assimilative impairment, which, while far short of that present in typhoid, must be corrected before an attempt to gain weight can be successful or before the attempt will be free from danger.

Besides faulty digestion from whatever cause and impaired functions of other organs of the body which contribute either directly or indirectly to the processes of nutrition there are other factors that contribute to the control of body weight which are too often overlooked. Chief among these, we may mention fresh air, sunshine, exercise, rest, sleep and mental influences.

I do not intend here to give these more than a passing notice. With the value of fresh air almost every one is acquainted. If the air one habitually breathes is such that it poisons the body or fails to supply the required amount of oxygen, health is impaired, nutrition is perverted and body weight suffers.

Exercise as a means of developing and building up the body has no equal. It is often possible by this means to add from ten to twenty pounds of solid, healthy muscular tissue to the body in a short time. Many attempt to reduce body weight by exercise, and while it can be done in this manner, failure is the usual result. The reason for this will be stated later.

It is now nearly a hundred years since the sun bath

began to be used by Nature Curists in promoting health and in curing disease. It was not thought of as a "drug" nor as a therapeutic agent and, therefore, confined to but one or two bodily conditions, but was looked upon as an essential factor in natural hygiene and, therefore, good in all conditions of life. It exerts a profound and far reaching influence upon the processes of nutrition both in plant and animal life and its absence weakens and destroys the body.

Rest and sleep are essential after each period of activity. These should be of sufficient duration to permit complete recuperation from the expenditures during the period of activity. If sufficient rest and sleep are not had to accomplish this one begins his subsequent activities just a little below the normal standard and as this practice continues and the standard is lowered a little more each day, his body suffers.

The profound effects exerted by various mental states upon the nutritive processes are coming more and more to be recognized. Worry, fear, sorrow, jealousy, anxiety, self-pity, etc., especially inhibit digestion, impair the body's secretions and thus disorganize nutrition. Hope, courage, cheerfulness, love, etc., exert an opposite influence. Mental overwork, although, exceedingly rare is as great an offender against life as physical overwork. Ambition, the desire for place, power and pelf, is usually the driving force back of mental overwork. Health is sacrificed on the altar of mammon and when one gets what he has given his life for he is usually unable to enjoy or to rightly use it.

In general, we may say that any habit or indulgence that impairs one's health, that deranges digestion and lowers one's powers of assimilation will cause him to lose weight and prevent a permanent gain in weight. These should all be ferreted out and corrected at the outset, if one desires to gain weight. Enervation can be overcome only by correcting its cause and, after this, taking a real rest in order to recuperate.

Every year many thousands of people go away from their work for a few days or weeks for the purpose of securing a rest. But they do not rest. They are afflicted with the idea that rest means change so they exchange their work for a few days or weeks of dissipation at the sea shore or some summer resort, or sightseeing. Late hours, dancing, swimming, drinking, eating, riding, hurrying to see this or that sight—everything else but rest. The result is, they are less fit for work when they return than when they left. As has been so truly remarked: "No one needs a vacation like the man who has just had one." The feverish haste, excitement, dissipation and late hours that are called vacations are not rest. It is change, rapid change, but, at the same time, a tremendous waste of nervous energy with no compensating return. One may easily "rest" himself into exhaustion in this way.

There are two classes of fat people—those who eat all they can hold every time they go to the table, and those who eat but little at the table but fill up between meals. This latter class "never eats much." They cannot see why they are fat or why they continue to gain in weight. There are, really, a few fat people who do not eat much if judged by conventional standards. That is, they consume less food than the average person does. But one thing is as certain as that two times two equals four: that is, no one who is not consuming more food than his body requires can gain weight. It does not matter how small you think your food intake is, if you are still gaining weight you are eating more than your body requires to meet the daily losses. If you are overweight and remain stationary in spite of the apparent smallness of your meals you are consuming—and digesting and assimilating it—about what food your body requires.

If you are to lose weight without the use of some weakening process you can do so only by consuming less food than your body requires and thus force it to utilize the surplus. Perhaps you have tried this before and found that by reducing your food intake one-half you did not lose any weight. You may actually have gained in weight. This but evinces that you were consuming more than twice the amount of food required by your body but you were not digesting and assimilating it. When you cut down the food intake this gave the nutritive organs a rest, improved nutrition, and you added a few more pounds. Many, who are underweight, are so because continually overloading the stomach with food cripples its powers of digestion. The very effort to gain weight by stuffing often prevents one from gaining. Such people gain rapidly when changed from a three-meal-a-day to the two-meal plan.

Exercise is often resorted to to force a reduction in weight. It increases the appetite, improves digestion and assimilation and thus often results in an actual gain. Exercise to be successful must be coupled with control in eating. If exercise increases your appetite and you do not curb your eating you will be found consuming more food than formerly. I recall one young high school boy who weighed nearly three hundred pounds. He took up track athletics, chiefly running, for the purpose of reducing his weight. Each day he would spend about one hour in running, putting the shot, etc., with, to his disappointment, a gain of several pounds in weight, in a few weeks. His mother supplied the reason when she said that since he had taken up athletics he ate almost twice as much food as before.

An increase in work or exercise creates an increased need for food, but if this need is supplied from without there is no chance to force the body to utilize its surplus weight. One may carry his exercise to the point of exhaustion, that is he may continue to overdo it and, thus, impair his health, thereby, securing a reduction in weight but this is not what is desired. Similarly, one may try the sweat cabinet method and make the baths of sufficient duration and frequency to impair one's health and thus occasion a loss of weight but the sweat bath route to reduction will not work otherwise. In the sweat cabinet one only gets out a little water, then he takes a drink and he weighs as much as ever. No method of reduction that impairs one's health in the process is desirable. Typhoid fever will reduce the fat person very rapidly but we do not advocate it as a desirable means of weight reduction.

Fasting is an excellent means of reducing weight but it is seldom one can fast and continue his or her work. The better plan is, perhaps, a compromise. That is, diet control plus exercise. This plan is sure and will not impair one's health as the sweating process or the over exercise or as the various drugs that are advertised to reduce weight. You want health first and you do not want to lose weight by any method that must injure your health in order to reduce your weight. If you are overweight and not as healthy as you should be the right method of reducing weight will, at the same time, improve your health. In every case the results will pay one for the self-control and self-denial it entails.

CHAPTER 14
Man Shall Not Diet With Food Alone

Man may be appropriately defined as a fad-chasing biped that wears clothes. The latter part of this definition might exclude some of the ladies, but they, at least, come in under the first half. Just now the diet fad is leading the parade and every one is "on a diet." Diet "experts" and "specialists" multiply like rabbits and the end is not yet. Diet, we have learned, will both prevent and cure disease, cure poverty, prevent wars, correct the divorce evil and inaugurate the millenium. And the ex-spurts have proven all this on the rats and pigeons.

For sixteen years I have been studying diet and the many theoretical problems that meet one in this study. I have watched the so-called science of dietetics grow more and more complex with the passing of each year. The chemists with their test-tubes once supplied us with our knowledge of food and food values. Nowadays the "biologists" with their rats, pigeons, chickens, etc., tell us what to eat and what to feed the hogs. The so-called science of dietetics is hopelessly chaotic. No two "authorities" and no two little echoes of the "authorities" are agreed on the principles that should underlie feeding. They disagree and dispute and try it out on the rats. Thus they find that many things are true and many things are false. If they ever experiment with buzzards, they will find that ptomaine poisoning is a myth, and that the rotting carcass of a hog that died of cholera is wholesome food. Rabbits will demonstrate that belladonna is good food, and the porcupine will show that prussic acid is harmless. Experiments on dogs will prove that bones are easily digested. We can prove anything on the lower animals; anything that it is desired to prove, if we only use a sufficient number of kinds of animals. But it is a well known fact among vivisectionists that what works on animals does not always work on man. The last experiment must be made on man, and here we meet with factors which frequently upset our most beautiful and logically constructed theories.

There is too much of this test-tube and rat-pen dietetics handed out by the "authorities" today. Too many diet problems are being worked out in the laboratory rather than in the human body. The chemistry of nutrition is overemphasized. Artificial problems are manufactured by experiments on normal animals that are not subjected to the many influences of man and are not victims of the many devitalizing habits of the "superior" animal. Not enough attention is given to the individual and to the many and various influences besides food that affect his nutritive processes.

It is all very well to study the chemistry of food and the chemistry of the body, the processes of digestion, metabolism, etc., but, this is only a part of the story, and, perhaps, not the larger part, at that. It is well, also, to know all the factors that influence physiological chemistry and know how and to what extent these influences are exercised. For it is not enough to eat a perfect diet; we must also be able to digest and assimilate it.

If nutrition is the sum total of all those processes and functions by which growth and development, maintenance and repair of the body and, by which, reproduction are accomplished, then proper food is not even half of nutrition. To be properly nourished means more than to "eat proper foods in proper combinations." It means being able to properly digest and assimilate that food and to adequately rid the body of waste and refuse. And into this complex process there enters many factors other than that of food and food combinations. It is often claimed that life is chiefly a matter of nutrition, although the reverse of this is true. For, in the absense of life, nutrition is impossible. However, that may be, nutrition is not chiefly a matter of food. A world of wisdom is contained in the Biblical statement that "man shall not live by bread (food) alone." There are many factors which profoundly affect nutrition.

The world is full of diet ex-spurts and "scientists" who are seeking to accomplish by diet, that which diet can never perform. For thousands of years drugs have been supposed to exert some mysterious and powerful curative effect upon the human organism. Drugs failed and those who have not been able to eradicate from their minds a belief in "cures," are seeking a diet to do what drugs were formerly supposed to do. The longer they seek the more dietetics resembles the allopathic materia medica.

There are special diets for all ages, conditions and occasions, but an almost total neglect of the many other factors that contribute to or affect nutrition. If a patient suffers from defective nutrition, it is assumed to be always due to a deficient diet, and he is prescribed for accordingly. The results are very frequently disappointing. An anemic person is fed food containing much iron, although his regular diet may contain many times more iron than his body requires. It is no exaggeration when I say that I have never seen a case of anemia cured by a diet rich in iron. Children with rickets are fed a diet rich in calcium (lime) ; a diet of sunshine is usually more effective.

I have come to the conclusion that most cases of defective nutrition, if not wholly caused by other factors than diet, are, at least, contributed to largely by other factors. And I know, from observation and experience, that no diet can eliminate these other factors. To make my meaning perfectly clear, I will use an illustration that every person can duplicate among his own acquaintances. A skinny, scrawny individual desires to gain weight, and although in most cases, he is already eating more than enough food to supply his needs, he increases his consumption of food. He continues to overeat for weeks or months, or until he makes himself sick thereby, and does not gain weight. He may even lose weight. Many do. In such cases it cannot be claimed that the individual lost weight or failed to gain weight because he was not eating enough food to accomplish the desired gain. Nor can it always be said that such failures to gain weight are due to the lack of some one or more of the food elements in the food eaten, or to the lack of some of those mysterious, occult, incomprehensible things called vitamines. For I have watched cases in which no such deficiencies were possible in the diet eaten. The trouble is not always with the diet, as the many and repeated failures of the diet ex-spurts amply prove.

The available supply of energy with which to carry on the nutritive processes is, perhaps, the largest factor. If energy is low, that is, if the person is enervated, nutrition cannot be normal. Enervation is produced by many things. Any habitual practice or indulgence, any influence that uses up nerve force in excess of the daily supply brings on enervation and thus lowers organic function. The result is, every process and function of the body suffers. Secretion and excretion are impaired, nutrition and drainage are lessened and poor health results. When secretion and excretion are impaired nutrition cannot be normal, digestion must always suffer. If elimination is checked the resulting retention of toxins in the body also interferes with nutrition.

The statement that "more and more science is coming to look upon digestive disturbances not as separate ailments for which you take some drug, but as a danger signal for something that is fundamentally wrong with your eating" may be correct as far as it relates to what "science" is doing, but it is incorrect in saying that digestive disturbances are chiefly the result of incorrect eating. For it is not always correct to say: "For clearly what causes these disorders of the stomach is what we put into it." More often than otherwise, what we put into our stomach is only one of many factors that lead to such disorders, and often, very often, our food and drink do not form the biggest of these factors. For nutrition is more than starches, fats, proteins, mineral salts, vitamines, calories, bases and acids; and digestion is not all chemistry.

The most perfect diet that can be devised will not nourish the body if it is not digested. If it is not digested it will undergo fermentation and putrefaction and poison the body. That person who is habitually eating beyond digestive capacity is working harm to himself, no matter how perfect his diet.

Feed the most perfect meal that can be devised to a normal person, and feed it to him in a moderate quantity and then let him become gloomy, depressed, filled with fear, anxiety, worry, sorrow, anger, self-pity, etc., and he will fail properly to digest the meal. Not only so, but his mental state will profoundly affect every other process in the body that either directly or indirectly effects nutrition. His mental state may be of such a character as to completely suspend digestion, or it may be of an opposite nature, and he will digest and assimilate a meal that breaks all the rules of the ex-spurts. This is done daily by thousands of people.

Take a cow that is giving two gallons of milk at each milking. Let her graze on the pasture in peace and contentment the whole day through. Bring her in at milk time with the usual quantity of milk in her udder. Now frighten her or make her angry or beat her, and you will do well to get half a gallon of milk. The mental state of the cow inhibits the secretion of milk. We know that the same is true of women. We know that the same is true of other secretions of the body. Whether the mental state is temporary or constant, it effects the functions of the body one way or the other.

Take a man with excellent digestion; let him work the whole day through and come home in the evening ravenously hungry. Feed him upon an ideal meal. Hand him a message saying his business has failed, and he is left a pauper, or that his mother or daughter or son has died suddenly, and he will not digest the meal. If he has not already partaken of the meal when he receives the message, his ravenous appetite is instantly gone. Or take this same man after he has partaken of the meal and put him at some severe mental or physical task and his digestion will be impaired, if, indeed, it is not entirely suspended. Or, if the man is already exhausted from overwork, digestion will be impaired. Exercise, work and play all affect nutrition. If they are not carried to excess, they favor nutrition, although, during their performance, they impede it.

Perfect gastro-intestinal digestion and an ideal diet are not alone enough to insure perfect nutrition. The other organs of the body, the lungs, heart, spleen, ductless glands, etc., must be able to do their part of the work. They must not suffer from an inadequate nerve supply or imperfect drainage. The organs of elimination must do their work well. Such factors as bodily comfort, sunshine, rest, sexual habits, etc., are also involved in the process.

It is not correct to say that if the organs of the body are properly nourished, they will always perform their duty well. For, we know that there are many factors that influence these functions. Besides this, we know that in the presence or absence of these other factors these organs cannot be properly nourished.

Sunshine affects nutrition. Perfect nutrition is not possible in its absence. In fact, in its entire absence most plants and animals soon die. Feed a child proper food, the best of it, in proper combinations and rear him in a dark cellar where no ray of sunlight ever penetrates and see if he will be properly nourished. Bind up his arm so that it is never exercised and see if proper foods will prevent its atrophy, or cause it to develop normally. Feed proper foods to a man in high fever or intense pain and you will find that instead of nourishing him it only poisons him. Proper food! When is proper food?

Heat and cold affect nutrition. Extremes of either inhibiting it; moderate heat or moderate cold favoring it. Breathing affects nutrition. The amount of oxygen consumed should be in proportion to the amount of food eaten. If the oxygen supply is deficient, nutrition suffers. Nutrition is affected by the general habits of life. Lack of rest, loss of sleep interfere with nutrition. Sexual excesses derange digestion and impair nutrition. The use of stimulants impair nutrition. The general condition of the body affects nutrition. In acute disease the constructive side of nutrition is practically suspended. In chronic disease nutrition is impaired. Enervation impairs nutrition. Checked elimination impairs nutrition.

Thus it will be seen that the physician who wishes to properly feed his patients, will have to consider more factors than just food. If he has a patient, for instance, who is below normal weight, and who wants to put on several pounds of healthy flesh; before the physician can prescribe a diet that will accomplish this end, he must first find and correct every influence that is impairing nutrition. If there is some disease present, this must first be remedied. If it is some profound mental influence, or sexual excesses, or over work, or lack of exercise, or loss of sleep, these must be corrected. If the patient is greatly enervated, he will have to be put to bed, as well, in order that through rest, he may recuperate. If the drug habit or stimulant habit is impairing nutrition, these must be broken. Perhaps a lack of sunshine or a lack of oxygen is impairing nutrition. Sun baths and more air are required.

The reader who thought that nutrition is wholly a matter of food should now perceive his error. He should know that an inactive skin, through its failure to do its share in keeping the bloodstream pure, impairs nutrition; that a diseased liver or panaceas impair nutrition; that weak lungs do likewise. He should know that before a patient can digest and assimilate the best of food, all such conditions must be corrected.

If there isn't the necessary nervous power back of the processes of digestion, assimilation and elimination the "thin, anemic and sickly looking" individual will not derive the hoped for benefit from his food. It should be borne in mind that the body's nervous powers are drained away in a number of ways . . . i. e. by sexual excesses, loss of sleep, over work, destructive mental emotions, the use of stimulants and excesses of all kinds. A number of changes may have to be made in the "daily routine" before sufficient nerve power can be had to properly digest and metabolize a meal.

Laboratory experimentors, who work upon normal animals and have none of the above enervating factors to cope with may experiment until Gabriel blows his horn and never learn these facts. They may continue to produce

and "cure" by diet alone, certain diseases and thus prove
that they are disorders of nutrition. But so long as they
exclude these other factors, they cannot know how profoundly these disturb nutrition in spite of an ideal diet.
If they experiment upon normal animals under otherwise
normal conditions, or if they study chemistry, and chemistry only, and do not consider the many factors that influence the body's chemistry, influences that are often not
subject to laboratory control, they can never give us a true
science of dietetics. For, no profounder truth was ever
uttered than that: "man shall not live by bread (food)
alone."

Feed the most perfect meal conceivable to a patient
with high fever or in severe pain, and his body will fail to
digest it. Feed such meals regularly to a typhoid patient,
and he will continue to lose weight rapidly. Yea, more, he
will lose weight more rapidly and suffer more severely if
fed in any manner than if permitted to fast. Feed a perfect diet to a patient suffering with catarrh or rheumatism,
or gout, and he will improve more slowly than when placed
upon a fast. Feed a perfect diet to one whose elimination
is impaired, from any cause whatever, and he will not be
able to show the desired results. Feed such a diet to a man
greatly enervated from overwork, loss of sleep, sexual excesses, use of stimulants, or from any other cause, and
failure will mark the results. Enervation and impaired
elimination, whatever their cause, impair nutrition and all
the processes connected with it, regardless of the diet eaten.

I do not write these lines to discourage the study of
diet. I do not intend to be understood as believing that all
diets are equally good, or that some diets are not better
under certain circumstances than others. I do not mean
that diet plays no important role in regaining and maintaining health. But I do maintain that dietetics is now in
a hopelessly chaotic state and that so long as our present
methods of investigation and approach are in vogue it will
continue in this state. With all our knowledge of amino-
acids, mineral salts, vitamines and calories, we know no
more about the practical feeding of patients and infants

than those early Orthopathic practioners who simply said: "FEED NATURAL FOODS."

This was all that was ever necessary. Just as we breathe natural air and drink natural water and do not refine and process, pickle and stew, fry, boil, bake and hash these before using them, and just as we breathe only when we need air and drink only when thirsty, and not because it is drink-time so we should eat only natural— that is, unprocessed, unrefined, unpickled, uncooked foods —and eat them, not because it is eat-time but because we are truly hungry.

Of course, the term natural food means more than merely uncooked plants and grains, fruits, nuts and animal products. And it is here that the experiments upon rats and pigeons lead further astray. We would not experiment upon a cat to determine the best diet for rabbits nor experiment upon deer to discover the best diet for the lion. No amount of experiments upon dogs can supply the poultry raiser with the best diet for ducks or turkeys. Experiments upon houseflies will never determine the best diet for the silk worm, nor will a century of experiments upon such plants as thrive only in an acid soil determine what soil is best for those plants that perish in an acid soil. We cannot tell by experiments on hen eggs what temperature is required for the hatching of trout eggs. Because some animals can be frozen, and after remaining in this condition for some time, be thawed out and still live, we do not think that we can freeze up our live poultry and keep them through the winter this way.

Why then do we continue to attempt to determine the best diet for man by experimenting on rats, pigeons, dogs, etc? We may talk about nutrition being fundamentally the same in all animals, but we know that there are differences and discriminations that demand attention. That class of foods that is natural for dogs, or pigeons, or for deer, is not necessarily natural for man. Man does not eat shrubs with the giraffe, nor grass with the goat. He is not naturally a beast of prey like the cayote or tiger, nor a scavenger like the vulture or hyena. To eat natural foods does not mean to eat the whole plant and animal kingdoms.

Life is not a mere one-sided affair. We cannot eat our way to health or breathe our way to health, or sleep and rest our way to health, or exercise our way to health, or think our way to health, etc. We must live our way to health and to do this means that we must give due attention to all the factors of life. After our diet is made perfect we will still need fresh air and sunshine, rest and sleep, exercise and work. Given all these and tea, coffee, alcohol, tobacco, opium, soda fountain slops, destructive mental habits and emotions, sexual excesses, and all other execesses will be harmful. Health can be had only by healthful living, and this is constituted of more things than just proper eating .

If nutrition is impaired, we must seek out the cause or causes that are impairing it and correct these. Such causes are legion. It is generally admitted that if disease is interferring with the process of nutrition, this must be remedied before nutrition can become normal. It is seldom realized that if enervation has impaired nutrition, the enervation must be corrected before nutrition can be normalized. If enervation is due to overwork, the physician prescribes good nourishing food, (meaning, thereby, the conventional diet. The average physician knows nothing of diet), and a tonic or spinal stimulation. He does the same thing whether the enervation is due to loss of sleep, or sexual excesses or the use of stimulants or from any other cause. If tea or coffee or tobacco have overstimulated and led to enervation, it is the common practice to ignore these; and if the patient asks concerning them, he is assured that these have had no part in producing the trouble.

Such practices lead to failure and this causes the physician to say he does not believe in diet. Well, neither do I believe in diet, in this way. I do not believe that diet can overcome the effects of sensuality in those practicing sensuality, or that it can overcome the effects of inebriety in those who drink, any more than I believe that drugs or serums can do so. I do not belitve that diet can cure the fatigue following work or exercise, but I know that the body can cure itself during rest. Just so, I do not believe that diet can cure the effects of habitual and long continued overwork, or that the influences of overwork on nutrition can be cured without sufficient rest from work to enable the person to recuperate.

The proper food road to health and strength is like a wall with only one side, like a house with only one wall. Proper food is important, but it is only one of the factors that enter into normal nutrition and the man or woman who makes this the sole factor in his or her health program is headed for failure.

I do not know why it is necessary for me to place so much emphasis upon these well-known facts, unless it is that the diet ex-purts have forgotten their physiology. They keep telling us that all we require to do to attain and maintain health and strength is to eat proper foods in proper proportions and combinations. One of these men says that you can gain or lose as much weight as you please and he proposes to accomplish the whole thing by diet alone. He declares that "there can be no possible excuse for being thin, anemic and sickly looking when by eating correctly two pounds or more can be added each week until your weight is normal" and in order to do this you need "make no change in your daily routine."

There are so many factors, both internal, external and eternal, that have a profound effect upon the processes and functions of nutrition, that the man who imagines that he can usher in the millenium, by the ears, merely by the magic formula of a diet prescription, is doomed to disappointment. If we are dealing with the sick, there are usually many important things that must be done before the patient can properly digest and assimilate the best of food. Suppose he is suffering with gastro-intestinal catarrh; he cannot properly digest a meal. We must first correct the catarrh. Or, suppose we have a patient whose digestion is excellent and whose lungs or liver or kidneys or pancreas or skin is impaired. These may not be able to perform the task the digestion absorption and assimilation of a meal entails upon them. Shall we change his diet and feed him so many calories per day because he *needs* them, wholly irrespective of whether he can *utilize* them or not? Or, shall we first correct the influences that have impaired the patient's organ or organs and give these an opportunity to repair themselves first, and then feed correctly? Obviously this latter plan is by far the most sensible. Although it is the least scientific. It is also the most unpopular, for it promises no miracles and offers no signs and wonders all of which "science" does offer. It demands of the patient a degree of self-control and self-denial that he is unwilling to exercise and it does not promise to overcome the effects of his trangressions of the laws of life with some mysterious vitamins, or electronic reaction, or blood washing bath, or mechanical adjustment, or some catchy metaphysical formula.

Living Life to Live It Longer

By

Herbert M. Shelton, D.P., N.D., D.N.T., D.N. Sc.

A Study in Orthobionomics, Orthopathy
and Healthful Living

1926

Republished 1962
By
Health Research
Mokelumne Hill
California

Kessinger Publishing's Rare Reprints
Thousands of Scarce and Hard-to-Find Books!

- Americana
- Ancient Mysteries
- Animals
- Anthropology
- Architecture
- Arts
- Astrology
- Bibliographies
- Biographies & Memoirs
- Body, Mind & Spirit
- Business & Investing
- Children & Young Adult
- Collectibles
- Comparative Religions
- Crafts & Hobbies
- Earth Sciences
- Education
- Ephemera
- Fiction

- Folklore
- Geography
- Health & Diet
- History
- Hobbies & Leisure
- Humor
- Illustrated Books
- Language & Culture
- Law
- Life Sciences
- Literature
- Medicine & Pharmacy
- Metaphysical
- Music
- Mystery & Crime
- Mythology
- Natural History
- Outdoor & Nature
- Philosophy

- Poetry
- Political Science
- Science
- Psychiatry & Psychology
- Reference
- Religion & Spiritualism
- Rhetoric
- Sacred Books
- Science Fiction
- Science & Technology
- Self-Help
- Social Sciences
- Symbolism
- Theatre & Drama
- Theology
- Travel & Explorations
- War & Military
- Women
- Yoga

We kindly invite you to view our extensive catalog list at:
http://www.kessinger.net

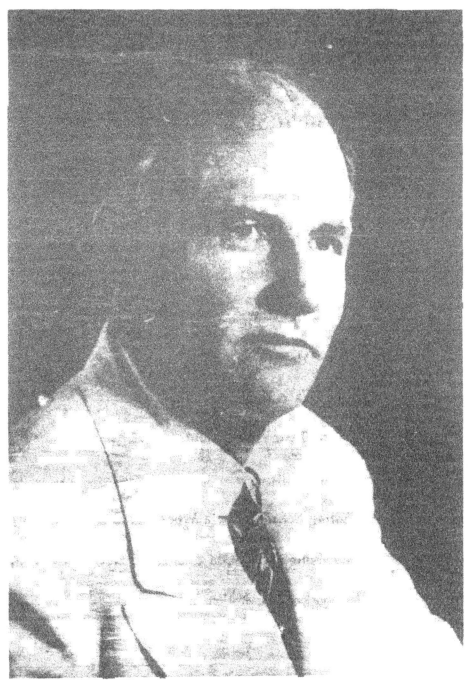

Yours for Health Truth and Medical Liberty
Herbert M. Shelton

INDEX

Part   **Page**

1. Man is Made for a Long Life............ 7

2. Findings of Biologists 12

3. The Body's Own Provisions for Nutrition and Drainage 19

4. How the Body's Efficiency is Impaired.... 26

5. Habits That Kill 36

6. Habits That Kill (Continued)........... 48

7. Habits That Kill (Continued)........... 61

8. Nature's Provisions for Living.......... 75

9. Temperance and Wholesomeness 84

10. The Reign of Health Law 91

11. Machine Made Long Life 107

12. Follies of "Science" 121

13. Medicine Shortens Life 130

Living Life to Live It Longer

MAN IS MADE FOR A LONG LIFE.

"Oppose the present age to theirs," says a recent writer, "and one finds that amulets are sold still as they were in Babylon, and Panaceas are yet in demand." He says of the world-wide and age-long quest for means of prolonging life and youth, "A faculty of learned men could labor for years and still not run down all the forms in which the wish of youth restored has taken shape. Europe, Asia—all the continents and all the islands have their versions, and in all lands there have been men to turn the hope to personal advantage."

Some have merely sought to prolong life. Others have sought to defeat the sentence "Dust thou art, and unto dust shalt thou return." But whichever they desired, the search was always for some formula, some magical and mysterious something with which to maintain youth and life. Theon, father Hypatia, had a plan for the transmutation of metals and a recipe for perpetual youth. Ponce de Leon died in Florida in search of the fabled Fountain of Youth.

Descartes, who died at the tender age of fifty four, invented a specific which would enable him to live five hundred years. Prof. Metchnikoff found sour milk to be the much coveted panacea. Sophie Lepple, who died a few years ago, had intended to live a thousand years. If she had lived about nine-hundred and thirty four or more years longer she would have accomplished her goal. Voronoff and Steinach have found the solution to the great secret in the transplantation of monkey glands. The young Greek, Christos Paresco, found it in a new bath. This bath, the wonderful biological blood-washing bath, derives its efficacy from a special patented and exorbitantly-priced shower head. It is purely and simply a fake commercial scheme.

Alcohol was once hailed as the *elixir vitae*. Its sale at present is prohibited by law in this country. One eminent biologist (?) is now seeking for the solution of the mystery with the X-ray. While this is a more powerful light than the lantern with which Diogenes sought for an honest man, I fear the learned biological dignitary will be compelled to employ a "light" of an entirely different nature before he finds the hiding place of youth and long life.

In his search for a means of prolonging life and youth, man has displayed the same lack of intelligence, the same credulity, and the same faith in magic, as he has displayed in his search for "cures" of disease. As Herbert Spencer so astutely remarked, man never adopts the right method until he had exhausted every possible wrong one.

Are there grounds for the hope of prolonging youth and life? Does a basis of fact exist upon which to rest our hopes? These, it seems, are the first questions that should be answered. Let us, then, look for a brief moment at some facts that may lend encouragement to our quest.

The great Naturalist, Buffon, stated:

"The man who does not die of disease reaches everywhere the age of 100 years or more."

Prof. Weismann of Friberg said:

"Death is not a primitive attribute of living matter; it is of secondary origin. There are animals that never die; for instance, infusoria and rhizopods, and in general all unicellular organisms."

The celebrated Dr. Wm. A. Hammond asserted that death is not a physiological necessity; that if balance between construction and destruction could be kept minutely and accurately balanced, we need never grow old and need never cease to live, so far as the theachings of physiology go.

Dr. Munroe, a renowned English anatomist, said:

"The human frame as a machine is perfect; that it contains within itself no marks by which we can possibly predict its decay; it is apparently intended to go on forever."

Dr. Morton, in his "Anatomical Lectures," declared:

"The human body as a machine is perfect; it bears no marks tending to decay, and is calculated to go on a hundred years, or we might say forever, did we not know to the contrary by experience."

A celebrated English physician, Dr. John Gardner, in a work upon longevity said:

"Before the flood men are said to have lived five and even nine hundred years, and as a physiologist, I can assert positively that there is no fact reached by science to contradict or render this improbable. It is more difficult, on scientific grounds, to explain why men die at all, than to believe in the duration of life for a thousand years."

These views do not differ materially from those at present entertained as will be seen later. The human body is a self-renewing, self-adjusting organism and does not manifest inherent inability to keep this process up indefinitely.

Animals live an average of from five to seven times the length of time they require to reach maturity. Man, as an animal, should do as well. Opinions differ about when he reaches complete physical maturity. These range from twenty years to thirty years. The average man does reach his full height by the age of twenty, but he is never fully developed by this time. If we assume twenty to be correct, he should live from a hundred to a hundred and forty years. If we take twenty-five as some estimate it, then his age should average from one hundred and twenty-five to one hundred and seventy-five years. Taking thirty as correct, his average age should be from a hundred and fifty to two hundred and ten years.

This is viewing man purely as an animal. But we find animals live almost wholly on the instinctive plane with instincts perfectly developed at birth, while man lives (or should live) chiefly on the intellectual plane, and has but few instincts. His intellectual development is never complete. Regardless of how long he lives and how much he develops mentally, there are undeveloped cells in his brain at death. This would seem to indicate that man's brain, and if his brain his body also, is designed for an indefinite existence.

The average length of human life in the United States is given today at fifty-five years for men, and fifty-seven years for women. In New Zealand it is given today at sixty-one and eight tenths years for women, while in India it is as low as twenty-two and six tenths years for males. About the middle of the last century it was estimated that half the human race dies in infancy. About twenty years ago a statistical juggler estimated that half the human race dies before its eighteenth year.

These figures seem to indicate an increasing life span. *But the increase is only apparent.* It is a matter of infant mortality. Hundreds of thousands of babies are now being saved by better care. The mature man of today is not so well off as the mature man of the past. He lives no longer, and finds the degenerative diseases such as cancer, Bright's disease, disease of the heart and arteries, diabetes, insanity, etc., rapidly increasing among the "middle aged." There has been no actual increase in the length of human life.

But even now, those who die in infancy, childhood, youth and after maturity is reached, including those who die in "old age," die not because they have lived to their fullest possible extent. They are not dying because they could not have lived longer. They are

This page was omitted in the original book.

This page was omitted in the original book.

rate of growth was, thereby, stimulated to such an extent that the tissues are said to have increased, in twenty-four hours, to forty times their original bulk. By this means he was able, not only to prevent the degenerative influences of the metabolic end products from gradually slowing down the growth of the tissues and finally resulting in their death, but also of increasing their rate of growth and making it possible, apparently, to continue his experiment indefinitely.

On Jan. 17, 1912, Dr. Carrel took a piece of connective tissue from the heart of a chicken and set about to maintain its life apart from the chicken's body. That piece of heart is alive yet (1926), and is, apparently as strong and vigorous as ever. Every day it is washed and supplied with a fresh nutrient media. The washing completely rids it of waste products. Kept clean and properly nourished it grows so rapidly that it is frequently necessary to subdivide it. Yet they do not seem to grow old in the sense that their vitality is diminished. On Nov. 21, 1925, it was announced that so rapid had been the growth of this piece of tissue, that had it not been cut down each day, it would have overspread the entire city of New York.

Burrows demonstrated that a chicken's embryo's heart-muscles beat rythmically when placed in an appropriate culture medium. Parts of the heart placed on the slides and fed with warm blood, soon began to build more tissue of their kind, and after a time they began to expand and contract like whole hearts within living bodies. One part, purposely made smaller that the other, pulsated reguarly with more speed than the larger piece, the smaller having 120 and the larger 92 pulsations per minute.

After three days the pulsations of the smaller piece dropped to 90 beats a minute, while those of the larger part dropped to 40. It was then washed clean and new blood supplied for food and the pieces again became vigorous and pulsated at a rapid rate. As they beat they increased in size, finally growing together and becoming one piece. The two parts which had been beating at different rates assumed a modified rate when they grew together and beat as one.

Both Carrel and Burrows discovered that cells which showed signs of what is called old age, require only to be placed onto a new culture media to become young again and to multiply and grow. Dr. Woodruff kept groups of cells alive for 8,500 generations without loss of cellular vitality.

Parts of the stomach, the kidneys, the lungs, the liver and other organs have been rebuilt by being fed with blood. Lung tissue added to the piece of lung, kidney tissue to the kidney, liver tissue to the liver, etc. Almost all parts of the body have been subjected to experiments of this kind, and have proven themselves capable of growth and repair under such conditions. Each part of the body renews and repairs itself, by its own intrinsic power to absorb nutritive material from the surrounding medium and assimilate, organize, and transform it into material identical with its own, and endow it with vital properties, if it is supplied with appropriate food.

Part of a newly-born rabbit was placed in coldstorage and allowed to remain there for a year. It was then placed on a slide, given food and warmth and it began to grow as soon as the proper temperature was reached. A piece of bone of a young pig began growing quickly, but a piece of bone from an old pig was slow in beginning its growth. Experiments have shown that parts taken from very young life begin to grow soon, those from middle life require more time to start growing, while those from old life require much more time.

The practice of grafting plants and trees is familiar to all. In fact, it is so common that everyone considers it a matter of course. In recent years graft-

ing of animal parts has been successfully accomplished.
For instance, pieces of skin have been put in cold
storage to prevent decay and, after they have been
there several months, have been taken out and fed
warm blood and they began to grow. New pores and
layers were built in perfect order, and all the intri-
cate apparatus involved in perspiration was constructed. Fresh pieces of skin placed on the denuded
flesh, where the skin was torn or burned away, grew
and united with the surrounding skin.

Pieces of bone have been taken from freshly killed
animals and fed with fresh blood with the result, that
they selected from the blood the elements necessary
to the building of new bone and rejected the rest.
Pieces of new bone have been grafted into the bones
of those who, from some cause, had had part of their
bone destroyed. The bone grew and united with the
surrounding bone.

During the war surgeons took many advantages of
the soldiers over seas and performed experiments
upon them by wholesale. How many lives were thus
unnecessarily snuffed out can never be known; nor
does it fall within the scope of this chapter to discuss
this phase of the subject. Rather, we wish here, simply to call attention to a few of the things that were
successfully accomplished with the few that were not
killed by the experiment.

If a part of a body was shot away or injured, a
new part from a recently killed soldier was supplied.
Often an organ from a recently killed soldier was
transferred to the body of a live soldier, whose organ
had been destroyed and he became "whole" again
Kidneys have been taken out and replaced by others
and even veins and arteries have been successfully
transferred from one to another.

Dr. Magitol removed a diseased eyeball from a patient and put it in cold storage for future use. Some
time afterward a patient came to him with a scar on

the eye caused by a severe quick-lime burn. He cut
out the injured part—the corner of the eyeball—then
cut a similar piece from the eyeball he had in storage and fitted it into the patient's eye. It grew and
the damaged eye was repaired without leaving, so it
is said, a scar.

Much fuss is made over the so-called recent discovery that when a person is declared dead, not every
part of him is actually dead. This "recent discovery
that when a person is declared dead, not every part
of him is actually dead. This "recent discovery" has
been known for many years. In fact, it is stated as a
truth in some of the older physiologies, written long
before the present "discoverers" saw the light of day.
However, it remained for recent experiments to prove
that parts of the body would, under favorable circumstances, continue to live and grow for some time after
the death of the body.

A piece of the spinal cord of a frog, for instance,
placed in a proper medium, kept warm and, protected
from injury, grew steadily and increased in size hour
by hour for two days and ten hours, or fifty-eight
hours, in the laboratory. It increased to many times
its original size. But these same cells resist the
anemia that results from arrested circulation, in
death, for about twenty minutes and then they too
begin to die.

Reflex actions secured upon the bodies of recently
killed animals, however, indicate that these do not die
suddenly at the end of the twenty minutes. It is
estimated that the brain cells begin to decompose in
three minutes after the heart ceases to send blood to
to them. But many cells in the body are still alive
and busily engaged in carrying on their life processes
even while the body is being lowered into the grave.

Professor Pozze of the Academy of Medicine, with
able assistance of other scientists, succeeded in removing the vital organs of a living cat and placed

them in a receptacle where he fed them with blood-food and maintained them at the normal temperature of a living cat. The organs carried on their regular functions for many hours; the stomach digested the food given it, the intestines moved in the usual way, the heart beat, the lungs breathed and the circulation was described as being perfect. However the ability to eliminate the toxic waste from the cells was very limited.

All the above enumerated experiments, and many more like them, demonstrate what was already known before—namely, that the cells of the animal body require, if they are to continue to live, grow and reproduce, proper nutrition, adequate drainage, a suitable temperature and protection from violence. Cells forming the bodies of the higher animals are not capable of independent existence under ordinary circumstances because of their specialized character.

Once the germ cells of the developing embryo become differentiated, they are incapable of returning to their former undifferentiated or germ-cell state. This is to say, muscle cells, when once they have become such, can never be anything other than muscle cells. To borrow from Delafield and Prudden (''Text Book of Pathology''), ''when differentiation has advanced so that such distinct types of tissue have been formed as connective tissue, epithelium, muscle, nerve, these do not again merge through metaplasia.'' There is no evidence that mesoblastic tissues can be converted into those of epiblastic or hypoblastic type, or vice versa. Once these cells have been differentiated and dedicated to a particular function, they can never become another and distinct type of cell with other and different functions. Therefore their dependence upon the body and their helplessness when separated from it.

However, these experiments serve to strengthen a certain fact of common observation which has been denominated The Law of the Cell. This "law" has been formulated in these words: *"Every cell in the body will continue to perform the functions for which is was designed throughout its entire life cycle provided its environment remains congenial to it."*

This Law would seem to indicate that if the cells of the body are maintained at all times in a congenial environment, man could live for many more years than he now attains, if indeed, he cannot live indefinitely. Of course, we have no means of telling how long man can live until the experiment is tried out by a sufficiently large number of people beginning at birth or before.

PART III.

THE BODY'S OWN PROVISION FOR NUTRITION AND DRAINAGE

The announcement that except for the daily paring of the piece of chicken heart kept alive for twelve years by Dr. Carrel, it would have overspread the entire city of New York, was not true. So great is the need for nutrition and drainage that had that piece of chicken been permitted at any time to grow beyond a certain size parts of it would have immediately begun to die of starvation and self-poisoning. Not even the daily washing and feeding of its outside surface by the scientists could save it. Special provisions would be necessary in order to convey the food to the cells on the interior and to completely drain away their waste. In the animal body this work is accomplished by a wonderful and complex arrangement of specialized organs and their various functions.

The organs of the body are perfectly adapted to life in the body. They are capable of replacing, by growth and reproduction, such as they undergo for the scientist in the laboratory, all worn out and broken down cells, while the body is capable of removing and expelling the injured or dead cells. By their powers of assimilation and self-maintenance, living organisms, preserve their condition notwithstanding the changes to which they are liable through the influence of external forces and their own natural decay. The stability and integrity of structure and function which they thus display is maintained by the continual formation of new cells and cell productions to take the places of those that are impaired and expelled. For this work of repair and self-maintenance to be performed at all, it is necessary that the cells composing the body be supplied with a proper nutrient media and have their waste promptly removed.

It is essential that they are supplied with the proper temperature also.

The organs composing the animal body make the medium in which its cells live. The body is also capable within reasonable limits of regulating and maintaining its temperature at the desired point. Such bodies are equipped with organs whose duty it is to take crude food substances from the surrounding environment and prepare it for use by the cells. Other organs carry it to and from the cells. Other groups of organs eliminate from the body or from the medium which bathes its cells in a continuously flowing stream, all the waste and poisons that have been formed by the activities and breaking down of the cells, or which have gained an entrance into the body from without.

Under ordinary circumstances the Ameba is supposed not to die. Barring death by violence, poisoning or starvation it is supposed to go on dividing and redividing forever. Conditionally it is supposed to be possessed of everlasting life. What are the conditions upon which its life depends? So far as these are discoverable they are: Appropriate food, water and oxygen, proper temperature and freedom from poisoning and violence. We might say its life depends upon a favorable or congenial environment, and that so long as its environment remains congenial it continues to function and reproduce.

The larger plants and animals are made up of cells assembled in vast numbers. When cells are thus massed as in the body of a worm, the situation of the cell differs much from that of the cell leading an independent existence. Its environment is made up largely of other associated cells. Comparatively few are in direct contact with the outside world; the greater portion being submerged among their brothers. They are shut in from food supplies, from the oxygen of the air and from water. A cell so situated would soon perish, were no special provisions made for its needs.

The cells composing an animal body are similar to, though more complex than, the ameba. All cells composing the body of any animal are of common descent, but they have taken on widely different characters and functions, this being made necessary by the conditions under which they are to exist. The Ameba, leading an independent existence, must perform all the activities essential to its existence—preparation or crude food locomotion, etc. In the multicellular animal this is changed. The specialization which groups the cells of such an animal into a number of classes each with definite work to perform also entails the dependence of each class upon the other. While the Ameba is self-sufficient those of the animal cannot continue to live under ordinary circumstances if separated from the body.

The association of cells into an organism necessitates the formation of special structures to perform special work and this in turn necessitates the assumption of special functions by the cells making up the various structures. Special function, as distinguished from the common or fundamental functions of cells, is the power to perform a special work in the body. Special functions are those which are not common to all cells and are not essential to the life of the cell *per se*, but are essential to the life of the organism. Special function varies greatly for the different cells, some as the bone cells serving as supports for other structures; others like the skin cells as protectors. Some, like the kidney cells excrete waste matter some of the liver cells secrete bile, others store up glycogen, etc. Fundamental functions are those that are common to all cells alike and are essential to the life of the cell *per se*.

The living thing grows, reproduces and multiplies its parts and extends itself by this repetition. To affect this it selects from matter in contact such elements as it has the capacity to arrange as parts of its own structure, and as promptly rejects and refuses all others—a necessary condition to the maintenance of its vital integrity. In the plant or animal, or wherever vitality reigns, assimilation and growth and refusal and rejection are its constant actions, and the energy of these acts must bear a constant relation to each other; for the vital endowment equally seeks its own welfare in either act. This process of self-formation from dissimilar materials which is wholly peculiar to living things, and, without which, none exist is by appropriation and transformation. Collectively this is called nutrition.

Nutrition is the sum of the processes concerned in maintaining the normal condition of the cell and includes growth and repair. So long as this is adequately accomplished the cells and the tissues which they form are able to perform their functions and to exhibit their own characteristic activities; to develop and maintain themselves. Development is the process by which each organ of a living body is first formed; or by which one already incompletely formed, is so changed in form and structure as to be fitted for the functions for which it is designed. Growth, which concurs with development and continues after it, is properly, the normal increase in the size of a part by the insertion or super-addition of materials similar to those of which it already consists. In growth proper, no change of form, structure or function occurs. Parts only increase in weight and size and, if they acquire more power, it is power of the same kind as before exercised. Maintenance is the process of repair and reconstruction by which the worn out or injured parts of a tissue or organ are replaced. Development, growth and maintenance are all accomplished by cell proliferation and, in the case of development, differentiation. What produces the differentiation is not known, probably never will be known, but it is known that the power

that determines the development of the embryo from
the germ or ovum to the nine months infant is identical with that which is the source of the constant preservation and renovation of the individual and of the
development and growth of the individual after birth.
The processes of cell life are carried on ideally only
in a nutritive medium which is in a state of solution, life being possible to cells only when their nourishment is in liquid form so they can assimilate it.
The Ameba, as was previously stated lives in water
or substances containing liquid. The cells composing
both plant and animal bodies likewise require a liquid
medium in which to live.

In all the larger forms there is a moving liquid medium which flows incessantly. In animals this medium is known as the blood and lymph, in plants as
sap. This medium bathes all the living cells in the
body and acts as a common carrier, supplying them
with food and oxygen and removing their waste. In
the higher animals the lymph only comes in direct
contact with the majority of the cells. From this
they draw their needful supplies of food and oxygen
and into it they discharge their waste. The resources
of the lymph at any point are very limited and are re-
plenished constantly from the blood stream which
passes close by in rapid movement in vessels whose
thin delicate walls permit the passage of material
both ways. The blood exchanges its fresh oxygen
which it has just brought from the lungs for the carbon dioxide from the lymph. It then carries the
carbon dioxide to the lungs and exchanges this for
more oxygen. At the same time it exchanges fresh
food for the waste of the cells and carries these
wastes to the excretory organs for elimination.

Just as the ameba appropriates food and oxygen
from the water or slime in which it lives and moves
and has its being and excretes its waste into this same
water or slime, so the cells composing the organs of
the animal body appropriate food from the lymph in

which they live and "move" and have their being, and excrete into this same lymph their waste.

If the nerve supply to an organ or part is destroyed it loses sensation and motion and perhaps it atrophies but it does not necessarily die. From this it becomes apparent that organic function is not possible in the absence of nerve supply. If nutrition and drainage are cut off from an organ or part its death is only a matter of minutes. This may serve to show the relative importance of nutrition and drainage as compared to innervation, but it must not be lost sight of that nutrition and drainage in the higher animals is wholly a matter of organic function and that under all ordinary circumstances normal organic function is capable of maintaining nutrition and drainage up to the standard demanded by healthy life. The preparation of food, the intake of air and water and their distribution to the cells and the removal of cellular waste and toxins are all accomplished by organs, the food, air and water being passive substances under the control of these organs.

Just as life, growth and reproduction, in the tissues used in the experiments already observed is a master drama of nutrition, drainage, and warmth under the control of the scientists in the laboratory, so, life growth and reproduction to the tissues in the body is a master drama of nutrition drainage and warmth under the control of the nervous system and the organs by means of which it accomplishes its work. If enervation is suspended it results in a train of pathological phenomena included under term death. Respiration and circulation and through the latter, nutrition and drainage, are suspended suddenly, if the cause is applied with sufficient force. If the cause is applied more gradually so that innervation is gradually suspended, in a few days, it may be, or in a few years it may give rise to any one or a number of the many pathological phenomena that have been classified as diseases and given separate names.

The tremendous importance of the nervous system and the vital organs through which it carries on the functions of animal life is thus made manifest. For it must be borne in mind that such is the interdependence of the various parts of the body upon each other that serious injury to one speedily effects the others. Nutrition and drainage are as essential to the nervous structures as to the muscular or glandular, etc. Oxygen is required by the nerves as well as by the muscles. If from any cause the lungs are damaged and oxygenation of the blood impaired the whole system suffers. If breathing is stopped entirely for a few minutes death of the whole body is the result. Damage to the heart suspending the circulation results in somatic death. Yet the sole object of the heart, and its accessory organs, the vascular system, is to distribute to the various parts of the body the nutritive material. Death comes because nutrition and drainage have ceased. Destruction or serious impairment of the kidneys, for instance, soon results in death from poisoning as these fail to relieve the blood of its load of toxins before its return to the tissues. The toxins soon accumulate in such quantities as to overwhelm the cells and stop all function.

The human body is adequately equipped with special organs the functions of which is to keep the cells supplied at all times with food, water, oxygen, warmth and to carry away from the cells and cast out of the body all waste and poisons that form therein or that gain admittance from without. That the normal organism is fully capable of supplying its cells with these conditions of continued active life requires no proof. *There is no sound reason for believing that the cells of the body could not live as long and as well in the body as in the test-tube of the scientist if the functions of life are not impaired.*

PART IV.
HOW THE BODY'S EFFICIENCY IS IMPAIRED

Biology, as at present taught, may be defined as an effort to support the mechanistic theories of spontaneous generation of life with subsequent transmutation of species. Prof. Pearl, of John's Hopkins University, who is one of the world's leading biologists says that the mechanistic and non-intelligent process of *Natural Selection* "makes each part (of the body) only good enough to get by." He assumes that while the long discredited Natural Selection produced certain organs that were capable of living indefinitely, a large part of the body is simply a makeshift and that death comes because these make-shift parts cannot endure the "strain" of living. They give down and this sooner or later results in death. More will be said about this in a future installment.

Hypothesis aside, every organ in the human body, if not impaired or defective, from birth, or, from causes operating after birth, is capable of performing much more work than is necessary for the life of the organism. The heart and lungs, for instance, are capable of greatly increasing their work if one is called upon to do a hundred-yard dash or even a ten-mile marathon with a trolley car or a bear.

The kidneys are capable of increasing their activities and taking up part of the skins work if for any reason, the skin fails in its duties. The skin, when one is subjected to great heat or to vigorous muscular effort, is capable of increasing its activities many times. The stomach, liver, intestines, bowels, etc., are all capable of doing much more work than the actual needs of life require. *The organs of a normal body are capable of carrying on the functions of life under all ordinary circumstances without strain, so long as they are not impaired by some cause or causes. The* real problem, therefore, is to find and remove the causes of organic deterioration.

If cells that are kept clean and properly nourished never grow old in the sense that they lose their vitality, and in the human body there are organs and functions that, when normal, completely rid the body of waste and toxins; and another process that, when normal, keeps the cells supplied with a fresh supply of nutrient material, what impairs these organs and functions so that the cells do grow old, do lose their vitality and die? It is assumed by the mechanists, who call themselves biologists, that this impairment is a necessary result of the community action of the cells of the body. This is only an assumption with no basis of fact to stand on.

Cells in the laboratory are killed by starvation and by poisoning. Why assume that their death in the body is due to other causes? The uneliminated products of metabolism, plus the breaking down of cells in disease, plus toxins absorbed from without are as capable of destroying cells in the body as in the scientist's test tube. Drugs, serums, vaccines, anti-toxins, etc., that are taken into the body, in any manner, for any purpose, kill cells and cripple organs. Starvation of the cells resulting from eating denatured food or from impaired digestion and assimilation is capable of killing cells in the body. It would, of course, be beneath the dignity of a so-called scientist to consider these things. First, they offer no mystery; and, second, their consideration might not be pleasing to state medicine and the "food" manufacturers. Scientists (?) must serve their masters.

We learned in the previous chapter that all the functions of the body are controlled by the nervous system—the nervous function being the only exception. It is a self evident fact that these functions are efficient or not depending on the power or weakness of the nervous system. With a full tide of nervous energy every function of the body will be vigorous and efficient. With nerve force inadequate, function lags —it becomes weak and impaired.

With impaired function—due to lowered nerve force, ENERVATION—The processes of nutrition and drainage are not conducted normally and, as a consequence, slow, gradual starvation and poisoning of the cells begins. The functional and structural integrity of the body suffers and the process of dying commences. How long it will require for dying to culminate in *somatic* death—that is death of the body as distinguished from death of the cells—matters little.

Nerve energy is a fluctuating quantity. It rises and falls from day to day, from hour to hour and from minute to minute, depending on the nature and degree of our activities and the nature of our environment. With every rise and fall of our nervous energies there is a corresponding rise and fall in functional efficiency. Those organs which, through heredity or abuse, are the weakest will suffer the greatest impairment of function when the nervous power is lowered. The degree of functional impairment may range from an imperceptible impairment to an almost if not total suspension of function as is frequently seen in shock.

Digestive powers are lowered. Secretion is not adequate to meet the needs of the food intake. Indigestion—or bacterial decomposition of food— with the formation of a whole series of toxins, some of which are absorbed into the body, occurs.

Bowel action is weakened resulting in constipation. Kidney action is impaired. Excretion and elimination through this channel lags. The liver and lymph glands are impaired. Their power to detoxify, through chemicalization, the waste and toxins in the body is weakened. The functions of the liver, pancreas and other glands of the body in preparing food for use by the cells lag. Elimination through the skin and lungs is impaired.   All this results in the slow, gradual accumulation, in the blood, lymph, secretions and cells of various toxins or poisons, "ARREARS OF EXPURGATION," as Dr. Jennings called them, and also in the slow, gradual starvation of the cells. Enervation impairs organic function and impaired function permits the slow gradual starvation and poisoning of the cells.   The process of dying which then begins is slow and gradual and may be prolonged over many years.

The accumulation of toxins, some of which are powerful acids gradually destroys the functioning cells of the various organs of the body—the liver, pancreas, kidneys, spinal cord, brain, heart, etc.   This gives rise to ascites, diabetes, Brights disease, locomotor Ataxia, paresis, paralysis, insanity and other brain and nerve diseases, diseases of the heart and arteries, etc.   The local irritations, congestions and hardenings caused by these toxins frequently give rise to tumors and cancers.

Earlier we learned that if cells are fed and washed daily they appear to be able to live indefinitely. They do not die or grow old in the usual sense.   When they die, and death is not due to violence, they die of starvation or poisoning.   The body is equipped with organs the functions of which it is to secure and prepare proper food for use by the cells and to carry away the toxins from the cells and eliminate them from the body.   We learned that due to ENERVATION, there is an impairment both of the nutritive and eliminative functions, followed by the development of TOXEMIA and by more or less STARVATION of the cells.   The body learns to tolerate these toxins, but this does not neutralize their destructive effects upon the cells of the body.   Just as the opium user learns to tolerate large doses of opium and these only seem to produce a feeling of apparent well-being but actually they undermine and destroy the body, so the TOXEMIA, while it is tolerated and does not appear to harm the body, actually undermines and destroys the body. Little by little, it undermines the body so that old age and disease creep upon us unawares. We are killed by the toxins we have learned to tolerate.

If it were not that the body learns to tolerate these toxins, if it always vigorously resisted and threw them off, then no chronic toxemia would or could ever develop. The body would either exhaust itself in its struggles against the toxins or we would be forced to reform our modes of living and conform to the laws of being. It is the power of toleration that deceives us and leads us to continue our disease building mode of living. It is toleration that kills us in the end. It is the power of toleration that enables us to harbor our worst foes. Toleration which is equivalent to the medical immunity is the cause of death, or, at least, it leads to death.

One of the evil effects of chronic toxemia is the slow, gradual and certain destruction of the functioning cells of the various organs of the body. They are slowly poisoned to death by the toxins the body has learned to tolerate. The body possesses power to replace such cells with new ones, but, owing to enervation and toxemia, this power is greatly reduced. Instead of replacing these cells with more of their kind, their places are filled with a functionless substitute of connective tissue cells which form what is called "scar tissue." It is the substitution of "scar tissue" for the normal liver cells that produces what is popularly known as hob-nailed liver. The same thing takes place in the brain, spinal cord, arteries, eyes, ears, lungs, heart, kidneys, pancreas, etc., forming part of that condition associated with "old age" which is called hardening or sclerosis of the tissues and organs. Any prolonged irritation, as by toxins, of an organ or part will result in overgrowth of connective tissue in an organ and thus cripple its efficiency.

Thomas Parr who was killed in England about four hundred years ago, at the ripe old age of one hundred and fifty-two years, was found, at the necropsy performed by Dr. Harvey, discoverer of the circulation of the blood, to have escaped this hardening process. His body was that of a young man. He should have lived another hundred and fifty or more years, had his physicians not been so anxious to save his life. They bled and purged and puked him and killed him to save him after the king had wined him and dined him into a mild acute disease. If you want to live long, keep your tissues soft and fresh by avoiding toxemia and beware of the drug-to-kill doctors.

Any toxin, whether formed in the body or taken in from without, is capable of bringing about this hardening process. The rapidity with which it is brought about will depend upon the amount and strength of the poison and upon the resistance the system can offer to the poison. Alcohol, tobacco, tea, coffee, condiments, salt and all drugs, serums and vaccines as well as overeating, fear, worry, anxiety, jealousy, theft, untruthfulness, etc., produce hardening of the tissues of the body.

The hardening process that takes place in the body as age advances seems to affect a number of people earlier than others. It is probable that there is a diathesis or tendency in such people to age early, and rapidly. As one very prominent orthopath suggests, it may be a case of the parents eating sour grapes and the children's teeth being set on edge. Certain it is that two people living in almost the same manner will not grow old together. One will age more rapidly than the other.

Imprudent living, of course, hastens the aging process in all. Those predisposed to early aging will be caused to age earlier by all kinds of stimulants and excesses,—tea, coffee, cocoa, chocolate, alcohol, tobacco, drugs of all kinds, sexual excesses, mental or physical, late hours, worry, fear, anxiety, etc., and indulgences of all kinds that overtax the nervous energies and bring on ENERVATION AND TOXEMIA.

All parts of the body do not age at the same rate. Witness those who have sclerosis of the liver but whose kidneys are relatively sound and whose eyes remain good. Even the arteries do not all age at the same rate. They may be hardened in spots or localities and relatively normal elsewhere. When the arteries become hardened and thickened they are rendered less capable of accomplishing their most delicate work—that of renewal of cell life and elimination. The hardening of the tissues always interferes with the processes of nutrition and drainage and impairs the functions of those tissues thus affecting other tissues also. The ears may undergo hardening, impairing hearing, while the eyes remain good or the eyes may undergo hardening while the ears remain sound.

Those portions of the body that are weakest, those offering least resistance to the toxins, are most vulnerable. Likewise, those that are subjected to the greatest irritation and are, therefore, filled with an excess of blood harden more rapidly than other portions.

Knowing the cause of this condition is equivalent to knowing how to prevent its development. If a certain mode of life brings on a hardening of the tissues of the body and a consequent impairment of their powers, no ex-spurt should be required to proscribe such a mode of life. If the irritation to the heart, arteries, liver, kidneys, brain, etc., is due to the use of alcohol, then certainly the rational and logical course is to cease consuming the alcohol. It were, however, better to avoid such influences from infancy.

Job of many boils and much grumbling, prophesied of a time when the old man should return to the days of his youth and his flesh should be fresher than the flesh of a child. I do not know how much Job knew of physiology and pathology but 1 do know that if we hope to live much beyond the average age of man today, we must retain the youthful freshness of our tissues. They must not be allowed to harden. We must avoid all influences and agencies that singly and combined bring about such conditions of the system as favor the hardening process that results in "old age."

Old age is not a time of life. It is a state of being —a condition of the body. It is the cumulative effect of a whole series of causes that operate to weaken and impair the body. We meet some of these causes almost from birth and as we grow older and our sphere of life broadens we come in contact with an ever-increasing number of them. Many fathers subject their infants to tobacco smoke almost from the day of birth. Babies are over-fed, over-clothed, drugged, coddled, and mistreated in many ways.

Some are "old" at thirty-five or forty. Others do not get "old" until seventy or after. It is not the length of time they live, but the manner in which they live that ages them. Those of least resistance and those of greatest offense against the laws of life age first. *Flesh that should be as fresh as that of a child is soon hardened and its functional powers impaired.* The process of aging goes on gradually, almost imperceptibly. Little change should occur in man's body after maturity is reached. If he should forget his age at thirty, he should have no difficulty at seventy or a hundred in convincing those who know him that he is only thirty. *It is a sad commentary upon our mode of life that at twenty-five he cannot convince those who know him that he is not thirty or thirty-five.*

If man conserved his energies instead of wasting them in riotous dissipations, if he maintained a serene and poised mental attitude, if he did not poison his body and over load it with food, if he ate properly and lived as he should, he would retain the youth-

ful condition of his tissues to an advanced old age
and escape the many pains and aches he now suffers.
MAN'S LIFE SHOULD BE BUILT ON THE CON-
SERVATION OF ENERGY, NOT ITS DISSIPA-
TION.

Peter Maffin's History of India contains an account
of Numside Cogna who died in 1566 at the age of
three hundred and seventy years. His teeth, beard
and hair were renewed four different times. A historian tells us that Belour MacCraine lived 170 years
in one house. The records of St. Leonard's Church,
London, show that Thomas Carn was born Jan. 25th,
1588, and died in 1795. He was therefore, 207 years
old. Kentigern, founder of the Cathedral of Glas-
gow, died at the age of 185. A Russian soldier died
in 1825 at the youthful age of 202. Don Juan Sa-
veire de Lima died in 1730 at the age of 198. A Hun-
garian whose name was Brown died in 1750 at the
age of 172 leaving a widow 164 and a son 115. Drak-
enburg, "The Old Man of the North," was born in
Norway in 1624 and died in 1770 at the age of 146.
He was a sailor for 91 years and was married the
first time at the age of 111. His first wife was sixty
years old. After her death, when he had attained
the safe age of 130, he proposed to a young girl of
sixteen summers and was rejected. Either he possessed but little wealth or the girl thought he had
started out to beat Methusleah's record.

Some of these ages are questioned, but there seems
to be no room for doubt about part of them. One
peculiar thing about many of these old men is the
way in which life seems to get a *"second wind."* A
third set of teeth is sometimes grown. The hair comes
out anew, and, it is said, the wrinkles in the skin
sometimes disappear.

In the spring of 1923 I had an apartment in the
home of an old Civil War veteran. He was 85 years
old and had grown grand-children, I had known him
over fifteen years. All except the sides and back of

his head had been as slick as a peeled onion since long before I first knew him. He had to wear glasses for many years. His hearing was bad. One had to shout in his ears. At the age of 85 he grew a nice crop of hair on top of his head. It was not gray hair either. His sight became so good that he discarded his glasses and daily read his newspaper without them. His hearing did not improve. When I left Texas that year, the old man was still hale and hearty and was working with more vigor than many of less age. Such examples point to possibilities that we will realize when we evolve a real knowledge and self control.

PART V.

HABITS THAT KILL

Man is very largely a creature of habit. He forms bad habits as easily and readily as he forms good ones. He finds the bad habits just as difficult to break as the good ones. For untold ages man has had the habit of forming bad habits; and as civilization grew more complex and opportunities became greater, man's bad habits multiplied. Bad habits are numerous and are shortening the lives of every one today.

In this article I propose to treat of bad mental habits. I am not going to write an article on psychology or metaphysics. I shall leave the first of these to the libertines and the latter to the speculators. I propose only to deal with what is known and not what is often said.

Happiness is man's normal state. Blue-law advocates who seek to have their vinegar ideas incorporated into law, seem to think that virtue means joylessness and its reward a crown of thorns. The adoption of their program would soon convert a fertile continent into a barren wasteland.

Joy and happiness are essential to health. There are few hygienic influences that are equally as conducive to health and long life as a cheerful, equitable state of mind. Cheer is to the body what the sunshine and dew are to the grasses and flowers. It promotes digestion, paints the cheeks, puts a bright sparkle into the eyes and lends a bouyancy and elasticity to one's tread. Any mental state that does not promote cheer, that puts a harshness into one's words and expressions, that blanches one's cheeks and dulls the natural sparkle of the eyes, exerts a depressing effect upon every function of the body and plays havoc with all the forces of life.

It does one little good to eat a perfect diet, if his mental state is such as to impair and prevent digestion. Gloominess and grouchiness lead to an early grave. Happiness, contentment and cheer should be cultivated with as much care and persistency as the gardener exercises in the cultivation of his plants.

The destructive effects upon the body of certain states of mind are as interesting as they are evident. The effect is often like an electric shock altering the feelings, deranging the body's functions, and affecting the individual's sanity as certainly as alcohol or opium.

Many people, particularly women, have a very bad habit of allowing their emotions to run away with them. Indeed, they seem to derive a kind of false pleasure out of the sham emotions which they purposely work up. A sham emotion is an impulse or sensation which is cultivated for its own sake. It is not intended to be translated into actions.

Anne Payson Call said of these: "Sham emotions torture, whether they be of love, religion, or liquor. Emotional excess is a woman's form of drunkenness. Nervous prostration is her delirium tremens." She made that statement over twenty-five years ago, before the ladies had acquired the other form of drunkenness.

Emotionalism is, indeed, a variety of intoxication, or, perhaps it is more correctly described as hysteria. It is the "rose pink sentimentalism" which Carlyle so abhorred as "the second power of a lie, the tissue of deceit that has never been and never can be woven into action."

Emotions or sensations should normally be translated into action. If they are cultivated for their own sake, with no purpose beyond this, they weaken and destroy both the mind and body. Intense emotions and sentimentalism work in much the same way as liquor, and have very much the same evil results.

Religious emotions, often used as a source of pleasurable thrills, are very destructive to the nervous system. They have resulted in insanity in many instances. Any religion which leads to emotionalism, hysteria, trance, catalepsy, etc., is not religion, but mania. St. Paul admonished all Christians to exercise the "spirit of a sound mind."

I once listened to a nationally known leader in new thought circles lecture on emotional drunkenness. This lady advocated going to emotional excess, saying: "It is necessary that we go to excess before we can be satisfied, and we must be satisfied with one plane of being before we can go on to the next." This doctrine is not calculated to build strong minds, bodies and characters, and does not do so among its advocates.

Self-control is the great law of mental hygiene, and he who has not learned to control his emotions is permitting these to cut short his life. Bear in mind that sham emotions, whether of art, music, love, or of some other nature, are as weakening as religious emotions.

Fear is the most destructive of all emotions. It benumbs and paralizes the body and wastes nerve energy as few other things do. It has often been the cause of sudden death in weak individuals. There is a striking similarity between great fear and freezing. In both cases the face is blanched, the teeth chatter, the body trembles (shivers), becomes cramped and bent, the chest in contracted, breathing is slow and comes in short gasps.

Fear greatly affects the heart. In one case of death of an animal, through fear, witnessed by me, the heart was ruptured.

The stomach ceases to function under fear. Dr. Cannon, noted investigator of the physiology and pathology of digestion, was once watching the movements of the intestines of a cat by means of the X-ray. One day during the course of his observations a dog barked near the laboratory, frightening the cat. The cat's intestines immediately became rigid and immobile, forcing him to discontinue his experiment for several hours. Fear had caused the rythmic muscular motions of the cat's intestines to cease altogether. Many experiments have shown that these same influences interfere with and impair the functions of the glands that secrete the digestive juices. Note the dryness of the mouth, because of suspended salivary secretion, in fear.

Not only are the muscles and glands involved in digestion impaired by fear, but the muscles and glands of the whole body are impaired. Human beings, due to their more highly organized nervous systems, are more quickly and more profoundly affected by emotions than are cats or other animals, and the results are more far reaching.

As another example of the effects of fear upon the secretion, there is the well known graying of the hair in those who have been profoundly shocked through fear or by some great horror. Men sentenced to death often become gray haired in a few days. I saw young men go to France with hair as black as graphite and return a few months later as gray haired as aged men. This loss of color by the hair is due to the suspension of the secretion of minute glands at the roots of the hair. Fear caused the suspension. Fear often results in a sudden and involuntary discharge of the contents of the bowels and bladder. Apprehension causes frequent urination and often produces a diarrhea.

There are many things people fear—death, the "hereafter" the "end of the world," poverty, the dark and a thousand and one things. It makes no difference in the results of fear, however, what one fears.

Worry is a baby fear. It impairs secretion and excretion and depresses all the functions of the body. The secretions are altered and nutrition is impaired. Poisons accumulate in the body. The victim gradually wastes away. None of the functions of the body are carried on properly under such a state of mind. The appetite is impaired and digestion is weakened.

Every time there is a panic in the stock market the stock brokers rush to their physicians to be cured of constipation or of a functional glycosuria (sugar in the urine.)

More often than otherwise things over which people worry are trivial and unimportant. Often too, they worry over things they think are coming, troubles that are just ahead, or losses they are about to sustain. Usually they derive all the misery and unhappiness out of these things they can before hand, then the thing they feared does not materialize. They do not have the trouble they anticipated, do not sustain the loss they so much dreaded. If the trouble does come, the misery they have suffered while anticipating it does not help them to bear up under it. On the contrary it lessens their power to meet and overcome the ''necessary evils'' of life; but multiplies them, while weakening one's talents and energies and preventing him from accomplishing his best mental and physical work.

Some years ago a prominent hygienist recounted an experiment which he performed while he was a medical student at Columbia University. In a large room several healthy dogs were confined. One of these was placed in a large open cage in the center of the room, while three of four others were permitted to wander about the room at will. The dog confined to the cage whined and worried and made every effort to get out to his friends. After several days, careful analytical tests were made. These revealed that the loose dogs remained in good health, but the dog in the cage developed, among other things, a well marked case of glycosuria—sugar in the urine. Numerous repetitions of this test, always with the same result, eliminated the possibility of error.

The reader will see in this experiment and its results, the power of worry to impair those functions of the body that are concerned in the preparation of sugar for utilization. Numerous tests have revealed that it will do the same thing in human beings, only much more quickly. Life insurance examiners often make two or three urine tests when glycosuria is found, for they know that this condition may be due to fear, worry, anxiety, excitement, etc. If worry becomes habitual or chronic, then permanent impairment of these functions follow.

Sugar often appears in the urine during emotional states, nervous excitement or following a profound shock. Even so slight a nervous strain as accompanies the taking of an examination in school or college may cause sugar to appear in the urine. It may also cause diarrhea and frequent urination and loss of appetite.

Many sufferers have had their constipation, indigestion and other such troubles "cured" by "New Thought" or "Christian Science," after all other methods of treatment had failed, simply because these removed fear and worry from the sufferer's mind—something the other methods had failed to do—and supplanted them with hope and cheer. Much of the improved health of the last few decades is due to a more hopeful and less fearful religion—to more of hope, faith and love and less of hell, purgatory and fanatical persecutions.

Jealousy is a curious combination of fear, anger and the desire to have and to hold. There is no doubt that it is a strictly natural, normal manifestation and it is met with among the lower animals. It is truly, as Mr. Macfadden has termed it: "the green-eyed guardian of the family honor." It is this so long as it does not dethrone reason and intelligence. If it dethrones these it is a devastating pestilence.

The jealous person is fearful of losing, is angry at the thought of losing, and desires to have and to hold the thing he or she fears is about to be lost. There is, no doubt, a great mixture of wounded vanity and pride in the jealous manifestations. The jealous person usually suffers all the torments of Dante's

Inferno and often causes equally as much suffering to
others.

There is a marked change in the features and coun-
tenance of the jealous person. He rapidly develops
an intense hatred for those he fears, and this, added
to the fear, anger and self-pity already present, forms
a powerful combination of destructive emotions which
impair all the forces and functions of life. It is often
based on imaginary things or on a one-sided view of
life. It tends, when not controlled by reason and intelligence, to greatly magnify every real or imaginary injustice. Mole hills become mountains under
its magic influence. Misery, unhappiness, despair and
even death follow in its wake. Homes are wrecked,
love is destroyed or turned aside, and great injury
often done to innocent victims. Jealousy is truly a
consuming fire.

An old professor once performed some experiments
with the breath of man to determine the influence of
emotions on his functions and excretions. He passed
the breath of a man through a tube cooled with ice
in order to condense its volatile substances. Mingling
with this some iodide of rhodopsin he could produce
no demonstrable precipitate. He then performed a
modification of the experiment. The subject was made
angry and the process repeated. Within five minutes
after the man became angry a brownish precipitate
was produced. The professor concluded that this indicated the presence of a chemical compound occasioned
by the emotion. The compound, when administered
to men and animals, produced stimulation and excitement. The precipitate was then found to differ with
different emotions: extreme sorrow producing a gray
and remorse a pink precipitate.

We hear a lot more about the ductless glands today
than we know about them. However, we do know
something of their functions and of their extreme
importance and we do know that emotions are frequently the cause of their derangements. Anger is

among the emotions that have greatest effect upon these glands.

Someone has called self-pity mental consumption. It is the dry-rot of the soul. We frequently meet whinning, complaining individuals who feel that life has not given them a square deal. Instead of buckling down to hard work and earning the rewards of life, they sit around and feel sorry for themselves. Every such person feels his lot in life is the worst that anyone ever had. I say "feel" advisedly for this class of people seldom think.

The mental state of such "lone-lorn creatures" is difficult to describe, but its effects on the body are readily apparent. They do not regain their health until they are educated out of their self-pity. They do not enjoy life. They do not relish their foods. Everything they eat disagrees with them. Their bowels never function properly. They never sleep well. They are victims of constant introspection. They are continually discovering new symptoms, new pains, new worries. They lead a miserable life, indeed. And their misery is all due to the fact that they feel sorry for themselves and desire that others also feel sorry for them.

Grief is among the mental states that exert the most profound, far-reaching and powerful effects upon the body. Intense grief often kills outright. As in fear, in grief also, the hair has been changed from black to grey in a few days. The secretion of the mother's milk is checked and altered as surely and as quickly by grief as by lack of or by a change of food. Indeed, one of the immediate effects of grief is to reduce and impair secretion and function. Sorrow, as in disappointed love, often produces a wasted, weakened state of the body resembling consumption. Blighted love constitutes one of the most fruitful sources of indisposition.

Grief takes away the appetite instantly. A young girl's sailor sweetheart came into port. She waited a day or two and when he did not come to her nor communicate with her, attempted to drown herself. She was rescued by two sailors and her sweetheart, who had been detained on board ship by duties that had to be performed, was brought to her. He asked her when she had eaten and she replied: "Not since yesterday, Bill, I couldn't."

Grief had impaired or suspended secretion and taken away all desire for food. It would have been punishment to eat under such circumstances. Food consumed under such conditions would have fermented and putrefied and poisoned the body.

A young boy disappeared from home. He left a note telling his mother that she may never see him again. The mother was grief-stricken. Her very life was in danger. Her physician feared that if he did not return or send word of his whereabouts, she would die. Such is the power of grief to influence and impair the processes and functions of the body. It may cause collapse and death.

Secretion and excretion is impaired, elimination is checked, digestion is deranged, nutrition perverted, profound enervation is produced and toxemia grows daily. Weight is lost. Appetite is lacking. Disease and death may easily result.

That mental state we call hurry is also very destructive. You may have searched for something while in a hurry. You couldn't find it. You snapped your fingers, bit your nails, pulled your hair, danced and went through a lot of needless motions and then, later, when you were not in a hurry you easily found the object of your search. By hurry, you wasted both time and energy.

You go down the street in a hurry. At each crossing you are held up by the traffic. Between crossings the crowd annoys you. This all flusters and irritates you. Inwardly you boil. You try to shave in a hurry. You cut your face up and do not shave as quickly as commonly.

Watch the nervous twitching of your fingers and toes when you are in a hurry. Note the tenseness of your body, your restlessness and irritability. Then you will see why it wastes your energy. You will see why you leave out words in the letter you write in a hurry, why your tools slip and ruin the material you are working on or ruin your finger or leg. You will see that hurry cripples efficiency, spoils your work and wastes your life forces. You will then know why you should cultivate poise and learn to be deliberate. Hurry is incompatible with skill and not essential to speed.

Lying, stealing, cheating, gambling and all forms of dishonesty, produce enervation and hardening of the arteries. In all of these there is the fear of being found out. In gambling there is tension and the fear of losing. Before conscience becomes hardened there is the stinging lash of remorse and loss of self-respect.

Emil Coue had his patients hang a string of beads, as a rosary, around their necks, and count these in the old approved fashion while repeating to themselves the various formulas he had devised to favorably affect the minds of the sick. Many did receive some benefit from this kind of child's play, just as many thousands of others had received benefit from similar formulas coined by American metaphysicians in the years that have passed. But the average patient reverses the process. He may not use any beads, but their absence does not hinder his persistency in day by day recounting his symptoms and searching for new ones. He is not usually content, either, to tell them to himself and to the doctor, but pesters the life out of all his friends with a constant review of his troubles, real or imaginary. Often they get into such a habit doing this that they forget to stop when the symptoms are gone.

Now, all this is very depressing to the mind of the one who does the counting as well as to the one who does the listening; and a depressed mind depresses all the functions of the body, thus making the trouble worse than it would otherwise be. By thus constantly depressing your mind you drag yourself downward, and in no possible way does it help you. You should be healthy. If you are not, then reform your mode of living and forget the symptoms. Under healthful living the body will take care of these in as rapid a manner as possible.

Couering your symptoms in this manner is decidedly hurtful. So also is that of counting and dwelling on your troubles. The African Bulu says: "No rat counts his troubles—but his nuts." This is his way of saying that some people consume so much time talking over and counting their troubles that they have no time to enjoy the pleasures of life. They brood over their misfortunes so much that they forget their good fortunes.

The wood rat goes hunting for food in the darkness of night; perhaps it is raining and the wind is blowing strong, or it may be snowing. But the rat, when he returns, does not sit down and say to himself and fellow rats: "Woe is my lot in life. I had a terrible walk tonight in the dark. The wind blew, the rain fell and I could not see my way." Instead, the rat smacks his lips, counts the fruit and nuts he secured and thinks of the feast he is about to have.

Counting your troubles multiplies them. They grow bigger each time you go over them. They seem to increase in number as fast as they increase in size. This depresses the mind and functions of the body and detracts from the higher joys of life in proportion to the seeming magnitude of your troubles. Counting your troubles sours your disposition, confirms your pessimism and causes you to hesitate about answering the question: "Is life worth living?" Health cannot be maintained in this way.

Violent fits of passion will often arrest, alter or derange the functions of the body as quickly as an electric shock. Digestion may be wholly suspended by a profound state of fear, worry, anxiety or suspense. Fright, anxiety or even sudden joy are often immediately followed by diarrhea. Many students who have been exceedingly anxious about their examinations have experienced a diarrhea as a result. These same mental influences have all been observed to cause the appearance of sugar in the urine.

Mental shocks, anger, melancholy and all disagreeable or abnormal mental conditions render the secretions of the body more or less morbid. Anger quickly modifies the bile; grief arrests the secretion of the gastric juices; violent rage makes the saliva poisonous. Fear relaxes the bowels. It is claimed that many mothers have injured, and even killed, their nursing infants by furious emotions, which alter their milk. It is known that such emotions as fear, worry, jealousy, anger, etc., will reduce the secretion of milk and impair its food value to such an extent that the infant does not thrive on it.

These things should serve to emphasize for us the fact that the functions of the body are all under nervous control and make us see that any influence that impairs the nervous system or wastes nerve force will bring on disease and death.

Such mental habits and mental states may be appropriately termed HABITS that KILL, for they do shorten life and often kill quickly. Learn, then to control your emotions. Self-control is the great law of mental hygiene. Cultivate poise, cheer and contentment. Be of good courage. Cast fear and worry aside. Learn to love your fellow men. Be not quick to anger. Dismiss your troubles and think upon the better things of life. By so doing your health will be improved and your life prolonged.

PART VI.

HABITS THAT KILL

An isolated, untutored tribe living a hard simple life has but few bad habits. But civilized man has pushed out into almost every nook and corner of the earth and has not only carried his own bad habits with him but has adopted all the bad habits of each of the tribes with which he has come in contact. He now has many such harmful practices and their combined and cumulative effects are weighing down upon the health and lives of the multitude and gradually crushing them.

It is the constant falling of the little drops of water that wears away the granite boulder. It is the constant falling of the little flakes of snow that stops powerful locomotives and ties up the nation's commerce. So, it is the habitual repetition of injurious practices, however slight the injury resulting from one act may be, that wrecks health and life. No man or woman exists who has only one bad habit. We all have a collection of them. As the combined effects of this collection of bad habits accumulate weakness, disease, premature old age and an untimely death result.

In this chapter it shall be my purpose to discuss the most common "poison habits" and point out their office in shortening life. By the "poison habit" I mean those habits acquired by almost every one, particularly in civilized life, of introducing poisonous substances into the body, largely for certain effects which they learn to like.

To a normal person, the attractiveness of alimentary substances (food and drink) is proportioned to the degree of their healthfulness and their nutritive value. No normal person is ever misled by an innate craving for unwholesome food, nor by any instinctive aversion to wholesome foods. But all normal individuals are possessed of a natural repugnance to poisonous and injurious substances.

The instinctive aversion to any kind of poison can be perverted into an unnatural craving after that poison. Instinct is plastic. If the warnings of the organic instincts are unheeded, and the offending substance is again and again forced upon the body, nature, true to the law of self-preservation, seeks to prolong life by adapting the body to the poison.

All poison habits are progressive. The slave of a poison is conscious of a peculiar craving which is entirely distinct from a healthy appetite; an uncompromising craving for a once repulsive substance, each gratification of which renders it more irresistible. Only natural appetites have natural limitations. An appetite for peaches may be satisfied with strawberries, but an appetite for tobacco can be satisfied only with tobacco.

The seductiveness of every poison habit acquires strength with each indulgence, and that power is proportioned to the original repulsiveness of the poison. The opium habit holds its victims in a stronger grip than the coffee habit. Hashheesh is a more powerful master than tobacco. Tobacco is a more imperious master than tea.

But all these are progressive. The longer they are used the more is required to satisfy. Each indulgence is followed by a depressing reaction. The feeling of exhaustion is also steadily progressive and causes a correspondingly increased craving for a repetition of the stimulating dose, which forces the user either to increase the quanity of the poison used or else resort to a stronger poison. This is why abstinence is easier than "moderation." This is the reason one poison habit often leads to others. This is the reason, too, that one poison habit cannot be broken by substituting another and weaker poison for the ones used, and supplies the reason why "tapering off' on a poison habit is a failure.

About the only bad habit we acquired from the

North American Indian is the tobacco habit. Peyote eating has not found its way among us to any great extent. Quinine we acquired from South America and it is doubtful if the Indian was really responsible for this. Only a part of the North American Indians had tobacco. While the Indian was learning to drink the pale face's "fire water," we who boast of our civilization and contemptuously refer to the Americans as savages learned to use his tobacco. It was like two tramps sharing the same bed; one had cooties and the other had the itch.

Tobacco produces enervation by overstimulation—poisoning. The use of tobacco will cut down one's vitality twenty-five to fifty per cent. In any of its forms, the tobacco habit is a foe to the user. It is a virulent poison—nicotine ranking next to prussic acid in its deadliness—and kills those not accustomed to its use when given in small doeses. Its habitual use plays havoc with the nerves, unsteadying the hand and eye, impairing hearing and reducing efficiency. It stunts growth in the young, impairs digestion and produces "tobacco heart" in adults, and reduces strength and endurance in all. Due to this latter fact, athletes abstain from its use during periods of training for a contest. Repeated tests have shown that the use of tobacco lowers mental efficiency.

There are several ways of employing tobacco such as, chewing, smoking, dipping and snuffing. Much argument has been waged over which of these methods is preferable. Such arguments disregard the primary fact that neither method is desirable, useful, or necessary. However used, the first use is followed in the undepraved organism, by a violent systemic reaction against it. This manifests itself by such symptoms as nausea, vomiting, loss of appetite, diarrhea, dizziness, trembling and weakness of the body and limbs and sometimes prostration. As its use is repeated the reactions against it become progressively less marked, until finally, the organic instincts become so debased that they no longer protest. Rather, what was once abhorred is now called for, and the insistence of the call is in direct ratio to the debasement of the body and its instincts. One is now a willing and obedient slave to Lady Nicotine, just as truly as the opium addict is a slave to Morpheus, and the process of gradually and insidiously undermining the constitution goes steadily on until nature finally collects her debt and the account is closed.

The lining membranes of the mouth, throat and lungs become hardened, thickened and reddened. This hardening, toughening and thickening is the means resorted to to protect against poisons and irritations. It is part of the process of adaptation and really cripples the efficiency of the organs thus thardened. ADAPTATION TO ANY HARMFUL INFLUENCE IS ALWAYS ACCOMPLISHED BY BODY CHANGES THAT ARE AWAY FROM THE IDEAL.

Many absurd explanations have been given for the popular idea that cigarettes are more harmful than pipe or cigar. The true explanation is that they are not. Cigars are made of tobacco just as cigarettes are and have all the harmful effects of tobacco.

Cigarettes are usually inhaled, while the pipe and cigar are usually not inhaled. Cigarette smoke is weaker than cigar smoke, and the lungs learn to tolerate it more easily than they do the stronger smoke. The surface of the lungs is a hundred times greater than the surface of the mouth and their linings are much thinner. The nicotine of the cigarette is, therefore, absorbed in greater quantities than that of the cigar. Owing to their weakness and the habit of inhaling their smoke, cigarettes introduces more poison into the body than cigars or the pipe. Because they are inhaled, they also irritate the lungs more. The greater harm is not in the cigarette but in the manner of smoking.

Many, learning his, give up the cigarette and adopt

the pipe or cigar. Little is gained by this. The sensible method is to give up all forms of tobacco using. One can learn to inhale pipe or cigar smoke, and it is not possible to avoid inhaling some of it, even if one does not try to inhale it. As their use continues and the user grows more careless, more will be inhaled, perhaps unconsciously, but inhaled none the less. If we grant that owing to the manner of smoking them they are less harmful than the cigarette, we do not thereby rob them of their harmfulness. We should avoid all harmful practices, not just part of them.

Many have the vulgar habit of smoking in the house. The walls, curtains, rugs, carpets, bedding, closets, etc., become saturated with tobacco poisoning and those who live in the house, the wife or mother, the children, are forced to breathe day and night, air laden with tobacco. Their health suffers as a result.

Alcohol is a strong poison and its use in any form is inimical to the human body as, indeed, it is to every organized thing in existence. It is a product of the decay of organic matter occasioned by bacterial action. Only a small percentage of it is required to arrest the action of the bacteria themselves. It is for this reason that it is employed as a preservative.

Whether ardent spirits, malt liquors, wines, cider or other alcoholic drinks are used, the alcohol they contain is poisonous. In small doses it acts as a *stimulant*, in larger doses its effects are those of a *depressant*. It is highly irritating to every organ and tissue of the body and there is not one of them that is immune to its destructive influence. It coagulates the protoplasm of the cells of the body, just as it coagulates, or cooks, the white of an egg. This coagulation impairs and destroys the cells.

The normal cells are then replaced by a substitute of connective tissue cells forming what is called "scar tissue." This may occur in the brain and spinal cord resulting in paresis, paralysis, insanity and other nervous diseases; in the liver producing sclerosis and ascites; in the heart and arteries producing hardening and other troubles in these; or it it may occur in the lungs, kidneys, muscles or any other organ of the body. The functioning powers of these organs are gradually destroyed and the individual's resistance to other disease influences is lowered. The death rate and case rate in pneumonia is much higher in alcohol addicts than among abstainers.

"Moderate" drinkers are not immune to these effects. They receive their full share of them. In fact, the habitual "moderate" drinker receives more injury from alcohol than the occasional drinker who gets drunk when he does drink. It is used as a stimulant to digestion, but finally wrecks digestion.

Men slightly under the influence of alcohol are claimed to be able to do more work than when not under its influence but they do not do it as well. Mind, hand and eye are not so accurate, under alcoholic stimulation as when sober. All functional stimulation deteriorates the functional results. Stimulation never assists the body in the performance of its functions. For instance certain things stimulate milk production, but the milk is of poor quality. Condiments stimulate the flow of digestive juices, but the juices are poor and ineffective.

Tea, coffee, cocoa and chocolate shall all be considered together because they all contain very much the same active principles and have very much the same effects. Neither of them have the silghtest excuse for existences as beverages. Tea and coffee contain no food value, while the unaltered flavors of all of them are obnoxious to every unperverted taste. Coca Cola which contains caffine might also be included in this list.

They act primarily as stimulants and secondarily as depressants, or sedatives. Like tobacco, opium, and alcohol they are habit forming, and they are habit forming to exactly the degree in which they are stimulating. And they are stimulating in the degree to which they are poisonous and unfitted for the real needs of the body. The bitter, nauseous tastes of all these substances require the addition of sugar or other substances before they can be used by the undepraved taste.

Dean Henry H. Rusby, of the Columbia College of Pharmacy thinks that alcohol is unjustly famous as a stimulant while coffee is insufficiently praised. He says alcohol is a depressant while tea and coffee are truly stimulating and enable the user to work beyond his normal strength. He admits, however, that one must pay the penalty for the use of these drugs and for the loss of sleep they cause.

It is the curse of all stimulants that they enable one to work beyond his normal strength. That is, they enable him to keep on working long after nature has called for rest. They do this, not by adding to the powers of the body, but by calling out the powers held in reserve. They act in the same way a spur does on a tired horse. Slowly, but surely, the reserve powers of the body are consumed under the influence of stimulants and physical bankruptcy follows. Coffee, tea, coca cola, cocoa and chocolate, because of their almost universal use, are great offenders in this respect. They produce ENERVATION and sleeplessness in proportion to their use. Those who use them become coffee and tea or cocoa inebriates. They are addicts as truly as the opium user. The habitual user of tea or coffee is tired, listless, irritable and suffers with headache and other discomforts when deprived of his habitual cup. Nervous diseases result from the employment of such nervines.

Give a stimulant to a man of full-resistance and he reacts to it with increased activity and an increased feeling of well-being. When the period of increased activity ends there sets in, due to the excessive expenditure of energy and substance, a period of depression. Rest soon restores full health.

All stimulation is followed by a period of depression equal in duration and intensity to the period of stimulation. Keep up this stimulation by habitual repetition and renewal of nerve energy fags. A permanent depression—a profound enervation—which forms the foundation for the development of any disease of the nosology, follows. There is a slowing down of the functions of the body. The processes of nutrition and elimination fail to meet physiological needs.

Stimulants stand at the head of the many causes of excessive expenditure of nervous energy. The increased feeling of strength which follows their use is due to the expenditure of power which they occasion and not to any power which they add. We are conscious of power only in its expenditure. A pure or uncompensated stimulant is any agent or influence that occasions or induces an increase in the activities of the body or any of its organs without supplying any real need of the body. All such stimulants should be avoided.

There are many very popular drug habits. Thousands daily take a purgative or a laxative to induce bowel action. Many thousands more employ drugs to aid digestion, or to brace up their nerves, or to tone up their system, or purify their blood. Many use patent medicines, others use proprietary remedies or their physician's prescriptions. The patent medicines are almost, if not quite, as bad as those prescribed by the physician and should be avoided along with the rest.

There never was a drug or drug remedy that had any business in the human body.

Speaking generally, drugs either destroy more or less of the tissues of the body or they occacsion a needless and wasteful expenditure of its vital energies. Most of them do both these things. Their effects upon the system are not altered, because they are prescribed by a physician. It makes no difference once the drug is in the system who prescribed it; the effects are the same.

I shall pass over the opium, morphine, heroin and such debasing drug habits—not because they are unimportant, but because no one doubts their destructive offices—and shall pass to more common drug habits that are supposed by many to be beneficial. Among these is the use of headache "remedies."

The habit of taking headache "remedies" is becoming a national pastime. The average person, apparently, suffers from frequent headaches, and, judging by the readiness with which they resort to the "remedies" they fear a few minutes of slight pain more than the deadly drug they introduce into their system.

They do not realize what a terrible price they pay for this short respite from pain and for the restless stupor, miscalled sleep, which they secure through hypnotic or narcotic drugs. Deadening sensation does not cure disease; pain is never cured by deadening the nerves. Cause is never corrected in such manner. The reader should know that there is no cure outside of correction of cause.

Every dose of such drugs lessens nerve force and thereby impairs the various functions of the body. When nerve force is lessened there is always necessarily a checking of elimination resulting in a retention within the body of its waste products. And these produce disease and death. Every headache "remedy" interferes with elimination, and thus perpetuates the condition for which it is given. They are also habit forming, and many of them have a very deleterious influence upon the heart and other organs.

Anything that "relieves" pain without correcting its cause does so by diminishing the power of the nerves to *feel*. It is the part of wisdom to find out what is causing the trouble and correct this.

Acetanilid is the chief ingredient in most of the

headache powders. Every year many cases of acetanilid poisoning are reported which result from the use of these powders. People buy them regularly and carry them with them wherever they go. It is easier to dope their nerves into insensibility when they have a headache than to live properly and avoid the suffering.

Acetanilid, like coffee, often produces the headache for which it is given. A person begins the use of the drug when he has a headache due to other causes. Nature ultimately overcomes the other causes when the headache should cease. But it does not. He now has a headache due to acetanilid. The headache can be permanently cured only by discontinuing the use of the drug.

Coffee users who miss their coffee have a headache. A cup of coffee "cures" the ache caused by the use of coffee. Tobacco unsteadies the nerves. A smoke or chew temporarily steadies them again. Like them, acetanilid "cures" the trouble it produces, only to make the trouble worse than ever.

Aspirin is commonly bought and used as a headache remedy. It is a dangerous drug which cripples brain, nerves and heart.

Bromo-seltzer, a powerful drug, which is freely dispensed from soda-fountains is a popular remedy for headache. A teaspoonful of the drug contains about seven grains of bromid. Half an ounce is usually taken at a drink. In such a drink one takes about twenty-four grains of bromid, ten grains of acetanilid and about three grains of caffeine—the poisonous principle of coffee. Several such drinks are often taken daily. Caffeine (coffee) and acetanilid have been discussed.

Bromid is a powerful drug. It is employed extensively in nervous diseases. It depresses the great vital centers of the medulla weakening and slowing respiration, slowing and weakening heart action and depressing the spinal centers. It is employed to "kill" pain and produce sleep (stupor). It never cures anything—isn't given with any idea that it will cure. It is a twentieth century express to insanity.

Cases of loss of memory of words, of direction, location, etc., are frequently reported in the public press. Such cases are growing more common, even among the young. The reports usually run about like this: "Of slightly nervous temperament and had not been well for some time." The rest is easy. The great remedy for nervousness is Bromid. Keep sandbagging the brain centers with this drug for a while and almost any mental trouble is possible. Of course, other nerve and brain paralyzing drugs may do the same thing.

Bromid is commonly employed in epilepsy. Skin eruptions (Brom-acne) frequently results from this. The pustular variety of Bromid eruptions is most common. Discolored patches of irregular sizes and shapes and solid elevations of the skin ranging from the size of a pin head to larger than a pea frequently result from the use of bromid. In children, small reddish-brown nodes grow, fungus like, upon the skin as a result of the use of this powerful drug.

The coal-tar products have come into general use and are taking their yearly toll. These include creosote, phenacetin, antikamnia, antipyrin, and acetanilid. They are used as sedatives, pain killers, sleep (stupor) producers, and for reducing body temperature. They are popular in "nervous" headache, neuralgia, ataxia pains, gout, rheumatism and in certain female disorders.

One of their actions is to reduce the alkilinity of the blood and the number of red blood corpuscles. They depress all the vital functions and have a special tendency to produce heart failure. Their effects upon the nervous system are often terrible. Among the symptoms of coal-tar poisoning are listed despondency and loss of memory, nervousness, neuresthenia, paralysis and insanity. Our insane asylums are growing larger and more densely populated each year as the result of the use of these and other such drugs.

The cathartic habit is a growing menace. Cathartics, purgatives, laxatives, etc., are in frequent use. These produce their effects by their power to irritate the stomach, intestines and bowels. Due to this irritation they derange digestion and impair the functions of the whole alimentary canal. They produce and intensify constipation. They weaken the bowels. If their use is continued, atrophy and "falling" of the bowels and perhaps of the stomach and intestines results. They correct nothing, but cause much trouble.

Cosmetics contain various poisonous substances. Deaths and other serious troubles from lead poisoning have occured from using powders containing lead. Hair dyes, shampoos, skin bleeches, and other toilet preparations contain poisons that are absorbed to weaken and kill the cells, often they kill the whole body. Many are poisoned by poisons used in preparing and dyeing furs, etc.

The candy habit is rapidly supplanting the alcohol habit since the enactment of the Volstead joke. The fact that candy can be made to take the place of booze should cause thoughtful people to take notice. Candy is a highly concentrated form of energy and acts as a powerful stimulant. It has a strong affinity for water and creates an abnormal thirst. It possesses a "desire" for oxygen and robs the tissues of part of the oxygen, taken into the body. It is a denatured product, and when taken, leeches the blood and tissues of part of their salts. The candy habit "grows" on one, like the cigarette habit and is, in my opinion worse than the latter.

The shoe polish, floor polish, varnish, coal-tar dyes, flavors, preservatives, etc., that are contained in candy, cold drinks, "beverages," canned goods, sulphured (dried) fruits, etc., are frequently poisonous and many are being harmed by them today.

The yeast fad is harming many more. Yeast is a ferment. When taken by those with impaired digestion, and these are the ones who are using it, it converts the stomach into a gas tank. It sets up fermentation producing alcohol and carbon dioxide. At first, this produces better bowel action and the alcoholic stimulation makes one feel better. Ultimately, bowel action is made worse and alcoholic poisoning becomes apparent.

Excuses, not reasons, for the use of all these things can easily be found. In fact, I doubt if there was ever a period in history when more excuses for evil doing were advanced than today. It is a mark of "broadmindedness" and of "intelligence" to do these things. One is a "narrow" bigot or Babbit if he does not. One is only exercising his personal liberty in committing slow suicide by such means. Personal Liberty! What crimes are aften committed in thy name!

PART VII.

HABITS THAT KILL

Dr. P. Le Comte du Nouy, assistant to Dr. Alexis Carrell, of the Rockefeller Institute, stated, when embarking for Europe a few years ago:

"I am taking with me the secret of eternal life. It is this: Bathe and feed the cells daily."

This was the "secret" revealed by all the experiments that have been performed on living tissues taken from animals and man. But this secret only reveals the immedite cause of the death of the cells of the body, POISONING and STARVATION. The remote causes of death, that is, those causes that impair nutrition and drainage through lessening organic efficiency, are not revealed by these experiments and are not contained in this *secret*. The "scientists" of the laboratory and test-tube do not seem to be aware of the existence of these remote causes. *Living is left out of the formula.*

They must come back to the old proposition that *"the wages of sin is death,"* that *"when sin is finished it brings death,"* that *"death by sin passed upon all men,* for ALL HAVE SINNED AND COME SHORT OF THE GLORY OF GOD." I am not a preacher. But I am certain that through our habitual transgressions of the laws of life we all fall far short of the fullness of life for which we are designed. I recall that sin is defined as the "TRANSGRESSION OF THE LAW." Our habitual transgressions of the laws of life impair the processes of nutrition and drainage and thus shorten our lives and fill them with aches, pains and weaknesses. For this reason "man shall not live by bread (food) alone, but by every word (law) that comes out of the mouth of God."

Only a perfect and unceasing obedience to the laws of life will enable the processes of nutrition, drainage and elimination, in the human body, to perform their work so fully and perfectly, and continue to do so, that one may expect to live for an indefinite period, as do the tissues of animals in the test tubes of the biologists. This must begin at birth, or before, and will require not only healthy, vigorous, intelligent and well informed parents, who themselves live in harmony with life's laws and who train the child to do likewise, but will also require a better environment than most of us grow up under. A complete overhauling of our social and economic structure as well as a complete revolution in our mode of living will be necessary before the highest results can be looked for.

Man is adapted to his natural environment. He possesses a great power of resistance. He weakens his resistance by certain habits that have a debilitating effect upon him. Those who possess strong resistance may so weaken it that they fall easy prey to any unfavorable influence in their environment. Weather changes that have no appreciable effect upon the robust and strong occasion all manners of disagreeable symptoms and increase the severity of already existing ones in the sick and those of low resistance. The normal body, if not abused, is capable of adjusting itself to all ordinary conditions of nature. The author of nature did not intend that man, any more than the lower animals, should be the helpless victims of his native environment. That delicacy which like the hot house plant, is injured by every breath of air; and that rottenness of constitution which is the effect of indolence, intemperance and debauchery was never intended by the Author of Nature, and lays the foundation for numerous diseases and premature death.

In the early part of 1925 there was an eclipse of the sun. The astronomers figured out for us not only the day on which the eclipse would occur, but the very hour, minute and second. They told us just where the eclipse would be total and where not, even giving us accurate maps of the path of total eclipse. Here in New York City they told us that if we desired to view the total eclipse we would have to go above 110th Street. Those who did not go above that street did not see the total eclipse.

The astronomers could do all this because they knew that neither earth, moon nor sun would or could turn aside in their courses or vary from their path of travel. They knew that the movements of these heavenly bodies are governed by fixed and unerring law and that they could not violate the laws governing them. We know the same of chemistry, mathematics, etc.

Some have developed the idea that life is not subject to fixed and inexorable law; that it is governed by chance and haphazard. This is not so. The laws of life cannot be violated with impunity. Despite the growing tendency to doubt it, this is a moral universe. The world and all that herein is, is founded on laws as certain and inflexible as the law of gravitation. We must live by these laws or be killed by our infractions of them.

Through many infractions of the laws of being man dissipates his precious energies and undermines the processes and functions of life. One of the choicest means of expending energy is through excesses of various kinds.

All excess is harmful. Excess means over-indulgence in the normal or wholesome things of life. The word excess is not correctly applied when used in reference to tobacco, opium, alcohol, etc., for this would imply that the use of these up to a certain point is normal and wholesome. Excess is more than the needs of the mind and body. It cannot be said that anything over the normal needs of the mind and body for tobacco, alcohol, etc., is excess for, the mind and body have no normal needs for these things. Their use in any quantity is simply an unmitigated evil.

The human body is very largely a self-regulating organism. It is so constructed and arranged that if excessive demands are made upon it during youth and middle age, provisions for supplying these demands are made, so that there seems to be no injury done to the body. No generally recognized sign is given that the demands upon the body's forces are in excess and that its reserve fund is being slowly consumed. The greater the demands made upon the forces of life, apparently the greater the supply. However, no truth is more certain than that expressed by Sylvester Graham when he declared that: "An intensive life is not compatable with an extensive life."

The old song admirably expressed this fact in the words: "We never miss the water 'till the well runs dry." Solomon expressed it thusly: "Because sentence against an evil work is not executed speedily it is therefore fully written in the hearts of men to do evil."

Men are deceived by appearances. Because they are not knocked down every time they do a thing they refuse to believe it injures them. Because some one else has practiced a certain vice for a number of years without apparent harm, they conclude they can do likewise.

I recall a friend who died a few years ago. He was a young man—about 30 years of age. A man of large build and powerful frame and as full of energy as a freshly charged battery. But day and night he wasted his forces. No man I ever knew was more wasteful of his energies, and yet he was apparently unharmed. Then his trouble came on with apparent suddenness. He slowly wasted away for about nine months. His splendid reserve had been eaten away and his powers of recuperation were apparently unable to replenish it. Perhaps recuperation would have taken place if he had given up his wasteful indulgences and his physician had not added drug stimulation to these. But he was a slave to his indulgences and was unable or unwilling to free himself.

What is called overwork is excess. We work or play until we grow tired. If we do not stop and rest we soon become so tired we cannot continue. Nature has wisely arranged that under ordinary circumstances we cannot use up all the energy we possess. She holds back a reserve fund for emergencies. If we always rest when tired, there will always be a surplus of reserve energy to be used under stress or to maintain good health.

When nature demands rest it is the custom to give her a stimulant. Overwork is really overstimulation. Fatigue is a demand for rest just as thirst is a call for water and hunger is a demand for food. Stimulants of all kinds overwork the organs of the body, prevent sleep and enable us to go on with our work long after nature has hung out her fatigue sign.

Those who disregard nature's calls for rest, and go on in spite of it, are overworked. Ambition, the desire for fame, place, power and pelf, drives many to overstep the limits of fatigue and wreck their health in the pursuit of these baubles. The pursuit of happiness, or as it is practiced, the pursuit of thrills and excitement, overworks many more. Economic necessity goads many others onward into overwork. In any case, overwork is the result of forcing oneself to work when nature calls for rest, or, to put it differently, it is failure to secure sufficient rest and sleep to completely recuperate from one's daily activities.

An excellent example of the evils of overwork was supplied us by the recent example of Miss Gertrude Ederle, the first woman to swim the English channel. When she arrived in New York City the hero worshipers met her and cheered and marched and acted, in general, like hysterical savages, in her ''honor.'' They prevented her from sleeping all night. She was in a night club until far into the morning, dancing, eating, perhaps drinking, and being ''honored.'' For two days or more the yapping mob did not permit her to relax or sleep. She collapsed and was ordered to bed and callers barred from her room.

Two days later, while attending another boisterous

"celebration" in her "honor" she collapsed again. Wan and pale, with bloodless lips, dark lines under her eyes and a look of fatigue on her face, she had gone to the party to engage in its dizzy excitement. She is also said to have been under great emotional strain—joy, gratitude to the doting hero worshipers —for several days.

She was an athlete of ability. She possessed great physical strength and endurance, but the strongest give down before such abuse of body and mind. There are no iron constitutions. You may think yours is such, but you will learn, perhaps when you are beyond repair, that it is not.

Another form of overwork is that of keeping the body or parts of it tense at all times. To be constantly tensed in body and perhaps in mind as well, constitutes a ceaseless drain upon your nervous energies, and is often largely responsible for the troubles for which people run to doctors. Many people are so tense and nervous that they do not fully relax when they go to sleep. It prevents them from falling asleep quickly and prevents sound restful sleep when they do fall asleep. As a consequence they do not awake refreshed in the morning. The tensed person is always tired and exhausted.

The blood does not circulate freely through tensed muscles, the processes of tissue repair are impaired, waste matter is not carried away as rapidly as it should be and enfeebled health is the final result. When Paavo Nurmi was in New York City for two races on the same day in 1925 he lay stretched out on a table in peaceful sleep between the races. He was fully relaxed and therefore fully resting. In the same room the American athletes were excitedly jabbering and getting their rub downs. They were in a state of tension and were not really resting. They attempted to substitute the rub down for rest.

America is a busy world. We are always rushing, hustling, trying to get somewhere before we get started. This constant state of tension constitutes a terrible drain upon our nervous energies. Conservation is the secret of power. Relaxation is the means of conservation. Tension is a waste of power. It drains away your reserve. Your reserve gone you collapse just when it is most important that you hold up. Learn to relax—LET GO.

Another favorite form of excess is that of overeating. This is an almost universal practice. It usually begins in infancy when children, due to the ignorance of doctors, nurses and mothers, are fed too much and too often. As the child grows older the almost continuous eating is kept up. An imperious appetite is thus built up out of the early perversion of normal hunger and only rarely does anyone ever escape from its grip.

Eating beyond physiological requirements is a most prolific source of weakness, disease and premature death. Those who preach and practice the belly's doctrine of three squares plus and go by your appetite are always ailing. Man must acquire moderation in eating.

Overeating is a form of overwork. It overworks the entire digestive system in the effort to digest it. It overworks the eliminating organs which must dispose of the surplus nutriment. The heart is overworked in forcing excess nutriment through the body. The glands of the body are overworked in trying to make secretions equal the demands made upon them by the excess food.

That man or woman who habitually eats beyond digestive capacity sooner or later wrecks his or her digestion and is poisoned by the many powerful toxins that form in the digestive tract from the fermenting, putrefying mass of undigested food. More people are killed by feasting than by famine.

People do not seem to be satisfied to supply the normal demands of their system for food. Rather, they resort to condiments and dressings of various kinds to stimulate their appetite and enable them to eat more. A soldier once wrote home from India of his fellow English soldiers stationed there. "They eat and drink and drink and eat, and they write home that it was the climate that killed them."

If you are not hungry it is a crime against your body to eat. It is a crime against your own best physical, mental and moral interests for you to stimulate a false appetite by means of condiments, tasty dishes, etc. Alcohol, condiments, bitters, tonics, etc., all conduce to overeating and they one and all retard digestion. Absolutely no good comes of their use. Indeed, their continued use deranges digestion, destroys the ability to relish plain foods and leads to troubles too numerous to mention. Those who desire real health, health that can be depended on in emergencies, will avoid all spurs to appetite and eat only when truly hungry. If you cannot enjoy good food without the addition of salt or pepper or some other equally harmful and equally worthless "relish" wait until you can before eating.

Sexual excesses constitute a very common and very prolific source of disease, degeneracy and death. These may take any form from self-abuse to sodomy and other perversions. They may be practiced either within or without the pale of marriage and by both young and old alike. Both sexes, but particularly the male sex, are prone to these excesses.

What constitutes excess? The reply has been given: Anything is excess when procreation is not the end. Is this answer correct? It is true that in a state of pure, unperverted nature this is the invariable rule. Is it excess when used for other purposes? Yes, if our definition of excess is a correct one.

This answer would limit sex relations to the married and confine them to but few relations during life. I do not expect this answer to be regarded seriously by my readers. They will not be so restricted. Every animal possesses a sexual reserve for emergencies. It will not produce harm if this reserve is not over stepped. How far will this permit them to indulge! This I cannot answer. I can only advise extreme moderation.

The intensest pleasures are the costliest. Man should fight against the tyranny of pleasure. Plato, Spinoza, Descartes, Leibnitz, Kant, Berkeley, Hume, Hobbes, Spencer, Newton are but a few of the great thinkers who flourished on a Shaker system. And look at the ages of them! On the other side, as early victims of the "standard of pleasure" are Burns, Byron, Maupassant, Murger, Mirabeau and others. Epicurus advised men to eat moderately, exercise much and have nothing to do with women. It is suggested that his advice to women would probably have been the same.

Man is sexually perverted. He is the only animal that has his "social problem," the only animal that supports prostitution, the only animal that practices self-abuse, the only animal that is demoralized by all forms of sexual perversion, the only animal whose males will attack the females, the only animals where the desire of the female is not the law, the only one that does not exercise his sexual powers in harmony with their primitive constitution. This animal is driven by his perversions in all his sexual relations.

Even his and her so-called love life is based upon sexual perversion. Making love, or as it is now commonly called, "petting," is simply a means of arousing the sexual powers and passions. The petting, fondling, hugging, kissing, etc., that accompanies this orgy of animalism cheapens love, renders love almost impossible and keeps the purely animal powers ever active. The cultivation of sex thrills for their own sake, even when no sexual relations follow, constitutes a terrible drain upon the powers of life. It matters not whether this is indulged in within or without the pale of marriage.

In these days of promiscuous and unrestrained petting, it is no longer a secret that both sexes may, and frequently do, reach a sexual climax through petting alone. This is one reason for the great popularity of this form of masturbation.

"Petting," "spooning," "sparking" or "love making" as we call this manifestation is natural and serves a definite end. It is common to man and animals alike and in both serves the definite purpose of arousing the sexual energies and desires, and preparing the sexes for the function of procreation. It is this fact that makes it dangerous for young people who are frequently swept, by the almost uncontrolable desires thus aroused, into greater mistakes.

Custom sanctifies (?) petting orgies in married life but this does not deprive it of its enervating effects. Young men and women today openly indulge in this form of self-abuse and honest and sincere men and women defend the practice. It is unfortunate that a man may be both honest and sincere and at the same time be as ignorant as a child. When petting is not to serve its primitive purpose it should be avoided. This the pervert, man (both sexes), will not do, however. And in most cases, to caution moderation is simply waste of time. This habit, like all other habits grows on one and holds one in its vice-like grip.

Within recent years there has grown up a crop of writers on sex who have visited the reservations and brought back with them all the perverse forms of sexual relations they have found there, and through their books and lectures, have introduced these into society, some of them even advocating their use among the unmarried. This class of writers parade their filth under the proud banner of pretended science. They do not seem to be content with the amount of sexual perversion that already exists, and are bent on producing far more. An ally of theirs, in this corrupting work, is psychonalysis and pretended psychology.

Overclothing is a common means of weakening the body. Men are more prone to over clothe themselves than women. Present styles in women's clothes are far more sensible than men's. Particularly in winter do men overclothe themselves.

This business of bundling up like an eskimo begins in infancy. Fond parents weaken the reactive powers of their baby's skin by overclothing it. When the child grows older, his weakened powers of resistance cause him to feel the cold more than he normally should. He therefore keeps up the bad habit. The functional powers of the skin are weakened. It fails to do its full duty as an organ of elimination. It is unable to quickly and easily adjust the body to changes in temperature.

The failure of the skin as an organ of elimination throws more work upon the kidneys and mucous membranes of the body.

Dark clothing excludes the beneficial rays of the sun from the body and thus weakens, not only the skin, but the body as a whole. Sunlight is an absolutely essential factor-element in normal nutrition, as much so for the animal as for the plant. Man is by nature, a nude animal and the nearer he approaches this ideal the more healthful will he become. Clothing should be light and porous in texture and made of light colors or of white. A free circulation of air about the body is essential at all times.

Indolence is also a weakening habit of mind and body. Muscular exercise or work is as essential to physical vigor, strength and development as air is to life. Those of light occupations who neglect to exercise become weak, delicate and sickly. By an irrevocable law, growth of mind and body is acquired through exercise. It is a mistake to think exercise builds muscle only. It trains the mind and develops the heart, lungs and other vital organs. Indolence is a crime against the body. It produces weakness in every tissue in the body.

Breathing impure air is a source of weakness and disease. Pure air is best for life. Air that has been breathed over and over again is poisonous. All the excretions of the body are, normally, more or less toxic, and they become more so as health is enfeebled. The character of the exhalations from man's lungs differs with the varying states and conditions of his health. In diseased states these exhalations are laden with toxins of various kinds. Some investigators have reported finding a toxin in expired air similar to the ptomaines.

Do not force yourself to breathe over and over again the air from your own or the lungs of some one else. Have your bed room, living room, office and workshop well ventilated at all times.

The sensuous and voluptuous usually keep up their bad habits until a collapse of function forces a halt. Anorexia and nausea, perhaps vomiting, force them to eat less. Repugnance to smoke and drink forces them to cut down on these for a while. A breakdown forces them to rest. Functional collapse is due to enervation brought on by the HABITS that KILL.

Once these sufferers are able to be up and around they return to their bad habits. Repeated functional collapses do not teach them the way of life and health and, finally, chronic disease becomes their portion. They then seek for "cures" that will restore them to health without restoring them to sane living

These people do not desire to reform their modes of living. They do not care to discipline themselves. They are slaves to their habits. Almost anyone can give up habits for a few days or even for a few weeks, but to continue to live correctly for years is beyond the powers of the average individual. So enslaved are they by their habits that they declare they cannot see what one gains by abstaining from "all the good things of life" even if it does enable him to live a few years longer. Now if these bad habits really constituted "*good things of life*" nothing would be gained, not even increased length of life, by abstaining from them. We do not ask you to deny

yourself a single one of the good things of life. We
only ask you to abstain from harmful practices and
harmful excesses that enslave you. This will entail
no hardship upon you. But there is another and
even brighter side of this picture. To cease abusing
your body and mind will not only add years to your
life but life to your years. Instead of weakness, misery, aches, pains, disease, and suffering; health,
strength, joy and happiness will be yours. The highest and greatest joys of life are based on health.

There is a heedless class who declare they are
strong. They are masters of themselves. They harbor
the delusion that they shall always be as able to control themselves; that they shall be as free to choose
their course after frequent departures from the path
of virtue as they feel while they are yet only in con-
templation. They vainly imagine that when they
will, they can take their stand in unbroken strength
of soul upon the fartherest verge of harmful indulgence and say to the surging torrent of undisciplined
passions and desires: "Thus far shalt thou go and
no farther and here shall thy proud waves be stayed."

These people are not conscious of the growth of
their habits. They forget that habit is bondage. They
cannot see the end of their strength and foolishly
conclude it has no end. From master they are soon
reduced to slave. Heedless of the warning voice of
wisdom and experience they go recklessly on in their
mad pursuit of false pleasures.

There is another class who can be good for a brief
period and then must break over the traces and return
to their idols. "Just this once wont hurt me," they
say. And yet there is a first step in every career of
excess and dissipation. The Chinese proverb truly
says: "The thousand mile journey begins with the
first step."

Once a man or woman yields to the temptation to
do a thing, resistance is weakened and it becomes all
the easier to yield next time. One's powers of re-

sistance can be strengthened only by using them.
"Just this once" all too often grows more and more
frequent until a formidable habit is forged and the
victim of his own folly becomes bound to a practice
he did not intend to engage in. That "abstinence
is easier than temperance" is an old and true saying.

Let us learn that bad habits are always bad. The
repeated use or application of any substance which is
pernicious soon reconciles us to it. That which is at
first disagreeable and manifestly injurious, may become apparently neutral or even apparently salutary.
Such is the blinding influence of habit by which the
vital instincts are rendered insensible to constant irritation, if it possesses only a moderate degree of
force, so that, eventually, a craving or appetite is
formed for a substance or practice that is harmful
and foreign to the needs of the body.

Under the constant sway of such influences the body
is perverted and its functions subverted. The effects
ultimately produced must be commensurate with the
magnitude and duration of the harmful habit. In
the end, weakness, suffering and premature death
must result.

PART VIII.

NATURE'S PROVISIONS FOR LIVING

In the preceding chapters the following facts have been shown:

1. By virtue of the body's inherent and automatic powers of self-renewal, self-renovation and self-regeneration and its undeviating tendency to fullness of life, it is capable of a much longer existence and a much higher existence than men and women now live.

2. Disease, degeneracy and death come as the immediate result of poisoning and starvation of the cells of the body as a consequence of a combination of forces and influences which are largely under individual control and usually self-inflicted.

These facts serve to confirm the old statement that "man does not die; he kills himself." Men and women are dying far short of the age they are capable of attaining because they are engaged in committing slow suicide. So far, however, we have dealt chiefly with the negative side of living. It shall be our purpose in this chapter to tell you what you should do, if you would live to the fullest.

If you have ever watched a seed sprout and grow and then watched the tiny plant develop into a mature plant you will be able to fully appreciate the simplicity of Nature's requirements and the abundance of her provisions for living.

All that the seed requires in order to grow into a vigorous well developed specimen of its kind is proper soil (food) warmth, air, water, and sunshine. Given these simple conditions and it fulfills perfectly all the functions of its life. Deprived of any of them and it sickens and dies.

The minute germ in the egg, if it is to mature and become a full grown, well developed bird, requires these same simple conditions plus exercise after it has hatched. Deprived of any of these and it sickens and dies.

Puppies, kittens, calves, young whales, lions, etc., all ask for but these same natural elements of life. The human infant, likewise, requires these only if it is to grow into a healthy, well developed human being.

In all these cases beginning with the plant and bird and ascending up to man, freedom from violence must be added to our list of requirements. It should be observed, also, that where any element is not wholly lacking, but is deficient we have defective development, lowered resistance to disease, impaired functions and shortened life. Let us make one final addition—CLEANLINESS. This means, simply, freedom from poisonous filth.

Given a normal organism at birth and proper living conditions as summarized above, together with absence from injurious influences, and every baby born into this world will grow into a strong, healthy man or woman. But, observe, those same simple conditions that are the sources of the development of plant, animal and men from germ to maturity are the constant sources of the maintenance of these organisms after maturity is reached. Those same influences that impair or prevent development in the growing child or youth also impair the powers of life in adults.

Whether you have a good organism at birth will depend partly upon heredity and partly upon the nutrition you received from your mother. What that organism will become after birth, that is, whether it will reach up to its highest potentiality, or, fall far short of its inherent possibilities, will depend upon how you live. Of course there will be social factors that are not subject to individual control that may mar your life to a certain extent, but for the most part you and your parents and teachers will determine your life.

You cannot change your heredity. You cannot change your past. You cannot make society over.

But you can work for the betterment of these things for the future. Civilization has many influences in it that are inimical to health and life. But these are not inherent in civilization and can be eradicated. We can build for a better future and assure our children and grandchildren better conditions to grow up under. The standard of living can be raised; the conditions of life can be improved; not merely for the fortunate few; but for all.

How, then, shall we live?

1. *Cultivate poise and cheer.* Do not attempt to see the world through the rose-colored glasses of a sentimental Pollyana, but learn to take joy and sorrow, good fortune and misfortune with the same calmness and equitableness. Avoid worry, fear, anxiety, excitement, jealousy, anger, self-pity, etc.

2. *Exercise daily.* Daily physical exercise, preferably in the fresh air and sunshine, and, as often as possible, in the form of play, is essential to both mental and physical health. Avoid the strenuous life, however. Do not make the Rooseveltian mistake, and imagine that a strenuous physical life can offset gluttony.

3. *Secure plenty of rest and sleep each day.* Learn to retire early. Learn to relax and "let go." Earn your sleep by honest work, and avoid stimulants, and sleep will come easily and naturally. Do not turn the night into day. *Time is never wasted that is spent in recuperation.*

4. *Keep Clean.* This may refer to both mind and body. Do not indulge in frequent and prolonged bathing. Man is not a fish. Where time and work permit, a daily friction bath will keep the body clean without the use of water and that abomination of desolation, soap. If water bathing is indulged in, the water should be near the temperature of the body and you should remain in it only so long as is necessary to wash your body. Follow this with a brisk rub over the whole body.

Keep clean clothes, clean beds, clean houses, clean surroundings.

Keep the mind clean. Avoid lustful thoughts and desires. Do not become covetous, deceitful or corrupt. Nature penalizes you for all these things with hardening of the arteries and a shortened life.

5. *Breathe fresh, pure air.* Keep your windows open. Have your living room, bed room, office or work shop well ventilated. Get out doors as much as you can. If you live in the city take advantage of every opportunity to get out into the country.

6. *Get as much sunshine as possible.* This does not mean that you are merely to sit by the window, or that a walk in the sunshine heavily clad in dark clothes will be of great benefit to you. Your body needs sunshine just as it needs food and water. The direct and unfiltered rays of the sun should come in contact with your skin. Sun baths are best taken in the morning or evening when it is not so hot. They should be begun in infancy. In infancy childhood and youth more sunshine is needed than in adult life.

7. *Eat moderately of wholesome foods.* What are wholesome foods? All true foods that are fresh and that have not been processed and adulterated are wholesome foods. All foods that in the process of refining, manufacturing, pickling, canning, cooking, etc., have been deprived of more or less of their mineral elements and vitamine content or that have been adulterated and poisoned by bleaching, coloring, flavoring and preservatives are more or less unwholesome. All foods that have been raised in defective soil or in hot houses, or on manure fed lands, or lands fed on packing house fertilizers, or that are raised out of the sunlight, are more or less unwholesome. All foods that have begun to undergo decomposition are unwholesome. Avoid all such foods.

The diet should be composed largely of fruits and green leafy vegetables. Proteins, starches and fats should be eaten moderately. Eggs, cheese, meat and cereals, if eaten, should be eaten in great moderation.

The morning meal should be a fruit meal. No sugar should be added to fruit. Fruit is best eaten raw.

The noon meal should be light.

The evening meal should be the heavy meal of the day and should always be begun with a large raw vegetable salad.

No fried foods should ever be eaten.

The diet should be largely, if not wholly, raw.

After maturity is reached three protein meals per week are enough. Only one protein food should be taken at a meal. No starches or sweet foods should be eaten with the protein. Either acid fruits or a raw vegetable salad and cooked non-starchy vegetables should be eaten with these. Milk should never be eaten with proteins.

Starch may be taken four times per week. It should not be eaten with proteins nor with acid fruits. Take it with a raw salad and cooked non-starchy vegetables. Never put sugar, honey, jam, jelly, etc., on starch foods before eating them. Eat them plain. Take them dry and chew them well.

Eat only when hungry. If not hungry at meal time miss the meal. If you cannot relish your food wait until you can before eating.

If in pain, fever, inflammation, or mental and physical discomfort do not eat. If discomfort follows a meal miss the next one. If in fear, worry, anxiety, grief, anger, etc., wait until these have passed before eating.

Do not eat between meals nor in the evening before retiring. You can eat more than you require by eating three meals per day.

Chew your food well. Taste it fully before swallowing. Digestion depends upon taste.

Do not drink with meals nor for four hours thereafter. Fifteen minutes before meals and four hours after meals drink all the water called for by thirst.

If not thirsty don't drink. Don't try to drink six or eight glasses of water per day because someone told you you need them. Thirst will tell you when you need water.

Do not eat when tired. Rest a bit before eating. Do not eat a heavy meal immediately before nor immediately after hard mental or physical work.

Be moderate. Eat sensibly.

8. *Have an interest in life*. A purposeless life is marked for early dissolution. A purposeless life is not worthy of preservation. That man or woman who has no purpose in life is driven about from place to place; from discontent to despair.

9. *Get married*. Build a home. Rear a family. Statistics show that married people live longer on the average than single people.

Dr. George Robertson of the Edinburgh Royal College of Physicians recently stated that ''young men between 25 and 35 who remain bachelors die four years sooner than married men.'' He added that they also ''run three times the risk of becoming insane.'' It is, of course, not fair to charge all this apparent evil of ''single blessedness'' to the single life. We can only correctly interpret such figures when we understand why these men remained single. All normal, healthy men marry, or, at least, desire to. It is safe to assume that a great majority of those who remain single from choice are lacking in virility and are diseased perhaps in many ways. The thing that prevented them from marrying may also have been the things that caused their early death or that caused so much insanity among them.

Childless couples die before those with children. A childless marriage is usually more unhappy than where there are children. Home and children stabilize life.

Avoid contraceptives of all kinds. They are all harmful and all lead to sex gluttony. They are partly responsible for so much cancer of the womb in women. Don't build your married life on lust.

10. *Avoid all poison habits*—coffee, tea, cocoa, chocolate, tobacco, alcohol, opium, heroin, soda fountain slops and other drugs. These all weaken, poison and destroy the body.

11. *Avoid over clothing*. Overclothing weakens the body. It lowers resistance to heat and cold and impairs the powers of adaption to weather changes. It deprives the body of sun and air and keeps the excretions of the skin locked up against the body. You are literally wallowing in your own excretions.

12. *Avoid sexual excesses*. All sexual relations,—"petting," mental self-abuse, self-abuse and all indulgence—drain the nervous system of much of its powers. Conserve these powers.

13. *Avoid all excesses*. Build your life on the conservation of energy not upon its dissipation. Don't waste your forces in useless and needless expenditures. Be moderate and temperate in all things. If you waste your forces you impair your functions and build toxemia and impaired nutrition.

Do not become one-sided in your manner of living. You cannot become well and strong through exercise alone, or through diet alone, or rest and sleep alone. Fresh air and sunshine alone are not enough. Do not imagine that by breathing alone you can reach the heights. All these things are good, but life is more than exercise, or food and drink; more than thought, or rest and sleep. It is all these and more. Life must be lived as a whole.

Do not get the idea that you are an exception to the laws of life. There are no exceptions. The laws that govern life, health, growth development, disease and death in your body are the same laws that govern these same processes in the bodies of your neighbors. Physiological laws and processes are the same in Jones as in Smith. Both Jones and his neighbors are injured by the same harmful indulgences, practices, habits, agents and influences. Both are helped

by the same factors. Paste this in your hat. YOU
ARE NO EXCEPTION.

We must learn to view life as a struggle between
self-control and self-indulgence and must come to
realize that self-control alone leads to strength and
happiness. Self-indulgence leads to misery and destruction. The late Elbert Hubbard well said: "The
rewards of life are for service, its penalties for self-
indulgence."

There is absolutely no need for any action or habit
that impairs life and produces weakness and disease.
But people are so enslaved by their habits, so bent
on the pleasures of the moment, so lacking in self-
control that they cannot free themselves. Self-control is the world's greatest need. Self-discipline is
the only saving force. Our pleasure-mad and over-
stimulated age is almost wholly lacking in self-control.

Many will say: "I would rather live as I now do
and only live ten years than to live as you have outlined and live a hundred." They do not realize that
this is the despairing cry of a slave. These people
are hopelessly enslaved by their bad habits and thoroughly perverted in both mind and body. Mind and
body alike are dominated by their habits. They are
beyond redemption. They will declare they derive
more satisfaction from their pipe or cigar than from
anything else in life. Or they cry out, "Please don't
take my harem away." It is but a waste of time to
reason with such. One is always defeated in an argument with their appetites and morbid desires and
perverted instincts.

Their cry is "We live but once. Let us enjoy life
while we are here." We believe in enjoying life, real
life, life in the highest and fullest sense, not life on
the low groveling plane they mean. What they should
say is "We live but once, let us make it short and
snappy."

If these people would only die at the end of their

ten fast and merry years, little objection could be offered to their foolish "philosophy" and worse practices. But many of them do not do this. Instead, they hang on year after year, going from doctor to doctor and from institution to institution in search of a cure for the effects of the very abuses of their bodies from which they think they derive so much pleasure and satisfaction. They desire to be SAVED IN THEIR SINS, not FROM THEM. The "*satisfaction*" they derive from their pipe, or their gluttony or their alcohol or from their harem is a poor satisfaction. It is a poor substitute for the higher joys of real health based on wholesome living.

If you would live longer; live simply, live wholesomely, live right.

PART IX.

TEMPERANCE AND WHOLESOMENESS

Sylvester Graham used to say: "*A drunkard may reach old age; a glutton never.*" The truth of this statement is borne in upon us daily, hourly. Such outstanding examples of "good eating" as the late Wm. J. Bryan and Theodore Roosevelt and other men of public life come readily into mind. Our public men are wined and dined as a part of their social and political life and they soon become veritable gluttons, if indeed, they are not already such before they become public men.

Drunkards are often saved a glutton's grave from the very fact that their "booze" deranges and impairs their stomach and prevents them from eating. The use of tobacco also often prevents gluttony. Many men and women possess digestive organs that are stronger than the rest of the body and which, in the absence of intelligence and self-control, constitute a positive danger to their lives. Their over-indulgence in food works all the other organs of the body to death and wrecks the whole system long before their digestive organs begin to show signs of weakening. Such people may develop diabetes, Bright's disease, diseases of the heart and arteries, tumors, etc., as a result of over-eating and all the while they may be proclaiming to the world that their food never disagrees with them. They are laboring under the prevailing delusion that unless food causes distress in the stomach it produces no harm.

More people are destroyed by surfeiting than by starving; by feasting than by fasting. Simplicity of habits and moderation in eating are the prime requirements of healthful living. When the lives of old men and old women are studied, it is found that, while they have had their pet vices, they have led simple lives and particularly, have been moderate eaters. They may have used tobacco, but this, by putting a check upon eating, prevented them from killing themselves with gluttony. While, if they attained to old age in spite of tobacco they used tobacco in "moderation."

A few years ago Prof. Huxley, of England, the son of the older Prof. Huxley, took some young plenaria, or earth worms, and performed a very interesting and instructive experiment with them. He fed a whole family of these as they ordinarily eat. One he isolated and fed in the same manner, except that he forced it to undergo short periods of fasting. It was alternately fed and fasted.

The isolated worm was still alive after nineteen generations of his brothers had been born, lived their regular life cycles and passed away. The only difference in the mode of life and the diet of this worm as compared to that of his brother worms was his periodic fasts.

Professor Huxley explained that overfeeding clogs up the body and produces death. Habits of eating are formed during the period of growth when more food is needed and when the vigorous functions of life easily get rid of the excess. When maturity is reached and less food is needed, particularly of certain kinds, the habits of eating, already well formed, do not undergo any material changes. The individual continues to consume large quantities of food, eating as much building foods as during the period of rapid growth. This excessive consumption of food, clogs the body, over-works all its organs, and due to the acid-forming character of much of it, fills the body with powerful acids which destroy its vital tissues.

By fasting the worm at repeated intervals, the excess of food, that was clogging and poisoning the body, was used up and the toxins or acids were cleared out. The cells and tissues of the worm were kept soft and young and his system kept free of all encumberances. The result was that he lived over nineteen times as long as he otherwise would have lived.

Some interesting experiments, in which flat worms

were used, were recently performed by Prof. C. M. Child, of Chicago University. Prof. Child makes a specialty of studying the growth of complex animals. He found that the worm, like an overfed mule or an overfed man becomes fat, lazy and infirm. They begin to grow old. He took such fat, lazy and infirm, overfed worms and STARVED them for a long time. They grew smaller and smaller, living off the food stored in their own tissues, but did not die. After the worms had been reduced to a minimum size the professor fed them again and they grew again. But they started to grow as young worms. They were young worms, renewed by the starving process.

Farmers know that when they turn their overfed, overworked mules or horses out on the pasture for a season they lose their fat, become soft and undergo considerable regeneration. Then after a few days of work has hardened them again, they are in better condition for work than before put on the pasture. The rest and change of diet has worked great changes in their bodies. The diet on the pasture is almost wholly of green stuff with very little of the concentrated proteins, starches and fats to clog the channels of life and fill the body with powerful acids.

I would not claim that periodic short fasts would enable a man to outlive nineteen generations of his fellowmen, but I am sure that so long as man continues to play the hog periodic short fasts will enable him to get rid of his surplus accumulation and lengthen his life. Fat people do not reach old age. Neither do gluttonous people who are not fat. Abstemiousness is essential to health, strength and long life.

The case of Louis Carnaro, the venetian nobleman, is in point. A "fast life" of wine, women and late hours, such as was and is common to gentlemen or noblemen had brought him to the verge of the grave at forty. His physicians told him he had but a few months to live. Having more intelligence than his physicians he reasoned that if a life of indulgence and dissipation had brought him to this condition a life of abstemiousness and temperance would save him. He therefore abandoned his follies and adopted what was perhaps one of the most frugal diets of history with the result that he outlived his physicians. He lived to be a hundred years old and remained strong, healthy and in possession of all his faculties to the last.

His daily consumption of food after forty would not make a meal for the average man or woman of today. He ate but twice and sometimes only once per day. In addition to this frugal eating he took a fast each year.

Heavy eating causes rapid heart action just as heavy muscular effort does. The heart works faster if one is awake than if asleep; if excited than if calm. Light eaters who avoid stimulants have a heart beat of about 60 per minute. Heavy eaters and those who consume stimulants have a heart beat ranging from 72 to 95 or more per minute. The average of 72 beats per minute, that is considered normal, is too high and is the average standard for over-stimulated, overfed individuals.

But more rapid heart action is not the only evil of over-eating. All the functions of the body are conducted more rapidly than they should be until the over-work forces them to stop. This does not mean that the overfed man or woman is in better health or has more energy or endurance or more brain power. Rather the reverse is true.

The light eater has muscles of better quality. His strength and endurance are greater as shown by repeated tests. He thinks quicker, more accurately and clearly. The light eater has more reserve power and due to the fact that his light eating conserves and does not expend his powers in excessive physiological activity, he lives longer. He also escapes the aches and pains that fill the lives of the heavy eater.

Over-eating does not merely over-work the body, it also poisons it.

In our present state of hyper-civilization, we have developed another great evil that is responsible for much trouble and shortened life. One of the three causes of death is STARVATION—the other two being POISONING and VIOLENCE. There is a form of starvation and poisoning that results from eating —that is, from eating what was once food, but which has been rendered unfit for food by the refining, preserving, and cooking processes through which it has passed before reaching the table.

Most animals are able to walk at birth and their legs are straight and firm. These animals grow normally and their legs remain straight and firm if they are properly fed. But if fed on foods that have been deprived of part of their elements they suffer from defective development and become bow-legged or knock-kneed. A diet deficient in the elements of bone nutrition will accomplish this for chickens, calves, puppies, and human infants. Walking too early never caused bow legs. The author's baby sustained the weight of his body on his legs from the age of two weeks and was able with but little aid to do the deep knee bend several times when he was a month old. His legs are as straight as an arrow.

This faulty development is in many cases a case of partial starvation, due to a denatured diet. In some cases the partial starvation is due to lack of sunshine or lack of exercise or to faulty digestion due to over-feeding, coddling, too much excitement, and other causes. Starvation of this kind may actually be due to over-feeding. There are other troubles besides rickets that develop from eating a diet of denatured and adulterated foods.

White flour, degerminated corn meal, denatured cereal foods, white sugar, canned foods, pickles, sulphured dried foods, improperly cooked foods, are all denatured foods and should be avoided as far as possible. Meat is a denatured article. Meat-eating animals consume all the tissues of their prey and not merely the lean portions. They consume the blood, part of the bones and other portions that are usually rejected by the esthetic tastes of human vultures.

Meat is not only a denatured article of food when it reaches the cook but is further denatured in the process of cooking. Despite this fact many people must have meat with every meal and do not feel that the meal is complete without it. The meat eating habit, like salt eating, condiment using or the tobacco habit readily grows on one and soon results in the over-consumption of protein.

The over-consumption of cereal foods, particularly the denatured cereals is causing more trouble in this land of *"health food"* fads than any other food today.

Denatured foods not only fail to supply all the food elements required by the body but actually leech part of the body's own mineral reserve from its blood and tissues, particularly from the hair, nails and teeth, but from other tissues, as well. The result is that we are fast becoming a race of bald heads, glass eyes, false teeth and wooden legs. For a more detailed discussion of the results of denatured foods the reader is referred to the author's book "Food and Feeding."

This defective nutrition, particularly in childhood and youth, not only causes defects and troubles that persist throughout life, but affect also the offspring of the child after he or she has grown up. Upon this point Dr. Taliaferro Clark, expert in child feeding for the United States Public Health Service says:

"Underfeeding in certain essential food elements to a degree not necessarily accompanied by evidences of ill health or the production of pathological change, when continued from generation to generation, will cause marked changes in hereditary characteristics."

Dr. Clark quotes definite experimental proof showing that rats when fed for several generations on a slightly deficient diet, produce offspring that, even when fed a complete diet, do not thrive as well as rats that possess well fed ancestors. In addition to this he gives evidences from observation on human beings that reveal the same thing. It is evident that a defective diet, impairs the germ plasm to some extent and thus injuries the offspring. It is obvious, of course, that a defective diet eaten by the pregnant mother will injure the offspring. Proper feeding should begin, then with our great-great grand parents —or, to put it the other way around, if "civilized" peoples continue to eat denatured foods each succeeding generation of our posterity will be more defective and ailing and shorter lived.

The lessons the facts presented in this chapter teach may be summed up in a very few words.

1.   Abstemiousness and moderation in eating is of prime importance to health, strength and long life.

2.   All foods eaten should be natural foods, that is, foods that have not been processed, refined, preserved, adulterated and colored and cooked until they have had much of their food value destroyed and become a source of evil to the eater and his children.

PART X.

THE REIGN OF HEALTH LAW

So prone is man to look upon the conditions under which he is born and reared as natural and to look upon those things which the majority of mankind do as an average as the best for us to do as a whole that few are inclined to question the wisdom of the conventional standards of health and living, with a view to ascertaining if they best serve the physiological and psychological welfare of the individual and the race, but take it for granted that they do so. There is a happy delusion, a very convenient substitute for thought, that our present customs and standards represent the boiled down results of thousands of years of race experience and that they should not be tampered with. If it can be shown, historically, that a particular custom is old, this suffices to establish its value in the minds of many. Nothing could be farther from the truth.

Laboring under the delusions above noted, the doctor or health advisor who insists that his patients abandon certain of their pet vices and health destroying practices and indulgences, is justly considered severe. The doctor, however, if he is to be held responsible for the health and life of his patient, must necessarily be firm and insist upon obedience to natural law. The laws of nature are sharply defined, their penalties inexorable, if not always swift, and as an interpreter of her decrees, the doctor, under present thought, at least, cannot seem otherwise than severe. However it is not the doctor but nature that is severe. This being true, it behooves the health seeker to strive to understand God's rational order, that he may render an intelligent obedience to laws which cannot be broken, but, upon which, he only breaks himself in the attempt.

When we come to consider the means best suited to maintain life and health, youth, strength and beauty,

it is obvious that THE HIGHEST POSSIBLE
STANDARD MUST BE ACCEPTED. Critics often
point out examples of long lived, or apparently
healthy individuals who have habitually indulged in
many of the practices we condemn. They regard these
apparent exceptions as evidences that the condemned
practices are not harmful, or, at least, not very harmful. An excellent example of this kind of reasoning (?) was carried by many of the newspapers for
Feb. 26, 1924, in the form of an interview with one
Mr. Reuben B. Thomas, who was then 86 years old,
and who declared, that rules for health mean nothing,
that longevity "just happens." He was asked by the
reporter:

"There are many persons who would like to live to be as old
and active as you are. What would you suggest as a course
of procedure?"
To this, he replied: "My dear young man, do as you would
like to do, and if you are to become old, you will; if you are
to die, you cannot stop it."

This is fatalism with a vengeance. Mr. Thomas is
surely a good Presbyterian. He has transferred the
idea of fatalism from the realm of religion over into
that of hygiene and health. But, in this, he is not
alone. Every day I meet with young and old who hold
to this same view. They tell me that one will die
"when his time comes" regardless of whether his
course of living has been healthful or unhealthful, and
that he will not die before that time, regardless of
what his course of living may have been.
Mr. Thomas told the reporter the following story, to
illustrate his point:

"There was once a man who wanted to grow old. So he
started out, interviewing this man and that, asking how to
prolong his life.
'The first man he met, he asked: 'How am I to become
old?' And the man answered, 'Do not smoke, do not chew, do
not dance, do not eat everything, and go to bed at night at a
respectable hour.'
"The second man he met was an old sea captain 80 or 90

years old. The young man asked, 'How am I to grow old like you?' The Captain responded: 'I chew tobacco, I smoke a pipe, I have been drunk, I have been in fights, I have stayed out all night without sleep, I have caroused many times.'"

At this point Mr. Thomas is said to have smiled. He had proven his point. Long life, he had said, *"just happens,"* and had he not proven it by an appeal to folk lore? This is more than the doctrine of fatalism; it is the doctrine that law and order do not reign in the realm of life; it is physiological lawlessness, biological chaos. Mr. Thomas, a watch repairer, had worked at his trade for 68 years. He was still at it when the reporter interviewed him. He would not reason about watches as he did about life. He knows that any watch which receives proper care, will last longer and give better service than if it is treated as junk. Still, he holds that the body can be treated as junk, that one can *"do as he likes"* and if he is fated to become old, he will become old; he cannot kill himself before his appointed time; that, if he is not fated to live long, he can do nothing that will prevent him from dying early. Life and death just happen, and our voluntary habits have no effect for good or evil.

The above story, although, well representative of the popular notions entertained on the subject of health and life, bears on its face an obvious falsehood. There cannot be the slightest doubt that a few exceptionally powerful constitutions will endure to an advanced old age, in spite of the excesses and indulgences the second witness is said to have indulged in. But it would be impossible for two men with equally excellent constitutions, to reach an equally advanced age, with habits of life so opposite as that lived by the two witnesses in the story, without a very marked and apparent difference in condition and appearance of both body and mind. *It is not possible for two men of equally excellent constitutions to start out in life and follow such equally opposite courses and arrive at the same goal.*

That a life just lived as it happened, filled with numerous and various execesses, would enable a man to reach the hundred mark in as good mental and physical condition as another would be in, at the same age, who had led a temperate and well ordered life, is absurd on the face of it. To believe such, is to believe that life is subject to no law, that man is at the mercy of fortuitious circumstances or a capricious Providence that hygiene and sanitation are valueless, inebrity is as good as temperance, gluttony as salubrious as moderation, sensuality as healthful as virtue, impurity and nastiness as beneficial as purity and cleanliness, chaos, as approved as order. Are we to beilieve that there are no rules of health—no laws governing life. Or, are we to believe that, if such laws do exist, they are not binding, and that we may voluntarily set them aside when we will? Are the laws governing health any less real than those governing mathematics or chemistry. Do acts have no consequences in the realm of life?

Man is a pleasure seeking animal—ever intent upon present enjoyment, and will not consent to abandon harmful practices from which he derives a bit of fleeting pleasure, even for the sake of his future welfare. So long as he is favored with even a moderate degree of health, he rushes headlessly into the excitements of his various pursuits, pleasures, and indulgences; while nothing appears to him to be more visionary and ridiculous than precepts, admonitions and regulations, intended to preserve health and strength.

Man harbors the delusion that, if he enjoys health, he has within himself the constant demonstration that his manner of living, his habits and indulgences, are in harmony with the laws of life, at least, in his own constitution. So long as he is in the possession of, what ordinarily passes for health, he refuses to believe that he is in any danger of losing it; or, if he is in such danger, he does not think that anything in his mode of living can have anything to do with destroying or preserving it. He, consequently, refuses all advice contrary to his present enjoyment, and will not benefit by the experience and learning of others.

What are the results? Simply that, as a general rule, men and women, while in health, prodigally waste the resources of their constitutions, as if these were inexhaustible; then, after repeated violations of the laws of life have brought disease and suffering upon them, which interrupts their pursuits and destroys their comforts, they hurry to a physician for relief. Do they go to a physician to learn by what violations of the laws of life they have brought disease and suffering upon themselves? Do they seek to learn and to know how they may avoid such discomforts, difficulties and sufferings in the future? They do not. They regard themselves as unfortunate victims of fortuitious circumstances, visited with afflictions for which they are in no way responsible and which they could not have escaped had they tried.

In this idea, they are encouraged by their physician who comforts them with the advice that their trouble is due to a germ or a worm or a subluxated vertebra in their spinal column, etc. They seek the exercise of the physician's skill, in the application of remedies, designed to relieve their sufferings and remove their diseases, in order that they may return to their pursuit of false pleasures. The physician sells them immunity from the penalties of broken law in the form of drugs, serums, vaccines, antitoxins, adjustments, metaphysical formulas, electronic reactions, etc.

But the laws of life are not so easily side-stepped, and those who scoff at the laws of life and do as they please would do well to give some heed to them. There are no iron constitutions. A strong constitution will stand a lot of abuses before their effects finally make themselves apparent, but the strongest constitution that ever existed must ultimately succumb to repeated violations of the laws of our being.

Dr. Chas. E. Page, represents the matter thus:

" 'Nothing hurts me—I eat everything! (Next year): 'Nothing agrees with my stomach—I can't eat anything.' Thus the dyspeptic's ranks are kept full with recruits from those who 'don't want any advice about diet.' "

Dr. Page has not overdrawn the picture one bit. There is hardly an invalid, semi-invalid, and has-been-perfect-physically man or woman, in America today, that did not, at one time, say: "Nothing hurts me—I eat everything." All those who will recruit the great army of invalids as the present ones die off, are, today, following this same delusive idea. They are laughing at the idea of dieting, and are following no regular health rules. There are no copper lined stomachs. You may be able to digest pig-iron as you say, but *you are a fool if you try it*.

What is true of diet, is equally true of the other factors of life. Every day, the doctor is forced to listen to the tale of woe of the has-beens in the great army of haphazard livers, and it always runs something like this: "Doctor, I cannot do the things I once did. Once I could digest nails, now I have to eat baby foods. Once I could go all day and night without fatigue, but now I tire in a few minutes or hours. I cannot indulge as I once did without suffering." They thought they had cast-iron constitutions and copper-lined stomachs. They found they were made of flesh and blood and bones. THEY TRIED TO SEE HOW MUCH THEY COULD GET AWAY WITH INSTEAD OF TRYING TO LIVE IN THE HIGHEST SENCE. THEY ONLY GOT AWAY WITH THEIR HEALTH, STRENGTH, USEFULNESS AND LIFE.

But so long as they possessed a modicum of health, they could not be persuaded to observe the laws of life. Why should they "diet"? Were they not healthy? Why should they bother themselves about health rules and regulations? Was not their health

sufficient evidence of the healthfulness of their mode
of life? When they were well, was this not proof
that their haphazard courses of living agreed with
them? Why, then, should they have denied themselves the pleasures of the palate and the sensuous
enjoyment that comes of doing as one pleases? This
is the way men reason. How deceitful this reasoning
may be!

Present health is not always an indication that the
mode of living is a healthful one. Present health is
no guarantee of future health. There is nothing
more certain than that those who are called healthy
are the ones who become sick. It is equally as certain
that the course of living on which they maintain their
so-called health, is the one on which they grow sick.
When one of sound constitution and a powerful and
rugged body becomes an invalid or dies of acute disease, is this not sufficient evidence that his "healthful" course of living was not a healthful one? Or
shall we believe, that health and disease are subject
to no law, that they are subject only to the arbitrary
control of a capricious Providence or to the utter con-
tingency of accident? Are there no fixed and inexorable laws of life, by conformity to which, we can
avoid disease and maintain health with the same cer-
tainty with which we arrived at a correct solution in
mathematics if we follow the rules of mathematics?

A man is declared to be a "picture of health." This
is considered to be sufficient evidence of the healthfulness of his mode of life. If their "perfect picture of
health" dies suddenly, they exclaim: "How sudden!
The strong and healthy always seem to go quickly."
Not once do they stop to think that, perhaps, after all,
his health was as they expressed it, *a picture*.

*Popularly and professionally, if a man appears
well and feels well, this is enough. No matter if he
is on the brink of the grave, his most vital organs so
impaired and deficient in vital power that as soon as
they begin to falter the whole system is broken up*

and life becomes extinct. There is something basically wrong in the popular idea, fostered, though it is, by the medical profession, that one can be suddenly "attacked" by disease. It does not seem to be recognized that in the disease building process, a certain series of changes must necessarily take place in the body before any evidence of disease will be manifest, and that these changes require time. Physicians recognize the presence of disease only after it has advanced far enough to produce a physical sign. This is the reason those who sicken suddenly (?) and die quickly are said to have been a picture of perfect health.

Perfect organization and vigorous health is man's normal state. Everything short of this is a state of impaired health. From the topmost peak of bodily soundness to the lowest depth of impaired health there are several stages of transition. During the long period of "incubation" or period of descent into physiological depravity, the individual passes himself off as healthy and proudly points to his so-called health as an indisputable evidence of the healthfulness of his mode of living. But there is no escaping the fact that these "healthy" people daily become sick by the hundreds of thousands. Yesterday they were "pictures of perfect health"—today they imagine themselves to be in Dante's Inferno. But, if, yesterday, they were convinced, by their supposed good health, that their mode of living was a healthful one, their misery of today does not convince them that it was a disease building one. They do not believe that diseases are built. Instead, they think that they are "caught" or that they are sent upon us by a capricious Providence; that they are of spontaneous origin, or that when they become sick, they are undeserving victims of circumstances over which they have no control.

This land is full of hootch guzzlers who enjoy apparent health and who, declare, because of the fact that they are able to eat three square meals per day and force themselves through the day's work by stimulants, that their mode of living does not hurt them. Alcohol does not kill them instantly, therefore it does not harm them at all. So they reason. When they do become sick, as a result of the abuses which they daily heap upon their bodies, both they and their physicians are agreed that the trouble is due to a germ or to a subluxation in their spinal column.

The young hopeful who has hardly began his career as a user of tobacco, always declares: "tobacco doesn't hurt me and I can quit its use any time I desire." A few months or years later, when the same young hopeful has become convinced of the harmfulness of tobacco, in his case, he may be heard complaining that he cannot give up its use. He could quit, if he could get away where he would come in contact with no one else who uses the weed.

The tobacco user, the drinker of alcohol, the glutton, the sensualist, and all those who do as they please, nothing hurts them, scoff at the idea that there are any laws of life. So long as they are well they have the evidence, in their own bodies, of the harmlessness if their practices and indulgences. When, later, they sicken and die prematurely, it was germs, or exposure, or over work or "the will of God" or a kink in their spines, or some other equally ineffective cause that caused the trouble.

For this state of abject ignorance of the laws of life, which is equally as dense among those who have their parchments from the highest orthodox diploma mills as among the most ignorant and unlearned, the medical profession is largely to blame. In fact the medical profession willingly and knowingly perpetuates and propagates such ignorance. I have had many patients under my care from various parts of the country who had previously been under the care of medical men, and, who were still living and behaving as always. They were told by their medical advisors that they need not give up their use of tobacco, that they might continue their use of alcohol, if only they would use it in moderation, whatever that is, that they need give no particular attention to diet, and similar advice.

Why is this? Is it because medical men do not know the harmfulness of certain habits? By no means. It is wholly and simply because they have been taught that germs cause disease. They were never taught to trace a connection between repeated harmful practices and present ill health. The germ, not the unwholesome mode of living, is responsible for the trouble. For this reason, it is not necessary to reform the mode of life—all that is required is a few shots of this serum or a few doses of that gland extract or of some drug. If the symptoms are obscure and no germ be found, a Wasserman test is made. If this is negative, then the trouble is with the glands, and presto! a gland extract will soon overcome all the effects of evil habits while we continue their practice. It is like trying to sober up a drunk man while he continues to drink.

Those who ignorantly place their faith in the absurdities and vagaries of the germ theory may easily believe in sudden attacks of disease. They may believe that perfectly healthy individuals can be brought down suddenly, as a result of accidental exposure to a mysterious something, called contagion—something that conveys the germs into the patient's body. Such people may consistently laugh at the idea of following the laws of life; they may easily believe that health is a matter of accident; that perfect health and scrupulous hygienic living is not an effective preventative of disease.

Anyone, with common intelligence, can readily discern that, if health and rigid hygiene do not prevent disease, then, man is left a helpless victim of chance, a ready prey to the "devouring monsters," and must remain so until he discovers some effective barrier against the inroads of germs and worse. If a body pulsating with vitality and full of pure blood, is no guarantee against disease, so long, as, by hygienic living, it is maintained in this state, then health and hygiene are failures and man is, indeed, the helpless victim of circumstances beyond his control. If he possesses good health, it is simply due to his good fortune and not to his good behavior.

Those who hold to such a doctrine may laugh at the laws of life, and violate them continually, and, then if they possess a sound, vigorous constitution, they may abuse themselves a long time before the effects of these abuses show. But none but the fool can believe that even the most rugged constitution can be abused indefinitely without hurt.

Many medical men and most bacteriologists will admit that the truly healthy individual is immune to all or most germs; that his natural resistance to these must first be lowered before the germs can harm him. Now assuming, for the sake of argument, that germs are the cause of disease; what is it that breaks down one's resistance and permits the germs to move in? If two men are out hunting, and both are drenched for hours, in a cold rain, while the cold wind beats upon them, and one has pneumonia and the other doesn't even have a cold, is this difference in results a mere matter of accident? If the experience of the one proves that such exposures cause pneumonia, does not the experience of the other prove that they do not cause pneumonia or any other disease? If it be claimed that the pneumococci are the real cause of the disease and that the exposure only lowered the individual's resistance so that they could gain a foothold in the system, why did not it lower the resistance of both men? Or, if the resistance of one was already lowered, and that of the other was not, what lowered the resistance of the one? If this same man had previously passed through a similar exposure without contracting pneumonia or any other disease, what influences have been at work since to lower his resistance?

Is it not the logical proceedure to turn to these harmful practices for the cause of lowered resistance? Is it not just possible that some of these known harmful practices and indulgences have, by being constanly repeated, lowered his resistance? And if these things do cause lowered resistance, is it not more logical to correct these habits, and thus, allow the body to rebuild normal resistance, than to leave these habits uncorrected and attempt to build artificial immunity by drugs, serums and gland extracts? How can resistance be increased, without, first, correcting the causes or influences that have lowered it? It simply cannot be done. Medical men but display the extent of their ignorance, when they declare otherwise.

If it be claimed that medical men do correct these causes, I answer that, while it is no doubt true that some of them do, it is not the rule among them. Such causes are not even considered in the germ theory of etiology, and we have treated a sufficient number of patients, who had previously been under medical care, to know that, as a rule, they do not make such corrections. Not only so, but they themselves, are addicted to these same habits. A great majority of them indulge in tobacco, many of them indulge in alcohol at times and many of them use it habitually. They can be seen in all drug stores imbibing soda-fountain slops with the most ignorant; while, in matters of diet, they eat as haphazardly as any one. Many of them are drug addicts. The members of their families fare no better. It pains me that it is so, but I must admit that there is a large body of drugless men who set an equally bad example before their patients.

Disease ensues upon the accumulation, within the body, of toxins and impurities, due to faulty or impaired organic function. Function is impaired by any influence that lowers the vital powers of the body. Impaired function, lowered vital powers, the consequent accumulation of waste and impurities and, then, disease, *are all due to repeated violations of the laws of life. Health can be maintained as surely and certainly, by conformity to these laws of life, as disease can be built by disobedience of them.* In the realm of life there is an unceasing reign of laws more fixed than those of the Medes and Persians.

Health is potential in life; its realization depends upon the observance of a few simple conditions. We may observe these ignorantly and unknowingly, or, we may learn these laws and conform to them intelligently. Health based on an intelligent conformity to the laws of life is more certain and more dependable than the unknowing and accidental adherence to laws of which we are not informed. Let us learn these laws that we may intelligently order our lives for health.

We are told that since some men enjoy health and strength and live to an advanced age in a hot climate, some in a cold climate; some on one kind of diet and some on another; some under one set of circumstances and some under others; therefore, what is best for one man is not for another; what agrees with one disagrees with another, different constitutions require different treatment; and consequently, no general rules can be set down which are adaptable to every man in all circumstances.. The popular fallacy, as expressed in the aphorism, ''what is one man's meat is another's poison,'' covers the whole field.

But the processes and functions of one man's body are the same as those of another. They are governed by the same laws and subject to the same requirements. The anatomic structure and physiologic function of man is one. The human constitution is one. Any differences we see are in degree not in kind. Such differences are usually due to disease. The truly healthy man can do what any other man can and live under the same circumstances. It is possible, then, to set down a general regimen that will be best for all men and not just best for a few.

How shall we find this regimen? By studying the laws and conditions of life. We cannot easily find what is best by an appeal to the lives of those who have reached old age; for, if we do, we will find such diversity of ways of living as to hopelessly entangle us in a maze of contradiction. For instance, we find several individuals a hundred years old and all enjoying about the same degree of health and strength. We inquire of them and find they are of different and even opposite habits. Every one would contradict every other. We would not even know where to begin to find the road to long life.

Why? Because we must first know what is injurious to health and life and what is beneficial to these. To learn this we must study the laws and conditions of life. When we know these things we may again glance over our old men and this time we get a different view. It is not so contradictory after all. We find them all enjoying about the same mixture of good and bad habits and living under about the same mixture of favorable and unfavorable circumstances. We find a pretty nearly equal amount of what is salutary and conservative in the life and circumstances of each. One has erred in this direction and another in that. One has been correct in one thing and another in another thing. Or, some have lived better than others, but started life with weaker constitutions.

Now we take another glance. This time we visit the grave yard and watch the stream of dead souls into the graves. Are they old men and women? No; babies, children, young men and maidens, adults just past middle life; these make up the endless procession back to dust. The old man or the old woman is a very scarce item. People do not get old because they die too soon. Passing from the grave-yard we go to the city and country-side. It is from these the dead are being brought. We watch those that remain behind, how they live, what their daily habits and practices, their circumstances of life are. They are the same as those of the old men we found. It now dawns on us that this way of living is so deadly that only one in fifty thousand or so reaches the hundred mark. We see the wearing effects of this life upon all and we realize why our old men are worthless, why they are weak, tottering, helpless stragglers with feeble minds and impaired senses.

Nature does not require sacrifice of you. Obedience is better than sacrifice. It is no true sacrifice to give up that to which one has no right. One can sacrifice only by voluntarily surrendering that which is rightfully his. Nature does not require this. But she does require that you do not take that which is not rightfully yours. You may insist upon moderation in all things, including murder, theft, rape, incest, etc., but there can be no moderation in wrong doing of whatever nature. Moderation consists in the correct use of those things to which we have a legitimate right. We have a right to eat. Moderation in eating means eating to supply the needs of the body for food and when these needs are satisfied to stop. To eat for pleasure, or for sociability, or for some other fictitious reason, when no need exists for food, is not moderation—IT IS EXCESS. But man's body has no need for tobacco or alcohol. He cannot use these to supply any needs of his body or mind. Their use in the smallest amount is excess. Their use is punished according to the amount and frequency of such use.

Critics often point out examples of long lived individuals who have practiced many of the vices we condemn. But our aim is not to set up a standard that will enable an occasional individual, say one in fifty thousand, to reach a hundred or more years. We want a standard that will enable all of us to reach this point. Not only this, but we seek a standard that will carry us to the hundred mark or beyond in the full possession of all our mental and physical powers.

Mere longevity is not enough. Most old people come to old age in a weak, infirm and decrepit state. This is not desirable. We seek life, long life, in the possession of all its desirable qualities, with health, strength, grace and bouyancy, youth and beauty; with clearness of mind and in the possession of all our senses. To secure this we simply must avoid many practices that fail to kill a few before their hundredth year.

The simple natural processess of growth lead to superb health and a perfect equilibrium between the processes of waste and repair in the body. By this process the body is being renewed continually, it is constantly and eternally renewing itself. This process of renewal is automatic and perfect in its operations. We do not have to worry over it or try to bring it about voluntarily. We need simply to stop hindering it, for, so far as we know, the body is capable of keeping up this self-renewing process indefinitely. The power to establish and maintain a perfect equilibrium between the processes of destruction and reconstruction—waste and repair—is inherent. The *Fountain of Youth* is within you. But by your daily transgressions of the laws of life you are obstructing the fountain and preventing the normal flow of the waters of youth. Your standard is too low. You begin to grow old almost before you mature. The first few years of your life, infancy, childhood, girlhood and boyhood, adolescence, youth or maidenhood are filled with aches and pains, with weakness and disease, with failing sight and decaying teeth, with defective hearing and spouting noses. You were born to live, yet you begin to die almost before you see the light of day. Half of your number are cut off in death before their twentieth year, yea, an appalling number is cut off in the first year of life. This terrible death rate is not confined to the weaklings, the so-called "unfit," but carries off untold thousands of the physically strong and mentally alert.

PART XI.

MACHINE MADE LONG LIFE

Orthodox science, that is materialistic monism and so-called medical science, regard the human body as a machine every part of which is not equally strong because "we are products of evolution which is a haphazard process of trial and error called natural selection. The process makes each part good enough only to 'get by.' The workmanship of evolution is compared to that of the average automobile repair man—it works with good materials if these can be had, but if these are lacking will use the shoddiest. This is because evolution is a purely mechanistic process instead of being an intelligent one."

This pseudo-science says that in the human body the heart is stronger than the lungs and the brain will outwear either. Evolution stopped short of perfection in constructing the animal body, inventing a make-shift breathing apparatus and doing a faulty job in evolving the stomach and intestine, so that man dies, finally, because evolution bungled the works and left some organs so weak that they break down and result in the death of the rest of the organs. Dr. Pearl, eminent biologist of John Hopkins University, thinks that any omnipotent surgeon with the whole of nature's resources under his control could produce better systems of breathing and feeding. He considers that nature did not improve her original inventions because she was too busy producing other organs. She probably also had considerable trouble keeping her lungs and digestive organs alive while she produced the other organs.

Dr. Pearl found a suggestion in a pamphlet issued a few years ago setting forth some experiments by Profs. Fischs and Starlinger in the destruction of blood-cells by X-rays.

These men claimed to have ascertained that when the cells of the blood were exposed to X-rays of a certain intensity the weak cells were killed while the strong ones remained uninjured. After reading their account of the experiments Dr. Pearl reasoned: "Impaired cells can be killed by X-rays. Cells are potentially immortal. We should live forever—or indefinitely at least—if it were not for the impaired cells that break down the good ones."

With characteristic Allopathic thick-headedness, instead of asking what causes the impairment of cells, he assumed that this was due to the necessity of carrying on their functions in an organized body and set about the effort to find a means of destroying the impaired cells of the body without injuring the unimpaired ones. It is like the effort of medical men to find a drug that will kill all disease germs without destroying the patient. He is carrying out experiments with the X-ray. He says results so far are encouraging but it will probably take twenty years to say anything definite about it. He made the foolish mistake of imagining that an influence that kills weakened cells will not harm strong ones. The professor must know that the X-rays have no selective action. They do not exert their destructive effects upon impaired cells alone, but play with equal intensity upon the normal cells. The only reason the normal cells are not destroyed with the weakened ones is that they have more powers of resistance. Too many investigators and patients have received X-ray burns in normal tissue to allow such a statement to go unchallenged. Burns that refuse to heal, burns that are deep seated, burns that become cancerous and ultimately result in the death of the victim, result from the use of the X-ray.

Nature, herself, removes impaired and destroyed cells and replaces them with new cells. This process of cell renewal is automatic and constant. It fails to preserve life and youth only because something prevents the process from proceeding normally. What is that something that interferes? These "biologists" have assumed that it is a necessary consequence of the effort of the cells to function in a highly specialized body. "The necessity of functioning together in the body is what, sooner or later, causes a break and, eventually, death."

This assumption that enforced community action of the cells is the cause of death is the outgrowth of the hypothesis of organic evolution, which holds that man has been evolved from a unicellular ancestor. It assumes that originally all cells functioned as independent organisms and did not die, but when they "evolved" into complex beings with highly specialized organs and functions greater burdens were placed upon the cells than they were originally called upon to perform and these burdens place such a strain upon them that, sooner or later, they break. Death is the result of carrying on the functions of life.

If this assumption is a correct one, all this talk about prolonging life "indefinitely" or "forever" is superheated air. For it is obvious that if death is "the price we pay for having complex bodies" the only way we can escape death is by disorganizing our bodies and caring for each part in the same way Dr. Carrel cares for the cells from the chicken's heart. If death is "the result of trying to maintain cellular life in a complex, specialized body," life can be prolonged only by removing the necessity of maintaining cellular life under such conditions. *The body will have to be torn down.*

The cells of the human body are perfectly adapted to life in the body. The normal organ is fully capable of a full performance of its functions under all ordinary circumstances and of keeping itself in repair. Prof. Pearl says that the mechanistic and non-intelligent process of *natural selection* "makes each part only good enough to get by." Despite his statement, every organ in the body, if not impaired by disease influences, or if not defective from birth is capable of performing more work than it is called upon to do under the ordinary circumstances of life. The heart and lungs, for instance, are capable of much extra work if their owner is called upon to do a cross-country run with a bear. The kidneys are capable of doing much of the work of the skin, or the skin that of the kidneys, if either one or the other is temporarily impaired. The organs of a normal body are capable of carrying on the functions of life under all ordinary circumstances without strain, so long as they remain normal. The real problem, then, is to find and remove the causes of deterioration—a problem that is beneath the dignity of the "orthodox" scientist.

The present attempt of "biologists" to find a mechanical means of prolonging life again illustrates the truth of Herbert Spencer's statements that man never attacks fundamental problems until he has exhausted all the superficial ones and that he never tries the right method until he has exhausted every possible wrong method.

If the causes that impair cells are not found and removed they will continue to impair and kill cells. If the impaired cells are killed by means of an X-ray or by other means; the causes of cellular impairment, if not removed, will impair the normal cells that remain. If we assume that a means can be found that will kill all the weakened cells without injuring the normal ones, the sudden breaking down of thousands or millions of impaired cells, at the same time, will result in the production of large quantities of toxins that must inevitably impair the healthy cells.

We are told that:

"The break may come in the stomach group. The other groups try, as best they can, to accomodate themselves to the changed situation, but in time one or more of the other organs become impaired by the inability of the stomach group of cells to properly function, and the body dies."

What causes the stomach cells to break down? Can that cause be found and removed? If found and removed, and if the cells of the stomach are supplied with a new and clean nutrient media (blood and lymph), will these cells (like the ones used by Carrel and Burrows, when they discovered that "cells that showed signs of what is called 'age' need only be placed in a new culture-media to become 'young' again) multiply and grow?" If not, then we are wasting time in seeking for a means to prolong life. If a fresh, clean nutrient media will not produce the same result in the cells while in the body that it does in those cells when separated from the body, the present experiments are leading us astray.

Of course, Dr. Pearl is not to be daunted by the breakdown of an organ and its inability to repair and regenerate itself. He has a plan for overcoming this simple difficulty. A plan that reveals that the doctor should have been a mechanical engineer rather than a "biologist." A writer in the New York American some time ago said:

"In the light of Dr. Pearl's theory that we die an organ at a time, some doctors look forward to the time of amputating the entire intestinal tract of persons dying of intestinal afflictions and feeding the very empty individuals three times a day with a hypodermic needle, injecting all the chemicals necessary for his existence directly into the blood. Some mechanical device might be invented to do the work of the heart, just as the pulmotor now can do the work of the lung muscles."

We are told of the "magic properties of adrenalin" of the "mysterious tethalin" of the success of surgeons in engrafting pieces of bone and then treated to a bit of prophecy about the future when we will keep our grandfathers alive by "stowing them away in a glass culture tank, feeding them by hypodermic injection while the thermometer registers an exact degree of heat and scientific contrivances do the work of the heart or other failing organs."

Just what would be the advantage to grandpa or his children's children under such conditions is not

hinted at in the article but Dr. Pearl who is called
a biologist and a "distinguished scientist" is convinced that all this is possible and even probable. He
would make a better mechanical engineer than
biologist.

Feeding a man through his skin by hypodermic injections would be a masterpiece of materialism gone
mad. Shooting so-called "predigested" food into him
that has not undergone the absolutely necessary
changes through which it goes inside the cells that
line the intestines, as it passes through the intestinal
wall into the blood and lymph is a scheme that never
entered the head of any save an allopathic biologist
of the evolutionary brand. Such make-shifts for life
as hypodermic feeders, pulmotor breathing muscles,
mechanical hearts, animal "anti-toxins" gland extracts, and gonads from the goat or monkey and other such inventions and devices are about all one may
reasonably expect from materialism and its bastard
offspring, evolution, when these go to seed. But,
even, if such things were possible or probable they
would not be desirable. Mankind does not want to
make a yearly pilgrimage to the surgical shops for a
new pair of gonads and a weekly trip to the "biological" dispensary for repeated and progressively larger
shots of various gland extracts and anti-toxins. They
do not care to put themselves at the mercy of the
hypodermic feeders, nor lug a pulmotor around with
them everywhere they go. It would not be desirable
for them to carry a storage battery in their pockets
to keep their artificial hearts pumping blood. Grandpa does not desire to be stowed away in a glass culture
tank to be artificially heated and hypodermically fed.
When he reaches the point of absolute uselessness and
can no longer enjoy the most commonplace joys of
life he will not want a corps of highly-trained scientific social parasites to waste their time looking
after him. He would rather die and let the parasites
give their attentions to some useful and productive

labor. But if they can invent some mechanical or chemical substitute for the self-elected super-intellectuals who style themselves scientists, and, invent such sero-comic names by which to designate their occupational classifications, as biologists, etc., they will not require much time in which to solve the problem of long life and health.

So long as the self-styled scientist with his pretentions of great learning is permitted to seek for substitutes for natural methods and nature's requirements and is permitted to torture animals and men in cruel experiments upon them, we may expect the heartless brutes to offer such non-sensical schemes for prolonging life. These men are no more concerned with the causes of disease and death than they are with producing the phases of the moon. They are the legitimate offspring of the ancient alchemists. These ancients, who represented the "science" of their day and pretended a knowledge they did not possess, just as their modern descendants do, spent their lives in the search for an Elixir Vitae which would enable them to live several hundred years or forever; and in the effort to find a Philosopher's Stone which would enable them to transmute the baser metals into gold. The modern alchemist, calling theselves scientists, seek for some elixir of life in the realm of glandular extracts and hope to find some philosopher's "law" that will enable them to transmute one species into another and one force into another. They have but little conception of law and order, notwithstanding, they are constantly reminding us that this universe from the smallest "electron" and "atom" to the farthest star within the reach of telescopic vision is under the constant sway of inexorable law.

The fact that all the body does not die at the same time, which was known long before Dr. Pearl saw the light of day, is set forth as a startling conclusion reached by the doctor. This "startling conclusion" allows the doctor to decide that only one organ of the body dies at a time and then we are told that it has been scientifically demonstrated that the breakdown of these organs are "fated" to "happen," at certain ages. The heart, which we are informed, by His Wisdom, Nature made last, is the strongest and thus statistics "show" that "an almost negligable percentage of human beings die from disease of the circulatory system" until we reach ninety-five or a hundred when about 75 out of each thousand die from a breakdown of these organs.

How about the two makeship systems—the respiratory system and digestive system? 68 per cent of deaths in males and 40 per cent in females during the first year of life are due to diseases of the alimentary tract. In both sexes the respiratory system forms the danger zone from one year to four. Then diseases of the respiratory tract form the causes of death in 41 per cent of cases from the fifth year to the ninth after which the perecentage gradually becomes less until between fifteen and thirty it mounts upward again. Between the ages of 20 to 24 the percentage of deaths from respiratory diseases is 46 per cent among women and 52 per cent among men.

This preponderance of deaths from respiratory disease continues until about the fiftieth year when diseases of the digestive tract again assume the job of peopling heaven, carrying off about 21 per cent of the women who die. In men, the respiratory tract is the chief angel of death until they reach about fifty-five years. After this, and there are very few who reach this age, diseases of the circulatory system become masters of the ceremony.

Dr. Pearl assumes that the fault lies primarily with these organs, and not with the abuse that is heaped upon them. He does not know the nature of disease and therefore concludes that so-called diseases of these organs represent their breaking down. This leaves him to explain how "broken down" lungs, in pneumonia, ever recover and allow the individual to later die of circulatory diseases or how a "broken down" digestive tract in enteritis ever recovers and permits the individual to later die of cancer or Bright's disease. He does not know the cause of disease—the, to him, breaking down of organs—but assumes that the organs give down because the cells of which they are made cannot go on functioning in a complex body as they must if the body is to continue to live. He assumes that the deadly drugs, serums, ice packs, electric currents and surgical operations used by medical men on the sick really cure disease, instead of killing the patient, therefore he does not know that most of the deaths "due" to these diseases represent scientific and legalized manslaughter.

It is no doubt true that the treatment for diseases of the digestive and respiratory tracts carry off a larger percentage of the human family than diseases of any other system as a general rule, but deaths from other causes are far too numerous to make this a universal rule. Besides this fact, diseases, or "break downs" of these organs, are practically unknown among wild animals in a natural state and occur much less often among so-called savages than among civilized peoples. And this simply proves that these organs are not naturally weak; are not mere makeshifts. It proves that the primary trouble is not with these organs. Rather, it shows that our clumsy ways of abusing these organs break them down. And, be it remembered, that these groups of organs suffer more abuse than any other of man's organs.

The following three quotations from the article in the American will show how strongly an evolutionist thinks we are in the grip of heredity in this respect. In this matter of long life heredity is practically absolute, although in matters of evolution, heredity is so powerless as to let offspring vary so much from the parent form as to overstep the line of the species and become a new species. But to the quotation:

"It would seem that we inherit just so much strength and energy and barring carelessness and accidents, live approximately just so long.

". . . We may expect to live about as long as our ancestors had the habit of living; for science has about determined that heredity is the chief factor in determining the duration of life. Elaborate study of a number of family histories demonstrates beyond doubt that long life is handed down from generation to generation, provided a short-lived species of human being is not grafted on the family tree."

"So far, the best assurance of old age, on the best scientific authority, is the old age of our parents and grandparents. How much we can expect from the longevity of our ancestors is illustrated by the fact that if every 'preventable' disease could be controlled, the difference in the average life span would only be thirteen years. Dr. Pearl calls this computation 'the most striking demonstration that could be found of the overwhelming importance of heredity in determining duration of life.'"

The reader should know that this fellow science who has "determined" and "demonstrated" and "found" so many things to be true or untrue in so many departments of human endeavor, has no real or objective existence. He is a non-entity. When some one tells you that science has demonstrated thus and so, put it down that some man or group of men belonging to the present dominant school of thought have decided that a certain conclusion is in keeping with the hypothesis they seek to establish. Offspring inherit potentialities but they may never realize these. A man may potentially be slated for the century mark and die at thirty. He could transmit this potentiality to his offspring if he had any and his own early death would not rob his offspring of their potential possibilities. By this, I mean that. we cannot tell what man's potentialities are if he never realizes them. We may prove that long lived people have long-lived children but we cannot prove that short-lived ones do not possess the same potentialities for long life until we determine what carries them off at an early age. Until we do this all statistics can only show what now is, under present conditions, and not what can be or would be under entirely different conditions.

That there is a natural difference in the life span of various orders of animals which difference would continue even under the most perfect environment is, no doubt, true. For instance, dogs do not live as long as turtles, nor butterflies as long as dogs. Their inherent potentialities in this respect are different and we would not expect by any process to produce butterflies that could live as long as dogs or dogs that could live as long as turtles. But if we find that dogs or butterflies are not reaching the limits of their potentialities because of an unfavorable environment we can by correcting the environment enable them to reach their natural limits.

It is a mere begging of the question to say that long lived people have long lived children and short lived children are descended from short lived ancestors. Who "fixed" the life of the ancestors, who "fated" them for a long or short life? Suppose we trace them back to the beginning will we find an original long life strain and an original short life strain? Who decreed it thus? These fellows have all descended from John Calvin and have brought his predestination down to the realm of "biology" in the form of hereditary fatalism.

Nor is it possible to say how much the control of every "preventable" disease would add to the average life span until we first control these "preventable" diseases. Of course, if we assume that certain diseases are inevitable at certain periods of life and that, in spite of every effort to prevent these, they will continue to carry off at stated periods of life, a certain percentage of those born, then, we may get approximate figures, providing we know, in advance, which diseases are preventable and which are not.

But where is the man who can point to any disease and say definitely that "it is not preventable; everyone will develop this disease at a certain age or period

in life and die from it?'' No such man exists. And
no such disease exists. Seventy-five out of a thousand,
or even out of a hundred may die from it but the fact
that the remainder escape it proves that it is not inevitable. Again where is the man who can affirm that
all long-lived individuals and all short-lived ones
reached the limit of their possibilities? No one but a
scientist would attempt such a thing and he would,
even then, contradict his own conclusions based upon
his experiments, that the cells of man's body are potentially "immoral."

The body is composed of cells and their products.
It remains alive so long as the cells of all its organs
are alive. In the body the proper media for the life
of all its cells exists. It is obvious that it must have
some method whereby it controls the reproduction of
its cells, else we would never cease growing. This
method of control which seems to be largely if not
wholly glandular is normally able to balance the forces
of reproduction with those of destruction. Thus, so
far as can be really determined, life would seem to
be possible so long as the forces of destruction are
counter balanced by the forces of repair and reproduction.

Cells and tissues from the human or other animal
body continue to grow, reproduce and function so long
as they are properly fed, washed clean, kept warm and
protected from accident. In the human body they do
the same. The body is a self-feeding, self-cleaning,
self-warming and self-protecting organism. If Dr.
Pearl, instead of seeking an artificial breathing apparatus, an artificial heart, a method to feed hypodermically, and gland extracts and gonad transplanta-
tions, with which to prolong life, will seek the causes
that impair the functions and structures with which
the body accomplishes the self-regulating, self-adjusting actions, he would come nearer to a solution of the
problem of prolonging life. Vital organs and tissues
repair themselves under normal conditions, but it is

not necessary for one organ to die before its faulty function affects the remainder of the body. For instance, the pancreas is not dead in diabetes but its faulty function injures the whole system. The kidneys and bladder are not dead in cases of suppressed urine, but if this condition is not soon relieved the body dies. The bowels are not dead in constipation, but their faulty function injures the remainder of the body. The stomach and intestines are not dead in indigestion but their faulty function is ruinous to health.

Let us get back of faulty function and find out the causes for this and then we will be in a position to prevent the break down of our organs. Until we do this we are shooting in the dark without even knowing the general direction of our foe. *Starvation* and *poisoning* are the chief causes of the death of cells in the laboratory. Let us find how the cells in the body are *poisoned* and *starved*. Normally the body cleanses itself of poisons. Faulty function prevents this being accomplished thoroughly. Normally the body is able to digest and assimilate its own food and does not require the aid of a hypodermic needle. Faulty function and denatured diet prevent proper nutrition. Improper nutrition further impairs function and interferes with proper drainage. Improper drainage further impairs function and interferes with proper nutrition. With nutrition and drainage and all the subsidiary or accessory functions of the body impaired, destruction of parts is greater than re-construction or repair and, if this continues, death results. Death comes under such conditions, no matter how long lived your ancestors were nor how young you are. Let us then find out what impairs function and what foods are real foods and then we have the key to a long life. This will, however, point us to nature and her ways, and no "scientist" lives who would condescend to a recognition of the ways of nature. He would rather experiment in the vivisection laboratory until he finds an artificial and "superior" way.

As previously pointed out death is seldom, if ever, the result of "old age"—that is of having lived too long. Death usually comes as a result of destructive processes associated with disease, such as the decay of an organ, the rupture of a weakened blood vessel or treatment that suppresses nature's curative processes. These grow out of our faulty habits of living and foolish endeavors to overcome the effects of the habits by treatment. Death is almost always of our own making. Every death ever recorded was premature and a large majority of these was due to treatment. This will be made plain in the chapter on suppression.

PART XII.
FOLLIES OF "SCIENCE"

We are today witnessing a strange and misguided reaction, in quasi-scientific circles, against hygiene and sanitation. A number of quasi-scientific writers like Albert Wiggam maintain that hygiene, sanitation, medicine and religion are weakening and deteriorating the race and lessening its resistance to disease by saving the "unfit" and thus allowing them to propagate their kind. Some of these, like Paul H. De Kruif, recently of the Rockefeller Institute, go so far as to advocate the unlimited indulgence in alcohol, sex and other evils on the ground that these kill off the "unfit" and assure that only the "fit" will survive. Religion is condemned because it attempts to alleviate suffering and thus enables the unfit to survive. In all this foolishness there are three glaring mistakes such as only a self-styled intellectual is capable of making.

FIRST: there is the assumption that medicine can and does save life. Medicine is condemned because it enables the "unfit" to survive. This is claimed to be a reversal of the "order of Nature" as expressed in Herbert Spencer's discredited phrase *"the survival of the fittest."*

SECOND: there is the assumption that those evils that kill off the "unfit" and thus prevent them from propogating do not harm the "fit." This is the same inexcusable mistake that Dr. Pearl made in assuming that, while the X-ray kills feeble blood cells it does not injure vigorous ones. When one reads such nonsense one is forced to wonder just what advantage there is in a superior intellect, anyway. To add to their nonsense, they advocate "protecting" the "fit" with serums.

THIRD: There is the assumption that "fitness" to survive the deteriorating influences of the evils advocated is intellectual. All these men are self-con-

fessed intellectuals and super-intellectuals. The chief
fault they find with hygiene, sanitation, religion and
medicine is that these shield, protect and enable to
survive, the feeble-minded and moron. It is obvious,
however, that intellect is not a power against the effects of alcohol.

Alcoholic indulgence is advocated on the grounds
that it so injures the already enfeebled germ plasm
that the offspring of such parents will not reach maturity. Obviously intellect would not count in this
process. The resistance to alcohol is purely physical
or physiological. Aside from this the alcohol will
weaken both mind and body of the progeny of a line
of alcoholic ancestors. Intelligencia, thou art but ar-
rogant egotism, and incarnate sensualism!

The fault we find with medicine is not that it saves
the "unfit" but that IT MAKES THEM. The greatest deteriorating and degenerating influence in modern life is the practice of medicine as now carried on
by all the professed schools of healing, but especially
as practiced by the "regular" or allopathic school.

Not only are its practices evil but its tenents are
unethical demoralizing and encourage man in his
wrong living. This is also largely true of what passes
for religion. Religion holds out to man, as does medicine, promise of atonement. They both teach that
effects of wrong may be set aside. The super-intellectuals believe this also. They condemn medicine because it does set them aside and permits the "unfit"
to live. They do not see that medicine HAS NO
SUCH THEURGIC AND THAUMATURGIC POW-
ERS.

During the middle ages there arose the strange doctrine that all attention to the body detracted from
spiritual development. Filthiness of the body was
encouraged because it aided spiritual development.
The body was tortured in many ways to develop the
spirit. Man was supposed to mortify his flesh if he
desired to immortalize his spirit. Suffering in this life

guaranteed happiness in the next. The European races have not yet fully recovered from the evil effects of such a doctrine.

We are now witnessing a recrudescence of this doctrine; only now it is advocated by upstarts in the name of science. Hygiene and sanitation are evil. Not because they detract from spiritual development. But because they detract from the hardihood and intelligence of the race. They are racial, not spiritual, barriers. The Buddhistic doctrine of the worthlessness of terrestrial life was the foundation for medieval anti-naturalism and fanaticism. The hypothesis of organic evolution is the basis of the modern reaction against hygiene, sanitation and the humanities.

It is very apparent that these men have no remedy to offer for the prevalence of disease, degeneracy and premature dying. Theirs is another allopathic "remedy"—that of treating effects and leaving causes untouched. They want to really increase the causes of degeneracy in order that these may overwhelm the "unfit" before they can propagate. They are so short sighted that they cannot see that these causes would continue to produce a crop of "unfits" each generation. We cannot accept their proposed remedy.

What remedy does Dr. Pearl offer for these conditions? Nothing. In fact, he claims that little or nothing can be done about them and to prove it he has collected and "classified" the mortality records of widely different communities in Brazil, Great Britain and the United States and he finds that the mortality records are not so very different in this country, where so much attention is given to hygiene and sanitation, to what they are in other countries where the people are not so particular about "sanitation and other protective sciences." The difference in the death rate is wholly out of keeping with the effort we expend in hygiene and sanitation.

It never occurred to the doctor that there may be something wrong with our hygiene and sanitation.

He did not look for other salutary factors in the life of peoples in other countries which evened up the score. To do these things is not becoming the dignity of a "scientist" of the laboratory variety. Had he looked carefully he would have seen that our so-called hygiene and sanitation is nothing more than a war on germs, that it does not contain as much of the elements of natural hygiene as astrology does of astronomy. Yet he records some experiments which should have shown him the utter futility of the attempt to combat disease and death with a hygiene and sanitation that does not go beyond a war on germs.

In testing out Metchnikoff's theory that death is caused by intestinal bacteria, dogs that were kept in an absolutely sterile environment, fed sterile food and allowed only sterile air "showed the same disposition to die at the usual dog time as their flea-bitten, alley hunting brothers." Such facts should forever put at rest all the foolish vagaries that have grown up around the absurd germ theory. They should prove the utter worthlessness of all hygienic, sanitary and prophylactic measures that are devoted to a battle with the microbes. They should prove that germs do not cause disease and death, are not essential to life, or digestion and, for all future practical purposes, may be entirely ignored.

But do these men go this far? They do not. A writer discussing these things with particular reference to Dr. Pearl's book: "The Biology of Death" says:

"At present we carry within us all the germs that ordinarily produce death, and at certain periods in our life our weakest organs will nourish the first available germ as a means to break down according to schedule."

This language would seem to imply that these organs know the schedule and seek to break down. This in face of the obvious fact that millions do not break down according to schedule. In face, too, of the fact that the dogs in the above experiments persisted in dying on schedule time without the aid of germs. In face of the fact that the one universal tendency of all life is to maintain its vital and structural integrity.

This same writer says:

"Life insurance actuaries, who make a fat living guessing how long a given number of people will live, have reduced this principle (the hereditary transmission of long life) to a science, and admit that all the 'live right' propaganda in the world does not materially affect the death rate."

These same life insurance actuaries, however, are ready to assert that the alcohol habit shortens ones life expectancy and that over weight after fifty does likewise. If these evils help to break down the body, why not others also? If the death rate in pneumonia cases is higher among alcohol addicts than among abstainers why cannot that part of the "live right" propaganda that eschews alcohol produce some difference in the death rate? Do life insurance actuaries believe that to live wrong is to live as long as if we lived right? If they do, they are simply cursed with too much knowledge of the allopathic kind.

If Dr. Pearl and the Insurance actuaries think that respiratory and digestive apparatuses break down as quickly under proper care as they do when abuses are heaped upon them in the manner they are today it is only another evidence of the mind beclouding influence of conventional "science," especially medical "science." Nobody but a fool can believe that even the most powerful organism can be abused with impunity.

Still it may be true that the "live right" propaganda has not affected the death rate very materially. This is due to two chief causes.

FIRST: there are two kinds of "live right" propaganda. There is a false kind handed out by the allopathic school and other schools that are based upon the same fundamental propositions. This kind is taught in the public schools, spread abroad by the so-called Health Boards and Departments of Public Health Education, by the daily newspapers and popular magazines. The failure of this kind is amply demonstrated by Dr. Pearl's comparative statistics showing death rates in various localities of various countries. It has failed because it has been directed at the wrong things as was amply demonstrated by the experiments upon the dogs. Then, there is the "live right" propaganda that is carrying the message of natural health from natural causes and under natural conditions. This message hasn't gone very far, due to commercialism, and hasn't been well understood where it did go.

What is this popular "live right" propaganda? It is a lot of foolish advice to "drink lots of water," scrub the teeth, take a daily bath, take hot baths, take cold baths, take sweat baths, eat "plenty of good nourishing food," drink plenty of milk, eat eggs often, eat lots of cereal, take wheat bran with each meal, keep your bowels open, use antiseptics and germicides, etc. It cultivates a fear of germs and disease. It clamors for regular and repeated medical and dental examinations, early surgical removal of tonsils, gall-bladder, teeth; moles, warts, lumps, etc., frequent vaccinations and inoculations, etc. These things do not prevent disease—THEY BUILD DISEASE. The whole program is wrong and based on superstition and fear. How can such measures increase life?

SECONDLY: that part of the "live right" propaganda that has any real value has never been adopted by the public. Every one now scrubs his or her teeth once to half a dozen times daily because they have been taught the obvious falsehood that "a clean tooth never decays." Every one now bathes more or less regularly because they believe that "cleanliness is next to godliness." But this seems to apply only to external cleanliness. There are those who are miserable the whole day through if they do not have their regular bath, yet, who will make their stomach into a graveyard or a swill barrel or who will suck the rear end of a cigar, pipe or cigarette all day, or who will fill up on booze, soda fountain slops, candies, cakes, pies, and hash of all kinds. They are scrupulously clean on the outside and filled with all manner of corruption on the inside. The "live right" propaganda has not prevented women from taking up the tobacco and booze habit in recent years. The "live right" propaganda cannot affect the death rate until it is adopted. *One great obstacle in the way of its adoption is the medical profession.* Medical men not only do not live right themselves, but they scoff a those who do or who advocate doing so. Their henchmen; the life insurance actuaries, help them along in their folly by "admitting" that the "live right" propaganda does not materially affect the death rate.

We advocate adequate rest and sleep as essential to the highest degree of health and the longest possible life. But does this cause people to secure adequate rest and sleep? It does not. Here in New York, for example, thousands upon thousands of young and old consider it a hardship if they must retire before twelve o'clock midnight? It is no uncommon thing for them to be up until 2 or 3 A. M. They must indulge in activities and stimulants to keep awake. They soon exhaust themselves. What will be the effect on coming generations? Will two or three generations of this converting night into day not weaken the race? It will be argued by evolutionists that the body will adapt itself to little sleep and go on unharmed. Such are foolish. Do they not know that every adaptation to inimical influences is a deterioration? As we proceed up the mountain side we see the trees adapting themselves to the higher altitude and colder climate. But they grow smaller and more scraggy as we proceed until, when we reach the timber line, trees that are large, tall and stately in the valley, are small, twisted bushes. This is adaptation to unfavorable influences.

Some evolutionists have advanced the theory that sleep is not essential. They speculate about its origin and say that in primitive times the strong, vigorous and brave among our ancestors ventured out at night and were killed by wild animals while the weaklings and cowards stayed in hiding and acquired the sleeping habit—a survival of the unfit—and we have inherited their acquired character; that of sleeping. Sleep originated in blind chance and we will find a way to dispense with it. Some advocate serums, others advocate drugs to enable us to dispense with sleep.

When we simmer the whole thing down it amounts to the absurd proposition that life is subject to no law and that disease and death are chiefly matters of accident. Dr. Pearl, of course, has found two "laws" that govern disease and death, but none that govern health and life. He has found that the break down of certain organs is fated to occur at certain ages, and this is due to heredity.

What is considered short life must be due to causes that impair the germ plasm. Alcohol is known to do this. Deficient nutrition, although not deficient enough to cause distinct disease in the individual, if continued for a few generations weakens the offspring and shortens life. It is fortunate, however, that improved nutrition for a few generations will overcome this. The germ plasm is capable of regeneration as well as of degeneration. Indeed, it is probable that the highest powers of regeneration belong to the germ plasm. Correct living for a few generations, should eliminate the supposed hereditary short life. Wrong living over a few generations will shorten the life of the long-lived strains. Life goes up or down, depending on the conditions under which it exists. The inherent power of regeneration guarantees that under proper conditions the short-lived strains will become longed-lived. For, it is not thinkable that under present social and economic conditions and present modes of living these long-lived strains are unimpaired. A few generations, not of "live right propaganda" but of *really living right* will actually increase the length of human life.

PART XIII.

MEDICINE SHORTENS LIFE

The greatest cause of weakness, degeneracy and premature death, in modern life is the practice of medicine in all its branches. The means by which it brings about such results may be roughly classified under three heads, each of which will here be discussed in their logical order.

MEDICINE BOTH IN THEORY AND PRACTICE ENCOURAGES MAN TO LIVE IN A MANNER WHICH PRODUCES DISEASE. It is unethical in principle and demoralizing in practice. Medicine holds out to man the vain hope of immunization and cure. These two ideas are identical with those of atonement and forgiveness taught by religion.

To be immunized against a cause of disease is to be enabled to take this cause into your body at will without suffering the natural effects. Thus, if an agent were found that would immunize you against alcohol, you could drink to your belly's content without harm. There would then be no reason for abstaining from alcohol. If a serum could be found that would immunize you against the evils of sexual indulgence, there would no longer be any reason for good behavior in this regard. You could indulge as often as you pleased.

Now, so long as man believes he can be immunized against the causes of disease he will not avoid its causes. Our soldiers were "immunized" against typhoid in the late war. There was no longer any need for hygienic and sanitary precautions. These were neglected. Typhoid developed. Many cases and many deaths from this cause were reported. The surgeon general was forced to issue a circular to the medical forces of the army warning them that antityphoid vaccine was no substitute for sanitary precautions. He declared that the medical forces, believing in the protective power of the serum, had neglected the usual sanitary precautions. And this is just what I am attempting to point out—SO LONG AS MAN BELIEVES UNCLEAN LIVING CAN BE MADE SAFE HE WILL CONTINUE TO LIVE UNCLEANLY.

So long as man believes he can wallow in the mire without becoming dirty he will continue to wallow in the mire. All schemes of immunization encourage him in his desire to wallow. They encourage man in his harmful practices. He must learn that *every infraction of the laws of life must be paid for and no plan of immunization can prevent him from paying.*

The idea that disease can be cured is equally as demoralizing and debasing as the idea of immunization. A young lady asked me why she should follow healthful rules of living when she could do as she pleased, and then, when trouble resulted, she could take a pill and right the matter. If this thing could be done, then indeed, there would be no reason for living rightly. But it cannot be done. And it is well for man that it cannot be done. Pain and suffering are nature's automatic checks to wrong living. Were it not for these the human race would long ago have destroyed itself. If these could be "cured" then the race would soon destroy itself. The very belief that they can be cured encourages man in his gluttony, sensuality, excesses and dissipations. *The belief in cure is debasing and demoralizing.*

When Valentino was sick his physician told him he could smoke if he cared to. It is nothing uncommon to see men smoking in bed in hospital wards. Medical men never consider it worth while, in handling the sick, to correct any defects in their mode of living or to stop the "nerve-leaks." They imagine they can CURE disease and it is, therefore, useless to fritter away time correcting causes. Their practice is on the same level with the attempt to sober a man up while he continues to drink. It is like the effort to restore potency to the sensualist while he practices sensuality. Often they attempt to "cure" a disease with its cause or with some other cause of disease.

MEDICINE INTRODUCES INTO THE BODY CAUSES OF DISEASE, DEGENERACY AND DEATH. In this act it is a direct cause of shortened life and is responsible for many deaths. All the deaths ever recorded were premature and most of these were due to medical treatment. The whole practice of medicine is a crippling, killing process.

The medical profession once had a professional adage: "*Ubi Virus ubi vitus*"—"Our strongest poisons are our best remedies." Was a more delusive theory ever entertained? It was a strange doctrine that an agent that always tends to kill is to be used to cure the sick. Those agents that are known to lower the vital force of a well man, are known to make a well man sick, are chosen to restore the sick man to health; as if poison should be good in the violent stages of disease and not be good in health. As if it is not the nature of poisons to war against the powers of life and to spend their whole force against the vital energies in disease as in health.

Every poison known to all the kingdoms of nature —"All the dregs and scum of earth and sea"—have been and are being used in the effort to cure disease. Prove that a thing will kill the well man and the doctors will use it to save the sick. Prove that it will make a well man sick and they will employ it to make the sick man well. Prove that a thing is beneficial to the well man and they at once declare it ineffectual for the sick. Medicine attempts to reverse all the laws of nature and build health with the causes of disease.

Formerly the Allopaths contended that there is a law of cure which they called the "law of antipathies" and which they formulated thus: "*Contraria contrariis curantur*"—"Contraries cure opposites." They claimed they cured one disease by producing another. There can be no doubt about the fact that they produced *another*. Samuel Hahnemann gave this practice the name, Allopathy; meaning *"another suffering,"* because of their theory. The Hahnemannian school assumed the name Homeopathy—"similar suffering," because they held that the law of cure is the "law of similars," or, as Hahnemann formulated it; *"similia similibus curantur"*—"like cures similar." They attempted to cure one disease by producing a *similar* instead of an *opposite* disease. I may observe in passing that a "similar" disease is also "another" disease.

Whichever "law of cure" a physician held to, his means of cure were poisons. It was Dr. R. T. Trall who thundered that "THERE IS NO LAW OF CURE." And if there is no "law of cure" there are no means of cure but, as Trall declared, *there is a condition of cure and that condition is obedience.*

The medical profession is pouring the human body full of poisons of all degrees of virulence. The U. S. Pharmacopea contains a list of over 45,000 drugs that are regarded as cures for disease. Hundreds of others, not listed in its pages, are in use. Many vaccines, serums "anti-toxins," etc., are in use and many are being daily tried out in the eternal round of human vivisection that goes on in hospitals, dispensaries and state and charity institutions. All these poisonous substances of plant, animal and mineral origin are being sent into the body through the mouth; by the lungs, through inhalation; through the skin, by absorption; or, by being injected directly into the body by means of a hypodermic syringe; and, finally, they are intejected into the colon. Every one of them will produce disease and death. Not one of them is of any benefit to the body.

Surgery is also taking its toll. Organs are cut out and the body mutiliated on the slightest pretext; or, no pretext at all. Certain organs of the body are declared to be useless and a danger to life. The world is full of invalids and sufferers from nervous diseases who were made so by surgery. *Surgery removes the affected organ—it does not remove the cause of the weakness.*

Electricity, hydrotherapy and other means of torturing and stimulating the sick add to the degenerating and destroying means that are in use by so-called medical science in its vain efforts to "cure" disease. These are injuring and killing their tens of thousands.

Feeding the acutely ill, on the theory that they "MUST EAT TO KEEP UP THEIR STRENGTH," is responsible for much disease, suffering and dying. Feeding such patients poisons them and adds to their suffering.

BY SUPPRESSING THE HEALING EFFORTS OF NATURE, MEDICINE BUILDS COMPLICATIONS AND SEQUALEA, AND KILLS THE SICK. Practically all medical methods are aimed at suppressing symptoms. These are regarded as evil and the chief duty of the physician is to club them out of existence. But *symptoms are such only and not cause* and should receive no attention. The fool who directs his attention to the suppression of symptoms and ignores cause cripples and kills his patients.

A standard work on materia medica says:

"Disease is a departure from the normal, and the aim of the physician in giving a medicine is to change an abnormal function into a normal one." "A symptom is an abnormal manifestation of some function or other. Symptomatic treatment is the giving of a drug which will produce an effect just opposite to the effect produced by the disease."

His definition of disease is that it is abnormal action; while, his definition of symptomatic treatment implies the assumption that by disease is meant the thing that causes the abnormal action. Ignoring his evident lack of clearness in the matter, let us put these two definitions together and see what can be made of them.

Diarrhea is an "abnormal action." It follows a more or less prolonged period of constipation, or, some unusual dietetic indiscretion. Its purpose is to empty the digestive tract of a mass of fermenting, putrefying food. It is a protective or defensive measure. Now, symptomatic treatment would be the giving of a drug that produces "an effect just opposite to the effect produced by the disease." That is, to cure diarrhea, a drug would be given that produces constipation. They do, indeed "cure" one disease by producing another.

But what is the effect of checking the bowels? The decomposing food is retained in the body to poison and kill its cells. By suppressing the purifying effort of nature the physician has laid the foundation for serious trouble.

Suppose the patient is constipated—he is given a drug that produces diarrhea. Purgatives, laxatives, etc., are used for this purpose. How do they produce their effects? By irritating the digestive tract and causing it to increase its peristatic action. They also cause it to pour out much liquid and mucous in washing away the irritating drug. No power has been added to the body. None of the causes of constipation have been corrected or removed. What has really occurred? *The bowels have been further weakened and the disease made worse.*

A standard medical author declares:

"While these toxins of germs may be called the 'cause' of the elevation of temperature, yet the word 'reason' is better. Fever seems to be one of the protective measures of the body, a means to an end, and that end is a fight against the germ. The body seems to fight the germ better at a higher than at normal temperature, and so the fever is really rather a part of the defense than a direct result of the toxin in the sense in which the headache is such a result. We emphasize this point because so many persons think the fever is an evil and try to lower it by drugs. They can do this easily, but with no benefit—perhaps always with injury—to the patient. We like to see the temperature fall, as after a cold bath, but only when we are sure the reason for the fall is victory over the toxin, or that the total result of the bath is beneficial.''

He agrees with ORTHOPATHY about the beneficial nature of fever and deplores its reduction by drugs, as never beneficial, and perhaps, always injurious; but does not object to its suppression by means of the cold bath. He does not seem to realize that *when victory over the toxins has occurred the temperature will fall as naturally and spontaneously as it rose.*

The average physician is not averse to reducing fever with drugs. He looks upon it as an evil to be suppressed. It is a ''departure from the normal'' and a drug must be given that has an "effect just opposite to the effect produced by the disease.'' He administers a drug that reduces vital action throughout the system and down comes the temperature. Part of Nature's defense is thus broken and all her curative operations are reduced. The foundation is laid for much worse trouble. Complications develop. Sequalea follow. Perhaps the patient is killed.

This is symptomatic treatment. This is suppressive treatment. It cripples and kills the patient. The work on Materia Medica, previously quoted, says:

''The three most important purposes for which drugs and medicines are given in diseases are: (1) to avert collapse or death; (2) to eradicate, if possible, the cause of the disease; (3) to relieve pain or other symptoms of disease.

''Most drugs and remedies belong to the first and third classes. Very few drugs, of themselves, can eradicate the *cause* of disease. Remedies that act as curative agents on the *cause* of the disease are said to be SPECIFIC remedies. Example, quinine cures malaria by killing the malaria parasite in the blood. Remedies that simply *modify* symptoms, and most drugs are of this class, are called SYMPTOMATIC remedies. Example, morphia causes insensibility to pain, but does not cure the cause of the pain.''

Taking these three ''uses'' of drugs, in the order named, we have:

(1) Drugs that avert collapse or death. These are tonics and stimulants. They are the very causes of collapse and always hasten death. No drug can prevent death although any of them may cause it. This so-called use of drugs is based on the fallacy that life can be sustained on poisons—that the foes of life can be made to preserve it.

(2) Drugs to eradicate the cause of disease. This is based on the assumption that the cause of disease is some external thing or *entity* that attacks the body from without. It is a survival of the ancient belief in demons and evil spirits and is incarnated in the germ theory. Quinine is given as an example of this "class" of drugs. It is claimed to kill the blood parasite that is claimed to cause malaria. It probably kills all the parasites it comes in contact with; for, it is a protoplasmic poison. It kills men and animals, as well as parasites and will kill the patient long before it could possibly kill all the parasites that are claimed to be in the man's blood causing the malaria. *It does not cure malaria.* This I know, for a positive fact, as I have seen it fail too often both as a preventive and as a cure.

It depresses all the functions of the body and is frequently the cause of serious nervous and mental troubles and even death. It is employed as an antipyretic (a drug that reduces fever), because it depresses vital activity throughout the system and thus reduces heat production.

(3) Drugs that relieve or modify symptoms. Morphia is given as an example. It produces insensibility to pain by its paralyzing effect upon the nervous system, but does not effect the cause of the pain. Morphia is the principle narcotic of opium. The same authority, who offered morphia as an example of this third class of drugs, says of the effects of this drug:

"Small quantities of opium produce a condition of mental abstraction; large doses result in a drowsy condition. . . but, if still larger doses are given, sleep comes, sleep which is deep, merging into torpor as the poisonous dose is reached.''

''Morphine abolishes pain by depressing the areas of the cerebrum which govern sensation and thought . . . On the medulla it has the effect of depressing the respiratory centre and the vasoconstrictor centre.''

''Morphine and opium cause a contraction of the portion of the stomach which is joined to the intestine. After hypodermic injection morphine is soon found in the stomach and intestines, passing into these organs through the mucous membrane. A marked action in impairing the secretion and movement of the intestine follows the use of morphine and opium in man.''

I shall not deal with the syptoms of poisoning by morphine. These are simply greater degrees of the above and a few other effects. Indeed the above effects are symptoms of poisoning. Morphine: (1), Depresses the higher centers of the brain, producing drowsiness and torpor; (2), impairs or suspends thought; (3), paralizes sensibility; (4), depresses the respiratory centre, thus interferring with breathing; (5), causes a constriction of the arteries, thus interferring with circulation; (6), causes a contraction of the pyloric ends of the stomach; (7), impairs the secretions of the stomach, intestines and colon, producing indigestion; (8), impairs the movement of the stomach, intestine and colon—constipates.

These are but the most apparent of its effects. It depresses function throughout the body generally; directly, by depressing the brain centres and, indirectly, by interferring with breathing and circulation. It is used in *coughs* to ''dull the sensibility of the respiratory centre, so that the impulse to cough is not felt so frequently.'' It is employed in *''diarrhea, peritonitis, typhoid hemorrhage,* and in similar conditions . . . to check the intestinal movements and secretions.'' Its use is always to suppress some symptom and, in doing so, impairs every function in the body and, by this very action, lessens one's chances of recovery. People pay dearly for a brief respite from pain or other symptom. What is true of morphine is true of all drugs, or other means of suppression. It is true, as well, of all drugless means of suppression.

Every disease, and every symptom of disease, is beneficial in its action and represents vital effort in self-defense. Every method of treatment that is aimed at the removal or suppression of symptoms, and not at the correction and removal of cause, is evil and destructive. It is a combat against the body and the powers of life. *It does not cure, but kills.*

In concluding this chapter permit me to reiterate: THE PRACTICE OF MEDICINE IN ALL ITS BRANCHES IS, BOTH IN THEORY AND PRACTICE THE GREATEST CAUSE OF WEAKNESS, DISEASE, DEGENERACY AND DEATH IN MODERN LIFE. IT IS THE ONLY EFFECTIVE BARRIER TO HEALTH AND STRENGTH. ABOLISH MEDICINE IN ALL ITS FORMS AND HUMAN LIFE WILL INCREASE BY AN AVERAGE OF TEN YEARS IN A DECADE.

I THANK YOU.

CPSIA information can be obtained
at www.ICGtesting.com
Printed in the USA
LVHW061355050122
707670LV00036B/603